# Nonconvulsive Status Epilepticus

# Nonconvulsive Status Epilepticus

*Edited by*

Peter W. Kaplan, MB, FRCP

Frank W. Drislane, MD

demosMEDICAL

Acquisitions Editor: R. Craig Percy
Cover Design:
Copyeditor: Cate Murray
Compositor:Typographer Services
Printer:

Visit our website at www.demosmedpub.com



*Library of Congress Cataloging-in-Publication Data*

Nonconvulsive status epilepticus / edited by Peter W. Kaplan, Frank W. Drislane.
p. ; cm.
Includes bibliographical references and index.
ISBN-13: 978-1-933864-10-5 (hardcover : alk. paper)
ISBN-10: 1-933864-10-9 (hardcover : alk. paper)
1. Epilepsy. I. Kaplan, Peter W., 1951- II. Drislane, Frank.
[DNLM: 1. Status Epilepticus. WL 385 N812 2009]
RC372.N66 2009
616.8'53--dc22

2008034727

Special discounts on bulk quantities of Demos Medical Publishing books are available to corporations, professional associations, pharmaceutical companies, health care organizations, and other qualifying groups. For details, please contact:

**Special Sales Department**
Demos Medical Publishing
386 Park Avenue South, Suite 301
New York, NY 10016
Phone: 800–532–8663 or 212–683–0072
Fax: 212–683–0118
Email: orderdept@demosmedpub.com

Made in the United States of America
08 09 10 11 5 4 3 2 1

# CONTENTS

## V Nonconvulsive Status Epilepticus in Populations at Risk and by Age



## VI Management and Prognosis of Nonconvulsive Status Epilepticus

# PREFACE

In contrast with generalized convulsive status epilepticus, nonconvulsive status epilepticus (NCSE) usually has a subtle presentation and is often misdiagnosed and improperly treated. Like generalized convulsive status, however, NCSE can be a medical and neurologic emergency that warrants prompt and effective management as soon as it is detected. NCSE is rapidly gaining attention because of its many etiologic bases, varied clinical settings and protean manifestations. Management is still controversial, as are the varied prognoses.

After long experience and fascination with this field, and unresolved questions about the nature and management of NCSE, we have assembled a comprehensive monograph, *Nonconvulsive Status Epilepticus*. A panel of international authorities and colleagues have provided diagnostic and management insights for this mysterious, clinically challenging, and surprisingly common condition.

The purpose of this volume is to cover the full range of information on NCSE from animal models to the bedside, from neonates to the elderly, from the pleomorphic clinical features through the diagnostic dilemmas, ending with treatment options and prognosis.

The book is organized to cover multiple perspectives on age-related, genetic, syndromic, clinical, diagnostic, therapeutic, and prognostic considerations. It starts with chapters reviewing the history and a new classification of NCSE, reflecting a contemporary understanding of developmental, syndromic, and clinical aspects. Chapters follow on relevant epidemiology, electrophysiology, imaging, and pathophysiology. The next 2 sections cover the clinical features of focal NCSE arranged by the cerebral lobe involved and those of absence (generalized) status and electrographic status epilepticus in coma. Subsequent chapters are devoted to psychiatric and behavioral aspects of NCSE and to differential diagnostic considerations of its frequently unusual behavioral presentations.

An entire section is devoted to the different seizure types and NCSE syndromes according to age (from infancy to the elderly) and to special considerations pertinent to the management of NCSE in patients with specific risks, eg, mental retardation, and NCSE in patients in the intensive care unit—who are often comatose. The final section covers treatment principles and guidelines, along with individual chapters addressing prognosis in infants, children, adults, and the elderly.

We hope this volume will be helpful to neurologists, intensive care specialists, emergency room staff, mental health workers, fellows, residents, and students and that it will facilitate a comprehensive understanding and better treatment of the many forms of NCSE. We have enjoyed learning from the widely varied expertise of the many esteemed colleagues whom we were delighted to recruit and hope that this multidisciplinary contribution will provide physicians with a comprehensive source of information and opinion on nonconvulsive status epilepticus.

Peter W. Kaplan, MB, FRCP
Frank W. Drislane, MD

# CONTRIBUTORS

**Alexis Arzimanoglou, MD**
Associate Professor Neurology and Child Neurology
Epilepsy, Sleep, and Pediatric Neurophysiology Department
University Hospitals of Lyon
Hospices Civils de Lyon
Lyon, France

**Richard P. Brenner, MD**
Professor
Department of Neurology
University of Pittsburgh School of Medicine
Pittsburgh, Pennsylvania

**Krzysztof Bujarski, MD**
Fellow in Neurology
Thomas Jefferson University
Philadelphia, Pennsylvania

**Ada V. Chicharro, MD**
Fellow in Epilepsy
Department of Neurological Sciences
Rush University Medical Center
Chicago, Illinois

**Frank W. Drislane, MD**
Neurologist
Department of Neurology
Comprehensive Epilepsy Center
Beth Israel Deaconess Medical Center
Adhoc Professor
Department of Neurology
Harvard Medical School
Boston, Massachusetts

**Jonathan C. Edwards, MD**
Associate Professor and Director
Department of Neurosciences
Comprehensive Epilepsy Center
The Medical University of South Carolina
Charleston, South Carolina

**Michael Fischer, MD**
Department of Epileptology and Electroencephalography
Neurology Clinic
University Hospital Zurich
Zurich, Switzerland

**Nathan B. Fountain, MD**
Associate Professor
Director, Comprehensive Epilepsy Program
Department of Neurology
University of Virginia
Charlottesville, Virginia

**Diana Gomez-Hassan, MD, PhD**
Assistant Professor
Department of Radiology
The University of Michigan
Ann Arbor, Michigan

**Susan T. Herman, MD**
Assistant Professor
Department of Neurology
University of Pennsylvania
Philadelphia, Pennsylvania

**Edouard Hirsch, MD**
Professor
Department of Neurology
University Hospitals of Strasbourg and CTRS-IDEE, Lyon
Strasbourg, France

**Lawrence J. Hirsch, MD**
Associate Clinical Professor
Department of Neurology
Comprehensive Epilepsy Center
Columbia University Medical Center
New York, New York

**Jennifer Hopp, MD**
Assistant Professor
Department of Neurology
University of Maryland Medical School
Baltimore, Maryland

**Jeffrey Jirsch, MD, MSc**
Assistant Professor
Department of Neurology and Neurosurgery
McGill University Health Center
McGill University
Montreal, Quebec, Canada

**Barbara C. Jobst, MD**
Associate Professor of Medicine
Department of Neurology
Dartmouth-Hitchcock Medical Center
Lebanon, New Hampshire

**Andres M. Kanner, MD**
Senior Physician
Department of Neurology
Rush University Medical Center
Professor
Department of Neurological Sciences and Psychiatry
Rush University Medical Center
Chicago, Illinois

**Peter W. Kaplan, MB, FRCP**
Professor
Johns Hopkins University School of Medicine
Director, Epilepsy and Clinical Neurophysiology
Department of Neurology
Johns Hopkins Bayview Medical Center
Baltimore, Maryland

**Jaideep Kapur, MB, BS, PhD**
Professor
Department of Neurology
University of Virginia
Charlottesville, Virginia

**Christian M. Korff, MD**
Department of Neurology
Children's Hospital
Geneva, Switzerland

**Michael Koutroumanidis, MD**
Consultant and Senior Lecturer
Department of Clinical Neurophysiology and Epilepsies
St. Thomas' Hospital
London, United Kingdom

**Allan Krumholz, MD**
Professor
Department of Neurology
University of Maryland School of Medicine
Baltimore, Maryland

**Randa Y. Makhoul, MD**
Chief Resident
Department of Pediatrics and Adolescent Medicine
American University of Beirut
Beirut, Lebanon

**Mohamad A. Mikati, MD**
Professor of Pediatrics and Neurobiology
Chief, Pediatric Neurology
Departments of Pediatrics and Neurobiology
Duke University Medical Center
Durham, North Carolina

**Douglas R. Nordli, Jr., MD**
Director, Epilepsy Center
Children's Memorial Hospital
Associate Professor
Department of Neurology and Pediatrics
Northwestern University's Feinberg School of Medicine
Chicago, Illinois

**James J. Riviello, Jr., MD**
Professor
Departments of Pediatrics and Neurology
Baylor College of Medicine
Director and Chief
Department of Neurophysiology
Texas Children's Hospital
Houston, Texas

**David W. Roberts, MD**
Professor and Section Chief
Department of Neurosurgery
Dartmouth-Hitchcock Medical Center
Lebanon, New Hampshire

**Simon Shorvon, MD, FRCP**
Professor
Institute of Neurology
University College London
London, United Kingdom

**Michael R. Sperling, MD**
Professor
Department of Neurology
Thomas Jefferson Universtiy
Philadelphia, Pennsylvania

**Pierre Thomas, MD, PhD**
Professor
Service de Neurologie et UF EEG-epileptologie
Hôpital Pasteur
Nice, France

**Matthew C. Walker, MA, MB, BChir, FRCP, PhD**
Professor
Department of Clinical and Experimental Epilepsy
Institute of Neurology
University College London
London, United Kingdom

**Elizabeth J. Waterhouse, MD**
Professor
Department of Neurology
Virginia Commonwealth University School of Medicine
Richmond, Virginia

**Heinz Gregor Wieser, MD**
Professor
Department Epileptology and Electroencephalography
Neurology Clinic
University Hospital Zurich
Zurich, Switzerland

**Peter D. Williamson, MD***
Professor
Department of Neurology
Dartmouth Medical School
Hanover, New Hampshire
Benjamin Zifkin, MDCM, FRCPC
Department of Neurology
Epilepsy Clinic
Montreal Neurological Hospital
Montreal, Quebec, Canada

*Deceased

PART I

# GENERAL CONSIDERATIONS IN NONCONVULSIVE STATUS EPILEPTICUS

# CHAPTER 1

# THE HISTORY OF NONCONVULSIVE STATUS EPILEPTICUS

Peter W. Kaplan

The frightening aspect of convulsive seizures has, since ancient times, attracted the attention of observers, who have recorded their impressions on clay tablets, in ancient manuscripts, and in print. Throughout the ages, there have been many references to the appearance, causes, and treatment of seizures, as will be provided in further detail later in this chapter; withal, however, there has been surprisingly little mention of events that would seem to represent status epilepticus.

The striking aspects of seizures and epilepsy have been carried across time through the writings of early observers. Early on, several writers speculated as to the origin of seizures and epilepsy; for example, in the following quote, Hippocrates recognized that epilepsy is a disease of the brain:

> *... the man loses his speech and intellect, and his hands become powerless, and are contracted ... the eyes are distorted ... and they palpitate; and froth from the lungs issues by the mouth.*
>
> Hippocrates (1)

Five hundred years later, Galen categorized seizures into those referred to as *idiopathic*, which he speculated induced a dyscrasia of the humors of the brain brought on by cold; those arising from irritating substances brought to the brain, ie, *sympathetic*; and a third group that he attributed to a migrating humor from the limb to the brain. His description strongly resembles Hughlings Jackson's proximal ictal march.

In the Middle Ages, several writers, such as Georgius Zecchius in Basel (1586) and Vincentius Alsarius from Genoa (1617), wrote extended treatises on the subject of epilepsy and seizures. Many authors, including John of Gaddesden (circa 1280-1361), Bernard of Gordon (1305), Thomas Willis (1684), and Gerhard van Swieten (1744) (2), attributed epilepsy to supernatural forces.

Finding commentary on prolonged or repeated seizures is more difficult. An early reference to extended seizures can be found in the 25th and 26th *Sakikku* cuneiform tablets (obverse), housed in the British Museum, dating from 718–612 BC, and translated by JV Kinnier-Wilson (Figure 1.1).

> *If the possessing demon possesses him many times during the middle watch of the night, and at the time of his possession his hands and feet are cold, he is much darkened, keeps opening and shutting his mouth, is brown and yellow as to the eyes ... It may go on for some time, but he will die (3).*

Biblical references to Saul, when he was offering a prophesy at Ramah, were alleged by subsequent scholars to indicate that Saul was in status epilepticus (4). Somewhat later, a Latin scholar, Caelius Aurelianus wrote that "fits can recur ... even in the same day." "The attack (may) extend(s) into the second day."(5).

A particularly interesting account involves the ancestor of a colleague of Professor Gerhard of the Medical University of Innsbruck, Austria (personal communication). The colleague has childhood absence epilepsy with rare tonic-clonic seizures and 3-per-second spikes and waves on electroencephalography (EEG). As translated, the ancestor's condition (Figure 1.2) is described as follows:

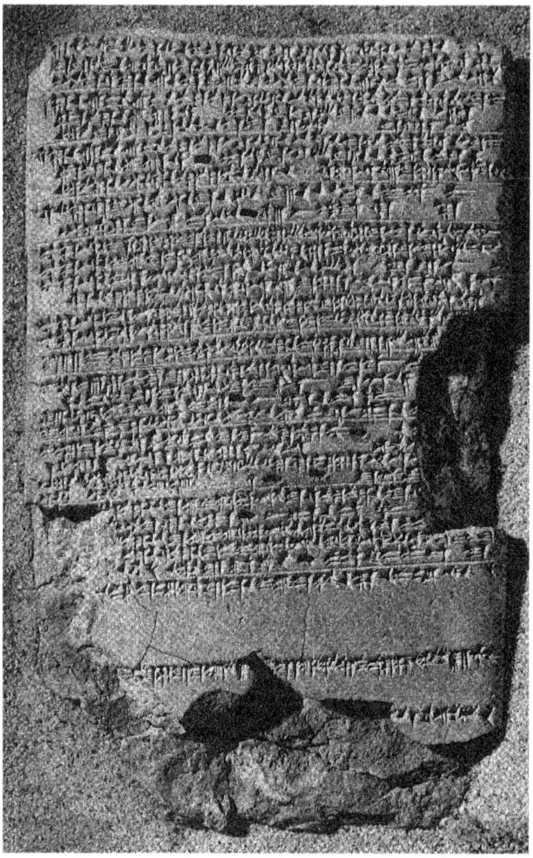

**Figure 1.1** Epilepsy tablet in the British museum. © The Trustees of the British Museum. Reproduced with permission.

*Oswalt (family name crossed out) citizen of Gmünd was in Altötting (a site for pilgrimage) a year ago ... his falling sickness ("hinfallerte Gichtern") has improved a little bit ... In the year 1501 he felt greatly sick. He lies down eyes open ... for as long as three days and many people came to him ... he did not see or recognize anyone ... a priest came and ordered a cap of wax ("Wachshaubn"—a remedy to treat epilepsy during this time) and he recovered. He praises and says many thanks to the Holy Mary in eternity ... June 1501.*

Is this the first documented example of familial/genetic epilepsy with nonconvulsive expression? And more recently, again referring

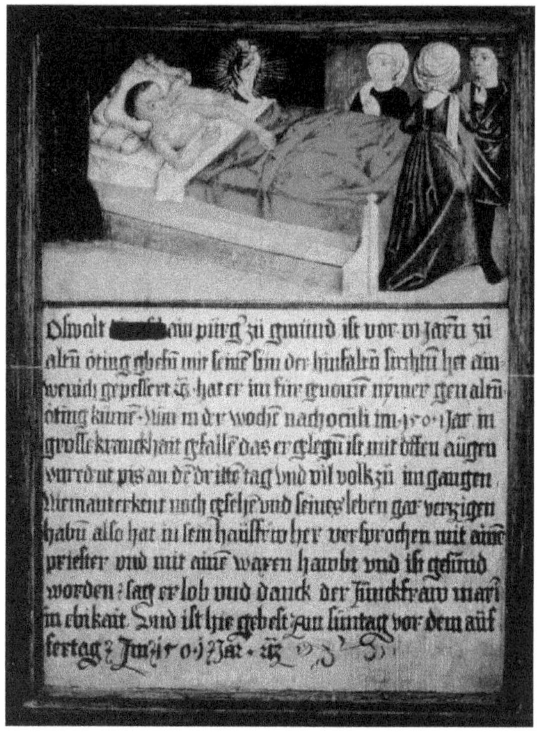

**Figure 1.2** Votif illustration from a Medieval German text of a patient who is possibly in a state of nonconvulsive status epilepticus (Courtesy of Bauer G. Innsbruck, Austria).

to sequential seizures, Thomas Willis in England wrote:

*... when as fits are often repeated, and every time grow more cruel, the animal function is quickly debilitated; and from thence, but the taint, by degrees brought on the spirits, and the Nerves serving the Praecordia, the vital function is by little and little enervated, till at length, the whole body languishing, and the pulse loosened, and at length ceasing, at last the vital flame is extinguished (6).*

Even in the late 18th and early 19th centuries, descriptions of status epilepticus were scant and few. For example, in England, with burgeoning medical observation, only occasional comment was made by Heberden, Lysons, and Good (cited by Hunter [7]).

The elaboration of the concept of status epilepticus as a manifestation of disease, however, was promulgated in France, with the coining of the expression *état de mal* appearing in written form in the university dissertation of Calmeil (8,9). In the excellent book on epilepsy, *The Falling Sickness*, Temkin quotes from Delasiauve's, *Traité de l'épilepsie*, "At the Salpêtrière we usually referred to them as [being] in an *état de mal*." Trousseau notes, "You, however, have heard of circumstances where fits have lasted two or three days, and ended in death. It is in these cases that one spoke of, at the Salpêtrière or at Bicêtre, of an *état de mal* (status epilepticus)." Calmeil claims that this usage goes back to the patients' use of the term: "It's what the patients among themselves called '*état de mal*' (status epilepticus)"; he distinguished between status epilepticus itself and the severity of seizures, delineating a sequence of seizures without pause that forebode a poor outcome (8,9). In English, status epilepticus was used when Bazire translated the clinical medicine lectures of Trousseau (10-12). Shorvon notes that 2 was largely unrecognized when Calmeil coined the term and that status epilepticus had not been distinguished from epilepsy proper (10). Prior opinion and writing reflected that status epilepticus had been seen as a distinct entity and not a state of repeated seizures, whereas Calmeil viewed it as the "maximum expression of epilepsy" (10), largely restricted to a convulsive state. Temkin's footnote on Hunter remarked that, "Hunter has shown that reports of this condition were very rare before epilepsy was studied in hospitals and remained rare until the introduction of potassium of bromide into the therapy of epilepsy" (9).

In 19th century Britain, cases of status epilepticus were described by Bright, Gowers, Hughlings Jackson, Horsley, Ferrier, Turner, Sieveking, and Coleman (10). Across the channel in Paris, there was also an increasing interest in patients with epilepsy, who often resided together in an asylum. The largest asylum in Europe was the Salpêtrière hospital in Paris, with 8000 patients. Physicians practicing at the Salpêtrière and Bicêtre included Calmeil, Pinel, Esquirol, Charcot, and Bourneville; along with Trousseau, working at Hôtel Dieu, they made many observations on their patients with epilepsy. Trousseau distinguished individual seizures from those "which are repeated in rapid succession and end in the death of the patient" and stated that petit mal seizures might recur in a fashion "that one seizure would become confused with the next, simulating a continuous seizure which might persist for two or three days," thus predating the EEG confirmation of absence status (see later in this chapter) (10-12). With the appearance in the same patient of petit mal and grand mal seizures, he suggested that this congruence was indicative of an epileptic proclivity, anticipating the syndromic approach to classification of epilepsy (10-12).

The physicians at Bicêtre and the Salpêtrière provided detailed clinical descriptions of status epilepticus. Bourneville, a pupil of Charcot, defined status epilepticus as a "serious complication" of epilepsy, with 5 stages. In Shorvon's summary, these are (1) the repetition, more or less incessant, of seizures that in consequence often become subintrant; (2) collapsus, which varies in degree of severity from transitory loss of consciousness to complete and irreversible coma; (3) hemiplegia, more or less complete, but transitory; (4) characteristic rates of pulse and respirations; and (5) marked rise in temperature, persisting in intervals between seizures and intensifying after the seizures cease (10).

In 1903, Clark and Prout reported on 38 patients with presentations that corresponded with status epilepticus " … composed of delirium, stupor or coma, cough or hiccough, and a variety of psychic states, which have for their basis cortical discharges … status comprising only psychic seizures, absences or vertigo" (13). They described the merging of individual convulsions into a state of coma, along with changes in respiration, temperature, and pulse, with seizure or status epilepticus durations from 2 to 9 days. There were alterations in pupil reactions, pulse, and eye movement and the eventual appearance of wasting and pressure sores. Final phases involved slowing of respiration and death. One patient is described as having more than 750 seizures in 12 hours, followed several days later by 500 psychic seizures, "a most unexplainable and interesting freak in the psychic phenomena of epilepsy"(13).

A historic reference to NCSE is harder to prove, as the diagnosis depends on the simultaneous appearance of seizure activity on EEG, a device that had yet to be invented when these observations occurred. It would be insufficient to prove NCSE based on only historic descriptions of confusional states even with clinical signs of NCSE, such as twitching of muscles of the face or limbs, cataplexy, or mutism, because several clinical states (such as encephalopathy, psychogenic unresponsiveness, or postictal behavior) may simulate NCSE. In early accounts of wandering confused persons, sometimes with visions or hallucinations (some of religious and zealous nature), the states were attributed, on occasion, to demonic or divine possession of the patient. Some patients were institutionalized in asylums built in France and England, with the increasing recognition that insanity and some forms of behavioral abnormality represented disease states (14). Accounts refer to a furor epilepticus for bouts of madness, often accompanied by violence. Terms used included *epileptic delirium*, *epileptic mania*, and fureur épileptique, which might appear after an ictal coma (14).

> *... the face is flushed, and the aspect of the patient is like that of a man under intoxication: he attempts to start from bed and run about, and on being withheld, vociferates and endeavors to overcome resistance. It continues commonly one, two, or three days, during which the patient requires confinement in a strait jacket, and then gradually subsides, and the patient returns to his previous state.*

Prichard (14) noted a state of epileptic ecstasy and somnambulism, as a patient was seen to wander in a confused state:

> *A more unusual circumstance in the history of epilepsy is the appearance of a species of somnambulism, or a kind of ecstasis during which the patient is in an undisturbed reverie, and walks about, fancying himself occupied in some of his customary amusements or avocations.*

An early user of the antiepileptic bromide cocktail was Sir Samuel Wilks (15), who wrote:

> *[I]n the condition which is popularly called "lost"; he is scarcely conscious of acts and conversation going on around him, yet he may continue walking in a given direction, showing that his movements must still, in a measure, be guided by his senses. He is in a dreamland, and is indeed in much the same state as a somnambulist. This condition under many varieties of form is called the status epilepticus, although the term is more usually applied to the case where the patient lies for a lengthened period in a kind of trance or stupor, as, for example, in the case of a man lately in the hospital, who after a succession of fits, lay for hours in a state of lethargy. In the milder forms it is one of great interest from a physiology point-of-view and seems to point to the possibility of a subconscious state, in which the brain is sufficiently active to control the spinal system and yet not awake enough to excite the feeling of consciousness. In reference to the influence of the brain on the muscles and necessity of consciousness to preserve their tone, the condition is one full of interest.*

Automatic behavior attracted the attention of Jules Falret (1824–1902) (16), who wrote about the petit mal intellectuel:

> *Such a patient might leave home or work, with clouded mind, dull in thought, subject to unprovoked anger and fits of despair ...; he was forgetful,*

> *had complete lapses of memory, headaches and étourdisement' (giddiness), noted luminous sparks, frightening objects and visions.*

In Germany, Höringer (17), in a thesis, noted:

> *(He) suddenly falls into a state of deep dreaming and stretches his hands in front of him. These together with his head and the upper part of his trunk begin to tremble. At other times he runs away during the attack and talks gibberish or he searches, as in a dream, in all of his pockets as if he were missing something, or he makes scrubbing or rubbing motions on his trousers; sometimes he answers if addressed during this dream state, but usually wrongly, and at its end he usually closes his eyes, seems to sleep for a few minutes, and then has no idea what happened.*

In Paris, toward the end of the 19th century, Charcot postulated that a state of somnambulism arose from seizures and, in his *Leçons du Mardi* at the Saltpêtrière Hospital in Paris, presented a case on several occasions

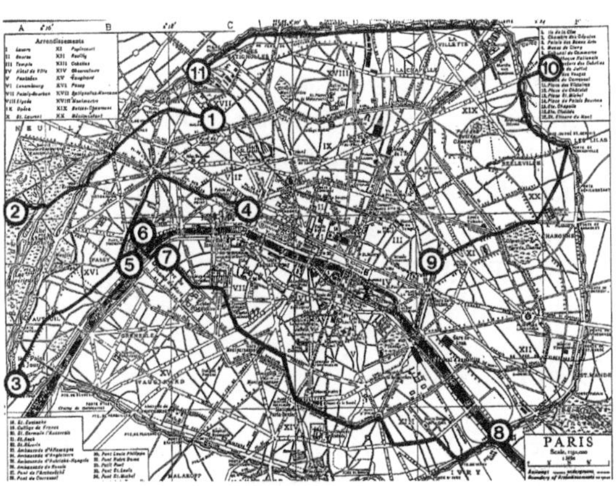


**Figure 1.2** Map of Paris in the 1880s. This shows the wanderings of a delivery man who may well have had bromide-responsive nonconvulsive status epilepticus. Reprinted with permission from Cambridge University Press (10).

(Figure 1.3) of a patient who exhibited such wandering behavior (18). The patient was a 37-year-old deliveryman who had found his way about Paris, wandering to Brest, where he was arrested on suspicion of theft, and it was only the intercession of Charcot that led to his release. The patient's wandering episodes responded to bromides, recurring when he stopped treatment. In London in 1901, Gowers (19) proposed that similar wandering states were postictal in nature, rather than an expression of the seizure itself.

> *After epileptic fits of moderate severity, the patient may pass into a condition of mental automatism, in which various acts are performed in an apparently conscious manner, but of which no recollection is afterwards retained.*

In his book *Epilepsy*, Gowers acknowledges Bourneville(19). He also describes a patient, in whose clinical course

> *the intervals between the fits become shorter, the coma deepens, the pulse and respiration become very frequent, and the temperature rises, it may be of 104°, 105°, or even 107°. Sometimes hemiplegia comes on after the condition has existed for several days. The patient may die in a state of collapse, death being apparently due to the violent and almost continuous convulsions, or, the fits ceasing, he may become delirious and present symptoms of meningitis, with rapid formation of bedsores, and may die in this stage. At any period, the symptoms may lessen, and the patient recover. A large proportion of the cases, however, end fatally.*
>
> *Fortunately, this severe degree of the status epilepticus is very rare, at any rate out of asylums for the insane. No instance in which death occurred has come under my own observation, although I have seen many examples of*

*a slighter degree of the condition, from which the patients have recovered.*

Treating these episodes was unsatisfactory. Gowers notes:

*[I]n the "status epilepticus," in which attacks recur with great frequency for several days, and in which bromide often fails entirely, I have known hypodermic injections of morphia, in doses of 1/16th of a grain to be of great service, and Sieveking has found it useful, given by the mouth, in the same state. But morphia is a remedy which can only be employed hypodermically in epileptics with extreme caution. If an attack occurs, and the post-epileptic coma coincides with the sleep induced by morphia, the patient's life is in great danger* (21pp193-194).

He states further:

*In the status epilepticus, bromide often fails. Inhalations of nitrite of amyl have been found useful by Crichton Browne. Chloroform inhalations rarely have a permanent effect. The remedies from which I have seen most good are repeated dosages of chloral, the subcutaneous injection of morphia, and the application of ice to the spine* (21pp290-291).

The historic descriptions of what might well have constituted NCSE were finally thrust into a provable domain when Berger put together a machine that could be used to record what had theretofore been theoretical: electrical impulses from the brain. In inventing the EEG, he enabled the measurement of brain dysfunction and its temporal correlation with clinical behavior.

The modern era of description and delineation of all types of seizures began with the Marseille colloquia of 1962 and 1964. The advent of EEG proved that NCSE derived from an epileptic brain and not from hysterical or nonepileptic fugue states. In 1945, Lennox (23) diagnosed absence status epilepticus with EEG correlate, and, in 1954, Penfield and Jasper delineated simple partial status epilepticus or aura continua in the form of recurrent sensory phenomena, commenting that they were "at least as common as continuing circumscribed movements"(24). This was followed by Gastaut and Roger in 1956, who described a nurse with complex partial status epilepticus that had lasted, possibly, several months (25).

In Germany, literature dealing with complex partial status epilepticus was focused on the phenomenologic description of this condition. A review by Wolf of his two cases and 7 others distinguished (as had Janz) a discontinuous form, consisting of multiple sequential seizures occurring at brief intervals (2 to 10 minutes), and a continuous form (26),categorized into (a) long-lasting sensory, somatosensory, or "psychic " seizures and (b) epileptic twilight states with psychotic signs and symptoms. Karbowski reviewed clinical and EEG features of 44 aggregate cases of his own and of others in the burgeoning literature of the time (27-34). (This summary of German contributions is courtesy of Profs. Wieser, Bauer, and Wolf.)

In the Marseille colloquia, better definitions for seizures and status epilepticus were produced, and, since then, increasing scientific and clinical attention have been directed at the physiologic underpinnings, neurochemistry, and pharmacology of status epilepticus. Newer techniques using blood flow, magnetic moments, and molecular spectra have provided functional imaging correlates of epileptic states (22), further enhancing our understanding of these conditions.

## REFERENCES

1. Lennox WG. Epilepsy and Related Disorders. Vol 1. Boston, MA: Little, Brown and Company; 1960:15-17,574.
2. Hippocrates. On the Sacred Disease. Adams, trans. Vol 2. 1849:850.
3. XXV-XXVI Tablet (obverse) 718-612 BC. British Museum, London, England. Kinnier-Wilson V, trans.

4. Temkin O, ed. The Falling Sickness. Baltimore,MD: The Johns Hopkins Press; 1971:149.
5. Caelius Aureliarus. On Acute Diseases and on Chronic Diseases. Drabkin IE, trans-ed. Chicago, IL: The University of Chicago Press; 1950.
6. Willis T. Pathologiae cerebri et nervosi generis specimen. In: quo agitur de morbis convulsivis et de scrobuto, 1667. Pordage S, trans. London, England: Dring; 1681. Cited by: Shorvon S, ed. Status Epilepticus. Cambridge England: Cambridge University Press; 1994:1.
7. Hunter RA. Status epilepticus: history, incidence and problems. Epilepsia, 4th series, 1 (1959-1960). In: Temkin O. The Falling Sickness, 2nd ed, revised. Baltimore, MD: The Johns Hopkins Press; 1971:162-168.
8. Calmeil LF. De l'épilepsie, étudiée sous le rapport de son siege et de son influence sur la production de l'aliénation mentale [dissertation]. Paris, France: Université de Paris; 1824.
9. Temkin O, ed. The Falling Sickness, 2nd ed, revised. Baltimore, MD: The Johns Hopkins Press; 1971.
10. Shorvon S. Status Epilepticus: its Clinical Features and Treatment in Children and Adults. London, England: Cambridge University Press; 1994: 2.
11. Trousseau A. Lectures on Clinical Medicine Delivered at the Hôtel Dieu, Paris, Vol. 1. Bazire PV, trans. London, England: New Sydenham Society; 1868.
12. Trousseau A. Clinique Médicale de L'Hôtel-Dieu de Paris, tome premier. Paris: Ballière et fils; 1868.
13. Clark LP, Prout TP. Status epilepticus: a clinical and pathological study in epilepsy [An article in three parts.] Am J Insanity 1903/4;60:291-306; 60:645-675; 61:81-108.
14. Prichard JC. A treatise on diseases of the nervous system. Vol. 1. London, England: Underwood; 1822:99-100.
15. Wilks S. Lectures on Diseases of the Nervous System. London, England: Churchill: 1878.
16. Falret J. "De l'état mental des épileptiques." Archives Générales de Médecine. 5th series 1860;16:661-679; 1861;17:461-49.
17. Höring CFF. Über Epilepsie [dissertation]. Unter dem Praesidium von Dr. W. Griesinger: Tübingen; 1859.
18. Goetz CG. Charcot the Clinician: the Tuesday Lessons. New York, NY: Raven Press; 1987.
19. Gowers WR. Epilepsy and Other Chronic Convulsive Disorders. London, England: Churchill; 1901.
20. Gowers WR. Epilepsy and Other Chronic Convulsive Diseases Together with the Border-land of Epilepsy. Birmingham, AL: The Classics of Neurology & Neurosurgery Library; 1986:193-194.
21. Gowers WR. Epilepsy and Other Chronic Convulsive Diseases Together with the Border-land of Epilepsy. Birmingham, AL: The Classics of Neurology & Neurosurgery Library; 1986:273-301.
22. Gastaut H, Roger J, Lob H, eds. Les états de mal èpileptique: compte rendu de la reunion européenne d'information électroencéphalographique. Xth Colloque de Marseille 1962. Paris, France: Masson.
23. Lennox WG. The treatment of epilepsy. Med Clin North Am 1945:29:1114-1128.
24. Penfield W, Jasper HH. Epilepsy and Functional Anatomy of the Human Brain. Boston, MA: Little Brown; 1954
25. Gastaut H, Roger A. Sur la signification de certain fugues épileptiques: état de mal temporal. Rev Neurol 1956;94:298-301.
26. Janz D. Die Epilepsien. Stuttgart: Thieme; 1969.
27. Karbowski K. Status psychomotoricus. Klinische und elektroenzephalographische Aspekte. In: Karbowski K, ed. Status Psychomotoricus und seine Differentialdiagnose. Bern, Switzerland: Hans Huber; 1980:39-71.
28. Ambrosetto G, Forti A, Spire JP, Tassinari CA. Studio elettroclinico di due casi di sato di male epilettico partiale. Bull Italian League against Epilepsy 1978;23:307-311.
29. Engel J Jr, Ludwig BI, Fetell M. Prolonged partial complex status epilepticus: EEG and behavioral observations. Neurology 1978;28: 863-869.
30. Mayeux R, Lueders H. Complex partial status epilepticus: case report and proposal for diagnostic criteria. Neurology 1978;28:957-961.
31. Oller Daurella L, Oller Ferrer-Vidal L, Russi A, Conill J. Los estados de mal de crisis parciales complejas. Bull Italian League against Epilepsy 1978;23:209-211.
32. Perri Di R, Messina C. Studio elettroclinico di due casi di "stato di male temporale." Bull Italian League against Epilepsy 1978;23:203-208.
33. Picornell Darder I, Conde M, Carbonell J. [Posttraumatic status epilepticus with only mental symptomatology]. Rev Electroencephalogr Neurophysiol Clin 1978;8:341-345.

# CHAPTER 2

# THE CLASSIFICATION OF NONCONVULSIVE STATUS EPILEPTICUS

SIMON SHORVON

There has been an interesting evolution of thought in this subject area, and any consideration of classification would best be embedded in this historical context; this is discussed in more detail elsewhere (1). When status epilepticus was first defined as a form of continuing epilepsy by Bourneville in 1856 (2), he confined the term to convulsive status. Although nonconvulsive forms of epilepsy and prolonged epileptic states had been well described by that time, their recognition as prolonged seizures had not been made explicit. This remained the position until at least the late 1930s when, with the advent of electroencephalography (EEG), it became clear that there were situations in which prolonged or continuous electrographic activity existed without convulsive seizures. In 1945, Lennox (3) first recorded absence (petit mal) status in his cousin, who had petit mal epilepsy, and coined the term *petit mal status*. Initially, all cases of nonconvulsive status were subsumed into this category, but it soon became apparent that not all patients with "nonconvulsive" status epilepticus (NCSE) had continuous generalized spike-wave on their EEGs, and not all patients with prolonged spike-wave exhibited petit mal status. A profusion of individual cases and small series were reported, each with different terminology (Table 2.1), and classification became labyrinthine and contradictory. In 1956, Gastaut described the first case of complex partial status epilepticus with EEG correlation (4).

A landmark in the conceptualization of status, and, in particular, in its classification and clinical definition, was the 10th Marseilles Colloquium, held in 1962. This meeting, convened by Gastaut, was the first devoted to the topic of status epilepticus. At the conference, 103 participants presented 267 cases of status, and a definition and classification were formulated (5). This was at about the time that the classification of epileptic seizure type was also being devised (again driven by Gastaut) and, in 1964, at the 13th Marseilles Colloquium, the first draft of the *International Classification of Epileptic Seizures* was presented, an approved version of which was finally published in 1970 (6). The classification of status epilepticus from the 1962 colloquium was eventually published in 1967 and mirrored exactly the newly evolved *International Classification of Seizure Type*. Implicit in this was, as Gastaut wrote later (7), the concept that there were *as many types of status as there were types of epileptic seizure*, and the classification of status epilepticus was then irrevocably yoked to the classification of seizure type.

The notion that "every seizure type had a status equivalent" persists to this day. This important statement cleared the way for an appreciation of nonconvulsive forms of status epilepticus and rapidly put order into the nosologic chaos that had developed; it provided a good superstructure for the consideration of status forms. However, a classification based on seizure type is essentially an artifact. Just as a seizure-type classification cannot account for epilepsy syndromes, so will a classification status-epilepticus based on seizure type perforce ignore the broader aspects of nonconvulsive forms, and this a very major drawback. According to the seizure-type formula, nonconvulsive status was divided into generalized (absence)—typical and atypical—and partial (simple and complex) status. This simply does not do justice to the variety of forms that actually occur nor to their widely varying pathophysiologic bases, etiologies, prognoses, or

**TABLE 2.1** PUBLISHED SYNONYMS OF ABSENCE STATUS EPILEPTICUS, 1950–1990

| |
|---|
| Petit mal status |
| Typical absence status epilepticus |
| Atypical absence status epilepticus |
| Spike and wave stupor |
| Etat confusionnel simple |
| Epilepsia minoris continua |
| Minor epileptic status |
| Epileptic twilight state |
| Prolonged epileptic twilight state with almost continuous spike-wave |
| Epileptic twilight state with spike-waves |
| Absence continua |
| Prolonged petit mal automatism |
| Status pyknolepticus |
| Centroencephalitc condition of prolonged disturbance of consciousness |
| Etat de mal generalise a l'expression confusionelle |
| Status psychomotoricus |
| Borderline petit mal status |
| Transitional petit mal status |
| Etat de mal frontal polaire |
| Temporal lobe status epilepticus |
| Complex partial status epilepticus |
| Psychomotor status epilepticus |

*These are just some of the terms used in the published literature between 1950 and 1990 used to describe prolonged generalized or partial nonconvulsive seizures. Derived from Shorvon (1).*

clinical settings. Indeed, a classification based on seizure type is a straitjacket that impedes intellectual development in this area and should be abandoned.

The limitations of the International League Against Epilepsy seizure-type classification were recognized quickly and resulted eventually in the second classification scheme—the International League Against Epilepsy's *Classification of Epilepsies and Epileptic Syndromes*, published in 1989 (7). No second International League Against Epilepsy *Classification of Status Epilepticus* has been proposed, but, in recent years, a number of alternative classifications have been suggested, which have loosened the classification from the constraints of a purely seizure-type schema; an example is the more extended classification proposed in this chapter. These classifications take into account the age, cerebral maturity, presence of an encephalopathy, epilepsy syndrome, and anatomical location—all of which are important considerations in devising a classification that can be useful clinically and for research purposes. These issues were widely debated at a workshop conference devoted to NCSE in Oxford in 2004 (9) and at the 1st London Colloquium on Status Epilepticus in April 2007.

## DEFINITION

It is the view of this author that, to a large extent, NCSE can be viewed primarily as a form of epileptic cerebral response that is largely dependent on the level of cerebral development and integrity, the presence or absence of encephalopathy, the type of epilepsy syndrome, and the anatomical location of the epileptic activity.

An unambiguous definition is of course vital for consideration of any condition, and, yet, because of both individual variation (for instance in brain development) and the issue of "boundary syndromes"(discussed later in this chapter), a clear definition of NCSE has remained elusive. The definition favored by this author, and one proposed and accepted during the Oxford conference on NCSE in 2004 (9), is as follows: *Nonconvulsive status epilepticus* is a term used to denote a range of conditions in which electrographic seizure activity is prolonged and results in nonconvulsive clinical symptoms. This derives from an earlier definition (1), and the wording is carefully chosen. Several points are worth emphasizing:

1. The definition is primarily dependent on the presence of electrographic seizure activity. This allows the inclusion, within the rubric of NCSE, of a range of "boundary conditions" in which such activity occurs but in which there are no obvious clinical "seizures." This is contentious—see below.
2. Electrographic seizure activity can take various forms. The inclusion of some patterns of electrographic activity within the rubric of NCSE is controversial. This is not discussed further here but is covered in Chapters 4 and 5.

## CLASSIFICATION OF NCSE

NCSE can be viewed primarily as a form of epileptic cerebral response that is dependent largely on the level of cerebral development, presence of encephalopathy, epilepsy syndrome, and anatomical location of the epileptic activity. Because of this, the classification of NCSE is best primarily subdivided by age. This primary subdivision is justified because many forms of NCSE at different ages are utterly distinctive (this is true of many aspects of epilepsy, but is perhaps nowhere so true as in NCSE) and also because many of the forms of NCSE described in subsequent sections of this chapter occur only at certain ages.

The form of NCSE also depends on the level of cerebral development or integrity, the presence of an "epileptic encephalopathy," etiology, and syndrome. These factors are all interrelated and combine to determine the final form of the status. In patients with profound or diffuse cerebral damage, the NCSE form is strikingly different from that of patients with integrated cerebral function, taking, in some cases, a distinctive form that depends on etiology (particularly genetic etiologies). The presence of a so-called "epileptic encephalopathy" also has an overriding influence on the form of status. The interaction of these factors is clearly seen, for example, in the strange forms of the condition that occur in hypoxic brain damage or in the Lennox-Gastaut syndrome.

Finally, the form of NCSE depends on the anatomical location of the epileptic activity—this is particularly important in relation to focal status, such as complex partial status epilepticus, in which relatively distinctive frontal and temporal forms exist, and in aura continua, in which the form depends almost entirely on the area of the brain that is activated.

In Table 2.2, a classification scheme is proposed in which the primary distinctions are by age. In Table 2.3 is given a summary of some features of each of these subcategories.

### NONCONVULSIVE STATUS EPILEPTICUS IN THE NEONATAL PERIOD AND INFANCY

There are a number of types of serious epileptic encephalopathy occurring in the neonatal and infant periods, which take the form of continuous or near-continuous episodes of NCSE. These are best subdivided by syndrome and etiology or by the presence or absence of encephalopathy.

- In West syndrome (10), with EEG changes of hypsarrhythmia, and other malignant epilepsies of childhood, such as Ohtahara syndrome (11) and severe myoclonic epilepsy of infancy (Dravet syndrome—a defect usually of the SCN1A gene [12]).
- Other cases are less specific, and the encephalopathy can be due to a wide range of etiologies, including infection, anoxia, and metabolic and developmen-

**TABLE 2.2** CLASSIFICATION OF NONCONVULSIVE STATUS EPILEPTICUS

1. **NCSE occurring in the neonatal and infantile epilepsy syndromes**
   1a. West syndrome
   1b. Ohtahara syndrome
   1c. Severe myoclonic encephalopathy of infancy (Dravet syndrome)
   1d. NCSE in other forms of neonatal or infantile epilepsy
2. **NCSE occurring only in childhood**
   2a. NCSE in early-onset benign childhood occipital epilepsy (Panayiotopoulos syndrome)
   2b. NCSE in other forms of childhood epileptic encephalopathies, syndromes, and etiologies, eg, ring chromosome 20, Angelman syndrome, Rett syndrome, myoclonic-astatic epilepsy, other childhood myoclonic encephalopathies
   2c. Electrical status epilepticus in slow-wave sleep
   2d. Landau-Kleffner syndrome
3. **NCSE occurring in both childhood and adult life**
   *With epileptic encephalopathy*
   3a. NCSE in the Lennox-Gastaut syndrome
      i. Atypical absence status epilepticus
      ii. Tonic status epilepticus
   3b. Other forms of NCSE in patients with learning disability or disturbed cerebral development (cryptogenic or symptomatic)
   *Without epileptic encephalopathy*
   3c. Typical absence status epilepticus in idiopathic generalized epilepsy
   3d. Complex partial status epilepticus
      i. Limbic
      ii. Nonlimbic
   3e. NCSE in the postictal phase of tonic-clonic seizures
   3f. Subtle status epilepticus (myoclonic status epilepticus occurring in the late stage of convulsive status epilepticus)
   3g. Aura continua with
      i. Sensory symptoms
      ii. Special sensory symptoms
      iii. Autonomic symptoms
      iv. Cognitive symptoms
4. **NCSE occurring in late adult life**
   4a. De novo absence status epilepticus of late onset
5. **Boundary syndromes**[a]
   5a. Some cases of epileptic encephalopathy
   5b. Some cases of coma due to acute brain injury with epileptiform EEG changes
   5c. Some cases of epileptic behavior disturbance or psychosis
   5d. Some cases of drug-induced or metabolic confusion state with epileptiform EEG changes

[a]*Derived from Shorvon (37).*
***Abbreviations:*** *NCSE refers to nonconvulsive status epilepticus; EEG, EEG electroencephalographic.*

tal cases. The form of NCSE in these conditions can be rather nonspecific, subtle, or fragmentary and does not conform easily to categorization by conventional seizure type. In severe myoclonic epilepsy of infancy, as an example, the periods of NCSE can persist for hours or days and can take the form of obtundation, sometimes with erratic small myoclonic movements. In Ohtahara syn-

**TABLE 2.3** NCSE—ETIOLOGY OR CLINICAL CONTEXT, FORMS, AND RESPONSE TO TREATMENT

| | Etiology or clinical context | Clinical form | Response to treatment or prognosis |
|---|---|---|---|
| West syndrome | Various | Infantile spasms with periods of NCSE with no clinical signs of ongoing epileptic activity | Poor |
| Ohtahara syndrome | Various | Tonic spasms | Poor |
| Severe myoclonic epilepsy of infancy (Dravet syndrome) | Genetic | Nonspecific | Poor |
| NCSE in other forms of neonatal or infantile epilepsy | Various | Nonspecific | Various |
| Early-onset benign childhood occipital epilepsy (Panayiotopoulos syndrome) | Idiopathic | Autonomic status epilepticus | Excellent |
| NCSE in other forms of childhood epileptic encephalopathies, syndromes, and etiologies, eg, ring chromosome 20, Angelman syndrome, myoclonic-astatic epilepsy, other childhood myoclonic encephalopathies. | Various, usually genetic or cryptogenic | Atypical absence and other nonspecific forms | Generally poor |
| Electrical status epilepticus in slow-wave sleep | Various, usually cryptogenic | No clinical signs but ongoing electrographic activity in sleep | NCSE usually remits but may leave intellectual deficits |
| Landau-Kleffner syndrome | Various, usually cryptogenic | Clinical correlate of electrographic activity is severe speech disturbance | NCSE usually remits but may leave intellectual deficits |
| NCSE in Lennox-Gastaut syndrome | Various, often cryptogenic | Atypical absence status epilepticus (see text) | Poor |
| NCSE in other forms of disrupted cerebral development (cryptogenic or symptomatic) | Various, often cryptogenic | Various | Variable |
| Typical absence status epilepticus | Idiopathic generalized epilepsy | Generalized absence | Excellent |
| Complex partial status epilepticus | Various—symptomatic or cryptogenic | Complex partial | Good |
| NCSE in the postictal phase of TCSE | Various | Confusion state with psychiatric features | Good |
| Subtle status epilepticus | Various | Coma with small irregular myoclonic jerks | Variable |
| Aura continua | Various—symptomatic or cryptogenic | Simple partial (sensory, special sensory, cognitive) | Good |
| De novo absence status epilepticus | Psychotropic drug withdrawal or idiopathic generalized epilepsy | Generalized absence | Excellent |

*NCSE refers to nonconvulsive status epilepticus; TCSE, tonic-clonic status epilepticus.*

drome, the EEG shows suppression-burst patterns, which can be almost continuous in both the waking and sleeping state (11).

## NONCONVULSIVE STATUS EPILEPTICUS IN CHILDHOOD

The cases of childhood NCSE are best classified according to syndrome or etiology, and the clinical form of the status often does not conform to a seizure-type categorization.

- The benign familial childhood epilepsies rarely result in status epilepticus, either convulsive or nonconvulsive. Occasional cases of NCSE in benign rolandic epilepsy are described, which take the form of tonic deviation or weakness of the face, speech arrest, sialorrhea, swallowing difficulties, oromotor apraxia, and partial loss of awareness (13). This state resembles the defects in the anterior operculumanterior culum syndrome (Foix-Chavany-Marie syndrome). The only benign syndrome in which NCSE is common is the Panayiotopoulos syndrome (14-16). In this syndrome, the seizures are often prolonged and classically take the form of "autonomic status epilepticus." The seizures are dominated by autonomic features and include nausea, retching, and color and pupil changes, and there is often associated forced deviation of the eyes. The median duration of seizures is two hours.
- A number of specific illnesses—usually those due to mendelian genetic defects, with onset in early childhood and due to a well-defined genetic defect—have prominent episodes of NCSE (17). Some of these syndromes exhibit NCSE with rather characteristic and distinctive patterns. For instance, in the recently identified ring chromosome 20 syndrome (18), the seizures often occur with only minor clinical or with a prolonged confusional state, with or without additional motor seizures. The ictal EEG pattern is of long-lasting, bilateral, paroxysmal, high-voltage, slow waves with occasional spikes. In Angelman syndrome (with the defect usually in the UBE3A gene), prolonged episodes of NCSE are common in which the child exhibits decreased alertness, hypotonia, and erratic myoclonia (19). The EEG shows high-voltage slow-wave bursts with diffuse spike-waves. In Rett syndrome, with the defect usually in the *MECP2* gene (20, 21), NCSE is also common and may not be recognized. Seizures consist of behavioral arrest, diminished movements, episodes of hyperventilation, or hand stereotypies. The EEG can show continuous partial or generalized activity.
- Electrical status epilepticus in slow-wave sleep. This term (synonym: continuous spike-waves of slow sleep)(22-25) refers to an epileptic encephalopathy characterized by the presence of generalized, 1- to 3-Hz, spike-wave discharges occupying 85% or more of the EEG of non-rapid eye movement sleep. There are no specific clinical signs during sleep. Overt seizures develop between the ages of one and 14 years, occur in daytime and at night, and can take various forms, both focal and generalized. Episodes of forms of status are common. The EEG pattern usually occurs in children with severe epilepsy and learning difficulty. Many of the children exhibit the symptoms of the Landau-Kleffner syndrome, and electrical status epilepticus in slow-wave sleep is also seen in some children with Lennox-Gastaut syndrome or benign rolandic epilepsy. There may be syndrome overlap or transitional cases.
- Landau-Kleffner syndrome. In this condition, almost continuous focal EEG activity is associated with a progressive aphasia, developing gradually over months or subacutely over weeks (24-26). This activity is associated with severe deterioration of verbal comprehension and expressive speech, and the children can become almost mute. Overt

epileptic seizures occur in about 75% of cases, and are usually mild, but 15% of cases have episodes of overt status epilepticus. Other features are hyperkinetic behavior disorders and learning disability. The speech defect is associated with repetitive high-voltage spikes or spike-wave discharges in the dominant hemisphere (or generalized discharges). Its inclusion as a form of NCSE is based on the postulate that the speech disturbance is directly due to the virtually continuous electrographic activity disrupting speech function. Alternatively, it could be considered that the speech and electrographic disturbance are both the result of an underlying pathologic process (not yet identified) and, thus, are not causally related. Whichever explanation is accepted, aggressive treatment of the electrographic disturbance is usually undertaken to improve speech function.

## NONCONVULSIVE STATUS EPILEPTICUS IN CHILDHOOD AND ADULT LIFE

The forms of NCSE in patients with childhood epileptic encephalopathies are very different from those without encephalopathy.

### *With epileptic encephalopathy*

- Episodes of NCSE are common in the Lennox-Gastaut syndrome (27). Two rather characteristic forms are atypical absence status epilepticus (ASE) and tonic status epilepticus. Atypical ASE is often "subcontinuous," with periods of hours, days, or even weeks in which the child is obtunded and slowed up, and exhibits variable behavior, motor, and tone changes. These episodes can be interrupted by tonic seizures and episodes of tonic status. These were first described by Gastaut (5). The tonic seizure can be precipitated by benzodiazepine therapy. Periods of normality merge into periods of NCSE, and the boundary between the two can be extremely unclear. The EEG in ictal and interictal states shows characteristically slow spike-waves, sometimes almost continuously, and the ictal and interictal EEG can be very similar.
- NCSE can also take atypical forms in other syndromes with prominent learning disability or disrupted cerebral development (either cryptogenic or symptomatic). There is no clearer example of the inappropriate nature of trying to fit all forms of status epilepticus into rigid seizure-type classifications than NCSE in people with learning disabilities of various degrees, forms, and etiologies. Episodes of NCSE are common, but their form and symptomatology are extremely variable, showing forms that are largely influenced by the level of cerebral development.

### *Without epileptic encephalopathy*

- Typical ASE. This is another classic form, first described by Lennox in 1945, and one of the early triumphs of EEG. It occurs only in the syndrome of idiopathic generalized epilepsy (28) and is described elsewhere in this volume (Chapter 12). Alteration of consciousness can be variable, although alterations are generally greater than in atypical ASE. The child appears out of contact, with delayed responses, altered speech, regressive behavior, drooling, gait disturbances, and episodic atonia, jerks of the face, head nodding, and eyelid myoclonia. The episodes are often terminated by a tonic-clonic seizure.
- Complex partial status epilepticus. This is a classic form of NCSE, first clearly delineated by Gastaut in 1956 (4), although perhaps first described by Hughlings Jackson. It is common, a fact recognized only in recent years, and has been extensively reported and studied. It can be divided anatomically into two

forms: limbic and nonlimbic. Anatomically, the seizures are as likely to arise from frontal as from temporal cortex and, in this sense, reflect a similar propensity for tonic-clonic status, but differ from complex partial seizures, which are more likely to be temporal than frontal in origin. Also characteristically, this form of NCSE "cycles" with fluctuating symptoms and alternating consciousness and impairment of consciousness. The typical forms of complex partial status epilepticus are described elsewhere in this volume (Chapters 8 and 10). Some cases of epileptic behavior disorders or psychosis are probably due to limbic status epilepticus, and this is discussed further in this chapter.

- NCSE in the postictal phase of tonic-clonic seizures (1). A particular form of NCSE seems to develop in the aftermath of some tonic-clonic seizures. It presents as a prolonged confusion state and can be differentiated from "postictal" confusion by the presence of on-going epileptic discharges. This is probably a not-uncommon event, although the exact frequency is not known. The clinical form is of a confusion state, often with some degree of obtundation and additional psychiatric symptoms, and that occurs in the immediate aftermath of a tonic-clonic seizure. This is quite distinct from the epileptic psychosis, which occurs without obtundation (and indeed is usually characterized by excited behavior), and that tends to develop after a lucid interval (see later in this chapter).
- Subtle status epilepticus. This is a form of status epilepticus that clinically and electrographically resembles myoclonic status epilepticus in coma, but the term is best confined to use in describing the similar clinical symptoms that sometimes occur in the late stages of tonic-clonic status epilepticus. The EEG shows periodic lateralized epileptiform discharges (PLEDs) or periodic epileptiform discharges (PEDs). The clinical and EEG progression from tonic-clonic to subtle status was first proposed by Treiman and colleagues (29, 30).
- Aura continua. This is a term used to describe simple partial status epilepticus without visible motor phenomena (31). It can be classified into 4 types depending on the region of cerebral cortex involved: (1) somatosensory (ie, simple partial status epilepticus arising in the central or parietal cortex); (2) aura continua that involve visual, auditory, gustatory, or olfactory symptoms (arising in the temporal or occipital lobe); (3) aura continua with predominantly autonomic symptoms (temporal lobe); and (4) aura continua with psychic or cognitive symptoms.

## NONCONVULSIVE STATUS EPILEPTICUS CONFINED TO LATE ADULT LIFE

There is one syndrome of NCSE that is confined to late adult life, de novo ASE of late onset (1,32). This syndrome occurs in patients without a history of absence epilepsy or with a history of seizures in long remission. It presents, as does ordinary ASE, as an acute confusion state with variable alteration of consciousness, ranging from profound stupor with catatonia and loss of sphincter control at one extreme through mental dullness and abulia to mild motor retardation. Moderate confusion is common, as are changes of affect or behavior. Commonly, the condition is misdiagnosed as dementia or acute psychosis. The EEG is diagnostic, showing continuous spike-wave discharges. The condition is often precipitated by psychotropic drug withdrawal (usually benzodiazepines) or abuse, and, when this is not the case, there is often a history of idiopathic generalized epilepsy.

## BOUNDARY SYNDROMES

Boundary syndromes are conditions in which it is not clear to what extent the symptoms are due to NCSE. This is a most interesting and controversial aspect of the subject area of NCSE. There are a number of conditions in which there is good evidence of ongoing electrographic epileptiform activity and, yet, in which the clinical symptoms are not conventionally considered to be "epileptic."There are 4 areas in which this is a particularly prominent issue.

A. Myoclonic status epilepticus in coma in the context of acute severe brain injury
B. Epileptic encephalopathies of childhood
C. Epileptic psychosis and behavior disturbance
D. Confusion states with epileptiform EEG changes (drug-induced or metabolic)

In each of these clinical situations, patients exhibit clinical symptoms associated with ongoing activity on the EEG (in some cases at least) that could be interpreted as NCSE. The question arises as to what extent the symptoms are therefore the *consequence* of this electrographic disturbance (and therefore due to NCSE). This is a difficult question for which there is no clear answer. The alternative explanation is that the EEG disturbance is an independent aspect, perhaps reflecting physiologic events that are not primarily epileptic (in other words the EEG findings are simply an epiphenomenon).

### *Myoclonic status epilepticus in coma*

This term is used to describe the clinical situation that can follow a severe acute cerebral injury (eg, hypoxic damage after cardiac arrest) in which a deeply unconscious patient exhibits EEG abnormalities such as PLEDs or PEDs, sometimes accompanied by clinically evident subtle myoclonic jerks. There are some who consider this state to be an example of NCSE and, conversely, others who hold that the occurrence of PLEDs or PEDs in this situation reflects "sick brain"' rather than some primary epileptic process. The distinction is important because it will greatly affect approach to treatment. Claims are made for improvement in the latter situation after intensive antiepileptic therapy, but prognosis is, in the experience of most, uniformly poor. In some cases, there seems to be good evidence that the primary process is "epileptic," but, in most, the evidence is equivocal. It is the personal view of the author, though, that the majority of cases are not epileptic (ie, a form of NCSE) but that the clinical picture reflects an agonal event ("sick brain") without truly epileptic features, and, thus, antiepileptic therapy is not indicated, but this remains a controversial area.

### *Epileptic encephalopathies of childhood*

Interpretation of the clinical and EEG changes in the epileptic encephalopathies of childhood is also complex. In a normal child, the occurrence of NCSE is usually very obvious and can be confirmed by EEG, but, in children with epileptic encephalopathies in whom cerebral development or integrity is disturbed and in whom the EEG is already severely abnormal, the distinction between the "interictal" and "ictal" state can be problematic. In the Lennox-Gastaut syndrome, for instance, there are episodes that may last hours or days during which the patient's mentation is slightly slowed but consciousness is preserved. There may or may not be additional signs, such as obtundation, altered mood and affect, irritability, loss of social interaction, loss of cognitive abilities, alteration of muscle tone, ataxia, delayed motor signs, dystonia, subtle myoclonic jerks, or increased sialorrhea. If these signs are marked, then there is no doubt that the patient is in an episode of NCSE, but, if these additional signs are mild, the periods may be referred to by caregivers as "off days," and the question of NCSE may be overlooked. The EEG in these periods, even if the additional clinical signs are marked, is not really much different from the EEG at other times and shows continuous and severe epileptiform changes, such as the presence of long bursts of diffuse slow (1- to 2.5-Hz) spike-wave activity, widespread in both hemispheres, roughly bilaterally synchronous but often asymmetrical. There seems to be a gradation between clear episodes of NCSE and normal behavior, and where the line is drawn between the two can be extremely unclear. In my view, these "off days" are likely to represent NCSE in the sense that the symptoms are likely to be due to nonconvulsive seizure activity in spite of the fact that the EEG does not show this. However, definition and diagnosis are difficult when symptoms and signs are simply a matter of degree.

*Epileptic behavior disturbance or psychosis*

This is in some ways the most interesting, and certainly the most contentious, and probably the most common boundary syndrome. The question of NCSE arises in those patients with epilepsy—usually limbic epilepsy—and in whom behavior disturbances, including psychosis, occur and are associated with increased EEG activity recorded in limbic structures. There are two situations in which this is possible: (a) the postictal psychosis that occurs typically after a cluster of tonic-clonic seizures and (b) true "interictal" psychosis. There is a good prima facie case for believing that the behavior changes are often driven by epileptic activity and amount therefore to NCSE. This is indisputable in relation to postictal psychosis and an intriguing possibility in relation to interictal psychosis. Wieser and colleagues also reported stereotactic EEG observations in patients with drug-resistant epilepsy during evaluation for surgery (33,34). A variety of behavior changes (particularly irritability and aggression), affective changes (particularly depression and anxiety), and psychotic symptoms (such as hallucinations and paranoia) occurred at times when ictal discharges were recorded from limbic structures by stereotactic EEG, often without a scalp EEG correlate. Others have reported similar findings. For instance, Takeda and colleagues provide an interesting report of a 25-year-old woman with intractable temporal lobe epilepsy who developed a postictal psychosis following a cluster of 18 seizures while undergoing intracranial EEG monitoring (35). The EEG during the psychosis showed continuous, and then improving, rhythmic spike-and-slow-wave discharges in the amygdala and other mesial temporal regions. When the psychosis resolved, the EEG returned to the baseline state. There seems little doubt in all such cases that the epileptic behavior change or psychosis is due to ongoing limbic seizure activity. These patients are obviously highly selected (those undergoing stereotactic EEG as part of evaluation for epilepsy surgery), and the intriguing question arises to what extent "interictal" behavior change or psychosis in all patients with epilepsy is due to NCSE. Heath performed one of the earliest studies correlating stereotactic EEG findings with psychotic symptoms in patients with epilepsy and found paroxysms of abnormal activity in the hippocampus, amygdale, and septal region occurring interictally and that were more pronounced during periods of psychosis (36). It is the view of the author that many such cases of epileptic behavior change and psychosis are indeed likely to be due to limbic NCSE and that NCSE in these cases is underdiagnosed.

*Drug-induced or metabolic encephalopathy*

In some confusional states due to drug intoxication or metabolic derangement, there may be myoclonus or "epileptiform" changes on the EEG or both. This is more common in patients with epilepsy, although it can also occur also without a history of epilepsy. There are many drugs that have been occasionally reported to precipitate nonconvulsive status, and, among the most commonly implicated, are tiagabine, valproate, and intravenously administered contrast media. Whether these are truly epileptic (a form of ASE) or some nonspecific form of encephalopathy is unclear. Certainly, clear-cut epileptic seizure activity is uncommon, in spite of the epileptiform EEG patterns. When the offending cause is removed, the state reverses, and the risk of subsequent ongoing epilepsy is small.

## ACKNOWLEDGMENT

The text of this article is based on a paper submitted for publication.

## REFERENCES


1. Shorvon SD. Status Epilepticus. Its clinical features and treatment in children and adults. Cambridge, England: Cambridge University Press; 1994.
2. Bourneville DM. L'état de mal épileptiques. In: Recherches cliniques et thérapeutiques sur l'épilepsie et l'hysterie. Compte-rendu des observations recueillies à la salpêtriêre. Paris, France: Delahaye; 1876.
3. Lennox WG. The petit mal epilepsies: their treatment with tridione. JAMA 1945;129:1069-1073.
4. Gastaut H, Roger J, Roger A. Sur la signification des certaines fugues épileptiques: état de mal temporal. Rev Neurol 1956;94:298-301.
5. Gastaut H, Roger J, Lob H. Les états de mal epileptiques. Paris, France: Masson; 1967.
6. Gastaut H. Clinical and electroencephalographic classification of epileptic seizures. Epilepsia 1970;11:102-113.
7. Gastaut H. Classification of status epilepticus. In: Delgado-Escueta AV, Wasterlain CG, Treiman DM, Porter RJ, eds. Status Epilepticus. Mechanisms of Damage and Treatment. Adv Neurol. Vol 34. New York, NY: Raven Press; 1983:15-35.
8. Commission on Classification and Terminology of the International League Against Epilepsy. Proposal for revised classification of epilepsies and epileptic syndromes. Epilepsia 1989;30: 389-399.
9. Walker M, Cross H, Smith S, Young C, Aicardi J, Appleton R, Aylett S, Besag F, Cock H, DeLorenzo R, Drislane F, Duncan J, Ferrie C, Fujikawa D, Gray W, Kaplan P, Koutroumanidis M, O'Regan M, Plouin P, Sander J, Scott R, Shorvon S, Treiman D, Wasterlain C, Wieshmann U. Nonconvulsive status epilepticus: Epilepsy Research Foundation workshop reports. Epileptic Disord 2005:7:253-296.
10. Riikonen R. The latest on infantile spasms. Curr Opin Neurol. 2005;18:91-95.
11. Ohtahara S, Yamatogi Y. Ohtahara syndrome: with special reference to its developmental aspects for differentiating from early myoclonic encephalopathy.
Epilepsy Res 2006;70(Suppl 1):S58-S67.
12. Dravet C, Bureau M, Oguni H, Fukuyama Y, Cokar O. Severe myoclonic epilepsy in infancy: Dravet syndrome. Adv Neurol 2005;95:71-102.
13. Gobbi G, Boni A, Filippini M. The spectrum of idiopathic Rolandic epilepsy syndromes and idiopathic occipital epilepsies: from the benign to the disabling.
Epilepsia 2006;47(Suppl 2):S62-S66.
14. Panayiotopoulos CP. The birth and evolution of the concept of Panayiotopoulos syndrome. Epilepsia 2007;48:1041-1043.
15. Koutroumanidis M. Panayiotopoulos syndrome: an important electroclinical example of benign childhood system epilepsy. Epilepsia 2007;48:1044--1053.
16. Caraballo R, Cersósimo R, Fejerman N. Panayiotopoulos syndrome: a prospective study of 192 patients. Epilepsia 2007;48:1054-1061.
17. Korff CM, Nordli DR Jr. Epilepsy syndromes in infancy. Pediatr Neurol 2006;34:253-263.
18. Inoue Y, Fujiwara T, Matsuda K, Kubota H, Tanaka M, Yagi K, Yamamori K, Takahashi Y. Ring chromosome 20 and nonconvulsive status epilepticus. A new epileptic syndrome. Brain 1997;120:939-953.
19. Williams CA, Beaudet AL, Clayton-Smith J, Knoll JH, Kyllerman M, Laan LA, Magenis RE, Moncla A, Schinzel AA, Summers JA, Wagstaff J. Angelman syndrome 2005: updated consensus for diagnostic criteria. Am J Med Genet 2006;140:413-418.
20. LaSalle JM, Hogart A, Thatcher KN. Rett syndrome: a Rosetta stone for understanding the molecular pathogenesis of autism. Int Rev Neurobiol 2005;71:131-165.
21. Bienvenu T, Chelly J. Molecular genetics of Rett syndrome: when DNA methylation goes unrecognized. Nat Rev Genet. 2006;7:415-426.
22. Tassinari CA, Rubboli G. Cognition and paroxysmal EEG activities: from a single spike to electrical status epilepticus during sleep. Epilepsia 2006;47(Suppl 2):S40-S43.
23. Tassinari CA, Rubboli G, Volpi L, Meletti S, d'Orsi G, Franca M, Sabetta AR,Riguzzi P, Gardella E, Zaniboni A, Michelucci R. Encephalopathy with electrical status epilepticus during slow sleep or ESES syndrome including the acquired aphasia. Clin Neurophysiol 2000;111(Suppl 2):S94-S102.
24. McVicar KA, Shinnar S. Landau-Kleffner syndrome, electrical status epilepticus in slow wave sleep, and language regression in children. Ment Retard Dev Disabil Res Rev 2004;10:144-149.
25. Galanopoulou AS, Bojko A, Lado F, Moshe SL. The spectrum of neuropsychiatric abnormalities associated with electrical status epilepticus in sleep. Brain Dev 2000;22:279-295.

26. Hirsch E, Valenti MP, Rudolf G, Seegmuller C, de Saint Martin A, Maquet P, Wioland N, Metz-Lutz MN, Marescaux C, Arzimanoglou A. Landau-Kleffner syndrome is not an eponymic badge of ignorance. Epilepsy Res 2006;70 (Suppl 1):S239-S247.
27. Markand ON. Lennox-Gastaut syndrome (childhood epileptic encephalopathy). J Clin Neurophysiol 2003;20:426-441.
28. Shorvon S, Walker M. Status epilepticus in idiopathic generalized epilepsy. Epilepsia 2005;46:(Suppl 9):73-79.
29. Treiman DM. Electroclinical features of status epilepticus. J Clin Neurophysiol 1995;12:343-362.
30. Chen JW, Wasterlain CG. Status epilepticus: pathophysiology and management in adults. Lancet Neurol 2006;5:246-256.
31. Wieser HG. Aura Continua. http://www.ilae-epilepsy.org/Visitors/Centre/ctf/aura_continua.html. Published May 4, 2001. Updated September 17, 2003. Accessed April 15, 2008.
32. Trinka E. Absences in adult seizure disorders. Acta Neurol Scand Suppl 2005;182:12-18.
33. Wieser HG. Depth recorded limbic seizures and psychopathology. Neurosci Biobehav Rev 1983;7:427-440.
34. Wieser HG, Hailemariam S, Regard M, Landis T. Unilateral limbic epileptic status activity: stereo EEG, behavioural and cognitive data. Epilepsia 1985;26:19-29.
35. Takeda Y, Inoue Y, Tottori T, Mihara T. Acute psychosis during intracranial EEG monitoring: close relationship between psychotic symtpomssymptoms and discharges in the amygdala. Epilepsia 2001;42:719-724.
36. Heath RG. Common characteristics of epilepsy and schizophrenia: clinical observation and depth electrode studies. Am J Psychiatry 1962;118:1013-1026.
37. Shorvon SD. What is nonconvulsive status epilepticus, and what are its subtypes? Epilepsia 2007;48(Suppl 8):35-38.

CHAPTER 3

# THE EPIDEMIOLOGY OF NONCONVULSIVE STATUS EPILEPTICUS

ELIZABETH J. WATERHOUSE

Although the epidemiology of convulsive status epilepticus has been the subject of several large-scale studies, documentation of nonconvulsive status epilepticus (NCSE) has been more challenging (1-6). There have been no systematic large-scale population-based studies that have focused solely on NCSE. There are several reasons for this discrepancy. NCSE is much more challenging to identify than is convulsive status epilepticus because the signs are much less obvious. It presents with a variety of subtle clinical manifestations and requires electroencephalographic (EEG) recording during the event for diagnosis. The definition and classification of NCSE have been subject to various interpretations, and no single system has been agreed upon (7-11).

Over the past decade, NCSE has been increasingly recognized. The use of evolving EEG technology has allowed increasing length of digital EEG recording, speedier methods for EEG review, and more widely available EEG monitoring. This increased capacity for NCSE surveillance, coupled with increased awareness of NCSE, and heightened diagnostic suspicion, allow NCSE to be diagnosed more frequently and more accurately than in the past, requiring reconsideration of historical low estimates of NCSE incidence.

## METHODOLOGIC CHALLENGES IN THE STUDY OF NONCONVULSIVE STATUS EPILEPTICUS

At present, the challenges inherent in NCSE diagnosis are overshadowed by the lack of conformity in its definition and classification. NCSE is not easy to study because it is not a single entity. A reasonable definition, "Nonconvulsive status epilepticus is a term used to denote a range of conditions in which electrographic seizure activity is prolonged and results in nonconvulsive clinical symptoms," has been proposed by Shorvon (9). This definition could be appropriately applied to a prolonged nonconvulsive ictal event in a person with a history of partial or absence epilepsy, as well as to coma in a patient with acute medical problems, no history of epilepsy, and an ictal EEG. Some would label both scenarios as NCSE, but others argue that the context and outcomes are distinct and that only the first depicts true NCSE (10). There is no standard for minimal duration of NCSE nor is there consensus on optimal classification, and both are necessary for large-scale data collection and analysis.

Attempts to apply traditional seizure labels such as "complex partial" or "absence" to NCSE in some comatose individuals have been unsuccessful because it is not always possible to determine the relative contributions of ictal activity and other etiologies of encephalopathy. Investigators have also objected to the terms "electrographic" and "subclinical" status epilepticus because such terms fail to acknowledge that the altered awareness is a clinical manifestation of ictal activity (12). Proposed NCSE classifications have been based on age, EEG pattern, and type of epilepsy (7,9,11). See Chapter 2 for further discussion of definitions and classification.

Case ascertainment of NCSE presents several challenges. Clinical symptoms may be subtle and may be mistaken for other medical or psychological conditions. Delay in diagnosis of NCSE makes it difficult to determine actual onset time, and, if time at diagnosis is used as onset time, duration is likely to be underestimated. NCSE must be confirmed by EEG, and, although EEG criteria have been proposed to distinguish NCSE from other encephalopathic patterns (12-15), there may be variability and subjectivity in EEG interpretation (16-17). An EEG pattern may be interpreted as triphasic waves by one electroencephalographer and as NCSE by another. Thus, EEG confirmation may lead to underdiagnosis or overdiagnosis of NCSE.

A variety of biases may affect the composition of the study population and NCSE incidence figures in population-based studies. One challenge that is inherent in studying NCSE is that EEG is required for diagnosis, creating the potential for referral bias. If the physicians who request EEGs have a higher index of suspicion for NCSE in a particular subset of patients (epilepsy patients, for example), that subset may be overrepresented, and the study sample will not accurately reflect the population at large. Another bias, one that is unavoidable, is that patients whose seizures are successfully treated within 30 minutes cannot, by standard definition, be included in status epilepticus studies, even if their seizures would have continued without treatment. Thus, the seizure episodes of patients included in status epilepticus studies may be skewed toward longer durations or toward refractoriness to initial treatment, and this has implications for outcome (18).

Shorvon has identified additional potential reasons why the incidence of NCSE may be underestimated in epidemiologic studies (9). The presence or absence of tertiary neurologic centers can lead to variation in incidence estimates due to ascertainment bias. Accurate diagnosis and characterization of NCSE require the availability of prolonged EEG monitoring. Around-the-clock availability of this technology is not the norm for all hospitals. If EEG is not available when the patient is symptomatic, NCSE cannot be documented, and NCSE incidence will be underestimated. Likewise, if a routine EEG shows electrographic ictal activity, but if the activity is not recorded for at least 30 minutes, the case is excluded, leading to underestimation of NCSE incidence (9). Recent population-based studies have been primarily hospital based and have not included patients with NCSE who were not evaluated in a medical care setting. Thus, some patients with epileptic encephalopathies and those treated in nursing homes, ambulatory settings, or at home were not counted, whereas those hospitalized with acute symptomatic illnesses or severe injuries were likely to be well ascertained (9). Finally, investigators have elected to exclude subsets of the population (neonates from the Richmond study, children in the Hessen study, and patients with postanoxic encephalopathy from the Swiss study), resulting in underestimation of cases (9).

## NONCONVULSIVE STATUS EPILEPTICUS AS A PROPORTION OF ALL STATUS EPILEPTICUS

An early study by Dunne and colleagues (19) estimated that NCSE comprises 20% of all status epilepticus in adults. More recent population-based studies of status epilepticus have found that 30% to 63% of all status epilepticus is nonconvulsive (Table 3.1). Differences in population characteristics and, possibly, differences in NCSE definition and classification likely contribute to this wide range. The highest proportion of NCSE occurs in the study from Hessen, Germany, which included only adults, with a mean age of 65 years (4). The frequent history of remote stroke, present in 36% of the population, likely contributed to the high proportion of NCSE. Remote focal ischemic lesions are associated with localization-related epilepsy, itself a risk factor for NCSE. Thus, an older population and the higher prevalence of both remote stroke and epilepsy are associated variables that may have contributed to the high proportion of NCSE in this study.

## ESTIMATES OF THE INCIDENCE OF NONCONVULSIVE STATUS EPILEPTICUS

Historically, NCSE was considered uncommon, and was described in case reports and small

**TABLE 3.1** NONCONVULSIVE STATUS EPILEPTICUS PERCENT OF TOTAL STATUS EPILEPTICUS

| | % of SE that is | Seizure type as a % of NCSE | | | | | |
|---|---|---|---|---|---|---|---|
| | NCSE | SP | CP | Absence | Myoclonic | Subtle | Other |
| Richmond, Virginia | 30 | 82.5 | 10.5 | 3.5 | 2 | | 2 cases electrographic, neonates under 1 month of age excluded |
| Minnesota, USA | 51.7 | 74.7[a] | See footnote [a] | 6.7 | 18.4 | | Adults and children |
| Germany | 62.7 | 21.3 | 69.1 | 9.6 | 0 | | Adults only, mean age 65, etiology remote stroke in 36% |
| French speaking Switzerland | 49.4 | 36.5 | 54.1 | 7.1 | 0 | 2.4 | Subtle not included, post anoxic myoclonus excluded |
| Bologna, Italy | 50 | 18 | 32 | 4.5 | 32 | | Adults only |
| Rural Italy | 52 | 43 | 43 | 0 | 14 | | Adults and children |

[a] *Simple partial and complex partial combined*

series of patients with epilepsy. In the early 1990s, annual incidences of absence status epilepticus (ASE) and complex partial status epilepticus (CPSE) were estimated at one per million and 35 per million, respectively (8). These figures were based on estimates of the prevalence of absence and complex partial epilepsy in the general population and the assumption that 1% per year of those with absence and 1.5% per year of those with complex partial epilepsy have an episode of NCSE. Since then, several population-based studies of status epilepticus have allowed updated incidence figures to be calculated. Shorvon has estimated that the overall population incidence of NCSE based on published studies is 5.6 to 18.3 per 100,000 per year (9). An indirect estimate based on extrapolation from nonepidemiologically based data is 32 to 85 per 100,000 per year (9).

Population-based studies that included all types of status epilepticus are summarized in Table 3.2. Where available, the proportion of nonconvulsive status epilepticus types is expressed as a percentage of all status epilepticus cases. Data specifically pertinent to NCSE were extracted, and an annual incidence per 100,000 population was calculated for NCSE as a whole and by status epilepticus type (Table 3.3).

## POPULATION-BASED STUDIES OF NONCONVULSIVE STATUS EPILEPTICUS

### RICHMOND, VIRGINIA

In the study of status epilepticus in the Richmond, Virginia, metropolitan area, data were collected prospectively from local community hospitals as well as from an urban academic tertiary care medical center (2,20). There were 204 status epilepticus cases in 166 individuals, and the combined incidence of all types of status epilepticus was calculated at 41 per 100,000 individuals per year. When the database was validated and correction was made for underreporting, the revised incidence was 61 per 100,000 per year. Among all ages combined, generalized convulsive seizures occurred most frequently, with generalized tonic-clonic status epilepticus comprising 29% of the cases, partial onset with secondary generalization comprising 42%, and myoclonic status epilepticus (MSE), 2%. Overall, 30% of cases were NCSE; 23% had simple partial status epilepticus (SPSE), 3% CPSE, 2% MSE, 1% ASE, and 1% electrographic status epilepticus in coma.

In the Richmond study, a history of epilepsy was present in 38% of children (aged one month to 16 years), 42% of adults (between ages 16 and 60 years), and 30% in the elderly (older than 60 years) (2). The crude annual incidence of NCSE per 100,000 was approximately 11.8 (SPSE, 9.4; CPSE, 1.2; MSE, 0.7; ASE, 0.5).

### ROCHESTER, MINNESOTA

A retrospective study of status epilepticus in Rochester, Minnesota, over two decades (1965-1984) identified 199 first episodes of status epilepticus and reported an incidence of 18.3 per 100,000(3). The numeric discrepancy between status epilepticus incidence in Richmond and in Rochester is attributable to methodologic differences (prospective vs retrospective) and population differences (21). Overall, 42.2% of the status epilepticus in the Rochester study was nonconvulsive. The age-adjusted annual incidence of the various types of status epilepticus, per 100,000 population based on the 1980 US population, was primary generalized, 4.6; secondary generalized, 2.9; partial only, 7.1; absence, 0.6; and MSE, 1.9 (3).

### HESSEN, GERMANY

This prospective study of status epilepticus in adults was based on reports from neurologists and other clinicians in the emergency department and intensive care unit (ICU) (4). Over a 2-year period, 150 patients with status epilepticus were identified, half of whom had a history of epilepsy. The age-adjusted status epilepticus incidence was 17.1 per 100,000, higher in the elderly and in men, and half of the patients had a history of epilepsy. The majority of patients

TABLE 3.2 RESULTS OF POPULATION-BASED STATUS EPILEPTICUS STUDIES

| Location | Year | N | Crude Annual Incidence | Adjusted Annual Incidence* | SP | CP | Absence | Myoclonic | GTC | Partial 2° Gen | Other/ Unspecified | Prior Epilepsy | Overall Case Fatality | Other |
|---|---|---|---|---|---|---|---|---|---|---|---|---|---|---|
| Richmond, Virginia | 1995 | 166 pts | 41 (absolute) | 61 | 23 | 3 | 1 | 2 | 29 | 42 | 1 (electro-graphic) | 42% | 22% | Neonates under one month of age excluded |
| | 1996 | 204 cases | | | | | | | | | | | | |
| Minnesota, USA | 1997 | 184 | | | 40.8[a] | | 3.3 | 10.3 | 28.2 | 17.4 | — | — | 19% | Febrile SE excluded |
| | 1998 | 199 | 18.3 | 18.3 | 38.7[a] | See footnote[a] | 3.5 | 9.5 "Incomplete myoclonic" | 29.1 | 19.1[b] | — | 18% | — | — |
| Germany | 2001 | 150 | 15.8 | 17.1 | 13.3 | 43.3 | 6 | 0 | 14 | 19.3 | 4 | 50% | 9.3% | 36% remote stroke |
| French speaking Switzerland | 2000 | 172 | 9.9 | 10.3 | 18.1 | 26.7 | 3.5 | 0 | 33.1 | Not reported separately | 18.6[c] | 43% | 7.6% | Post-anoxic myoclonic excluded |
| Bologna, Italy | 2003 | 44 | 13.1 | 10.7 | 9 | 16 | 2 | 16 | 9 | 41 | 7 | 39% | 39% | — |
| Rural Italy | 2005 | 27 | 16.5 | 11.6 | 22 | 22 | 0 | 7.4 | 7.4 | 37 | 3.7 | 41% | 7% | Total 2 deaths in study[d] |

**adjusted for ascertainment in Richmond studies, Age-adjusted in other studies.*

[a]*Combined simple partial and complex partial*

[b]*generalized with focal features*

[c]*tonic – 2.3%, clonic – 0.6%, hemiconvulsive – 8.1%, subtle – 1.2%, other – 6.4%*

[d]*1 myoclonic, 1 simple partial*

TABLE 3.3 ANNUAL INCIDENCE OF CSE AND NCSE PER 100,000 POPULATION[a]

| Location | All SE | CSE | NCSE | SP | CP | Absence | Myoclonic | Subtle | Comments |
|---|---|---|---|---|---|---|---|---|---|
| Richmond, Virginia | 41 | 30 | 11.8 | 9.4 | 1.2 | 0.5 | 0.7 | | |
| Minnesota, USA | 17.1 | 7.5 | 9.6 | 7.1b | See footnote[b] | 0.6 | 1.9 | | Febrile SE not included |
| French speaking Switzerland | 9.9 | 3.6 | 4.8 | 1.8 | 2.6 | 0.3 | 0 | 0.1 | Tonic and clonic SE included in CSE. Hemiconvulsive, subtle and "other" not included. Postanoxic myoclonic encephalopathy excluded from study. |
| Bologna, Italy | 13.1 | 6.5 | 5.7 | 1.2 | 2.1 | 0.3 | 2.1 | | Unclassified SE not included |
| Rural Italy | 16.5 | 7.9 | 8.6 | 3.7 | 3.7 | 0 | 1.2 | | Unclassified SE not included |

[a]*All numbers refer to calculated crude incidence, except for the Minnesota figures, which are age-adjusted*
[b]*SP and CP combined*

(74%) had acute or remote brain injury as the etiology of status epilepticus. Remote cerebrovascular disease was the most frequent etiology, likely contributing to the increased incidence in men and in the elderly.

## FRENCH-SPEAKING SWITZERLAND

A 1-year prospective study of status epilepticus in 6 French-speaking Swiss cantons identified 172 cases (1). Cases were referred by physicians in emergency departments, ICUs, and EEG laboratories and by local pediatricians and neurologists. The standardized annual status epilepticus incidence was 10.3 per 100,000, higher in the elderly and in children younger than one year of age. Overall, 48.2% of the cases were nonconvulsive, 18.1% SPSE, 26.7% CPSE, and 3.5% ASE. "Confusional" status epilepticus comprised 30% of the sample, and, of this group, 11.5% were absence, 19% were of temporal lobe origin, and 52% were of frontal lobe origin. The initial ictal focus could not be localized by EEG in the remaining cases.

## RURAL AND URBAN ITALY

Vignatelli and colleagues studied the incidence and short-term prognosis of status epilepticus in adults in the urban area of Bologna, Italy, and also in a rural area of northern Italy (5,22). The authors identified patients by prospective observation of the neurology ward, neurology consultation service, EEG recordings, emergency department admissions, and hospital admissions and by review of all epilepsy discharge codes. In the urban setting, the annual age-adjusted incidence of status epilepticus (all types) was 10.7 per 100,000. ASE occurred in 2% of the study population, SPSE in 9%, and CPSE in 16%. Overall, NCSE was more common in the rural setting, where it comprised 44% of status epilepticus, compared with urban Bologna, where 27% of status epilepticus was nonconvulsive. In the rural setting, the annual age-adjusted incidence of all status epilepticus was 11.6 per 100,000, with 22% SPSE and 22% CPSE, and no ASE documented. In both studies, approximately 40% of the study populations had a history of previous seizures.

## NONCONVULSIVE STATUS EPILEPTICUS AND AGE

When all types of status epilepticus are considered together, there is a bimodal distribution of incidence, with the highest incidence occurring in children less than one year of age and in the elderly (2). Age is associated with status epilepticus type, with partial onset status epilepticus the most common status epilepticus type in adults, and generalized convulsive status epilepticus the most common type in children under the age of one year (2, 3). The age-specific incidence of partial status epilepticus in those aged 80 to 85 years is 44.3 per 100,000 and is far lower in younger age groups, ranging from 0 for several age intervals in young adulthood and middle age (20-25, 35-40, and 40-45 years) to 10.9 per 100,000 for children between the ages of one and 5 years. After age 60 years, the incidence of partial status epilepticus continues to rise steadily (3).

## AGE AND NONCONVULSIVE STATUS EPILEPTICUS TYPE

In both adults and children, SPSE is the most common NCSE type, comprising 29% of all pediatric status epilepticus and 22% of all adult status epilepticus (20). CPSE is less common, comprising 0% of pediatric status epilepticus and 4% of adult status epilepticus. Partial onset with secondary generalization occurs in 36% of pediatric status epilepticus and 43% of adult status epilepticus. Partial status epilepticus frequently secondarily generalizes, and the final seizure type is generalized convulsive in approximately three fourths of all pediatric and adult status epilepticus cases (20).

Absence status epilepticus is rare in all age groups, accounting for 6.7% of status epilepticus cases younger than 20 years of age, and 1.5% of cases aged 20 years or older (3). Of the 184 nonfebrile status epilepticus patients identified in a study by Hesdorffer and colleagues,

6 patients, of various ages, had ASE. One patient was younger than one year of age, one was in the 5- to 10-year-old age range, two were between 15 and 20 years of age, and two were in the 35- to 50-year-old age group (3).

## NONCONVULSIVE STATUS EPILEPTICUS TYPE

The determination of status epilepticus type is based on clinical semiology, EEG findings, and, sometimes, response to treatment. Interpretation of descriptions of NCSE seizure types is complicated by changes in terminology over time. Initially, the term NCSE included only CPSE or ASE (23-25). The term ASE was applied to all cases of electrographically generalized NCSE that lacked focal features, leading to the impression that ASE occurred more frequently than did other types of NCSE (23). Long-term EEG monitoring has led to the recognition that generalized EEG ictal activity frequently demonstrates focal onset, or waxing and waning focal features, and thus would more appropriately be termed CPSE (26-28). There is no standard definition of NCSE, but today investigators tend to include SPSE, CPSE, ASE, unspecified electrographic status epilepticus, and MSE under the umbrella of NCSE, excluding primary or secondary generalized convulsive status epilepticus. See Chapter 2 for information on the classification of NCSE.

Hospital-based series have described the varying distributions of NCSE types. A 1987 study identified 113 patients with status epilepticus over a 28-month period. Status epilepticus occurred in 0.2% of all admissions to the Royal Perth Hospital and 7% of the seizure admissions. Almost 20% of status epilepticus was nonconvulsive, and the majority (82%) was labeled ASE, including 6 de novo cases and 12 with a history of epilepsy. The remaining patients, all elderly, had CPSE (19). More recent series have found a significantly lower proportion of ASE, if any. A study of patients referred for EEG to evaluate alteration of consciousness or possible NCSE did not identify any ASE. Probable or definite NCSE occurred in 37%, and, of these, 57% of were CPSE, 39% were subtle generalized status epilepticus, and the remainder were myoclonic (29).

In population-based studies, NCSE types comprise 30% to 63% of all status epilepticus (Table 3.1). Data from epidemiologic studies of status epilepticus are presented in Tables 3.1 and 3.2. Table 3.1 lists the proportion of NCSE accounted for by each type of status epilepticus. Partial status epilepticus accounts for 50% to 92% of all NCSE. In the Richmond study, SPSE was the most common type, but, in Germany, Switzerland, and urban Italy, CPSE was the most common NCSE type. In rural Italy, SPSE and CPSE occurred equally, whereas, in the Minnesota study, both types of partial status epilepticus were combined into a single category.

Table 3.3 lists annual incidence of convulsive status epilepticus and NCSE types. Most studies have demonstrated a higher incidence of convulsive status epilepticus compared with NCSE, although the studies from rural Italy and Switzerland had a higher incidence of NCSE. Annual incidence for all NCSE ranged from 4.7 to 11.8 per 100,000. SPSE incidence ranged from 1.2 to 9.4 per 100,000, whereas CPSE incidence tended to be lower, ranging from 1.2 to 3.7 per 100,000. The incidence of MSE ranged from 0.7 to 2.1 per 100,000. ASE had the lowest incidence of all NCSE types in all studies, ranging from 0 to 0.6 per 100,000.

## NONCONVULSIVE STATUS EPILEPTICUS AND SEX

Age-adjusted annual incidence of status epilepticus (of all types) in males was almost double that of females (23.2-26.1 vs 13.1-13.7 per 100,000) in two population-based studies (3,4). In rural and urban Italy, however, the age-adjusted status epilepticus incidence was higher in women than in men. The authors attributed this finding to a more severe baseline neurologic condition of elderly women compared with men, due to a higher risk of dementia or worse clinical condition following stroke (22).

There are few data regarding incidence of NCSE by sex. In rural Italy, 74% of the 27 status epilepticus patients studied were women. Of the 14 patients with NCSE, 86% were women. Women comprised 80% of the SPSE (4 of 5 cases), 80% of the CPSE (also 4 of 5 cases), and 100% of the MSE (2 cases) (22). Whether or not sex is a risk factor for poor NCSE outcome is unknown. The relative risk of death within 30 days was significantly lower for women (RR = 0.4), compared with the risk of death for men. To avoid the potential confounding influences of age and etiology, the authors analyzed a subset of subjects over age 65 years, with etiologies limited to hypoxia or stroke, and found that the short-term risk for women remained lower than that for men, but statistical significance was not reached due to the small number of cases (30).

## NONCONVULSIVE STATUS EPILEPTICUS ETIOLOGIES

Considering all types of status epilepticus, the most common etiology is low antiepileptic drug levels, present in one third of cases (20). Acute symptomatic causes account for one third to one half of all status epilepticus (1,3,5). Approximately 40% to 50 % of patients in population-based studies including all types of status epilepticus have a history of epilepsy (Table 3.2). A series of 45 patients with NCSE also found that approximately half had a history of epilepsy (31). NCSE in this clinical context may be a manifestation of incompletely controlled epilepsy, low antiepileptic drug levels, or other provoking factor.

Status epilepticus etiologies vary according to age. More than half of childhood status epilepticus occurs in the setting of fever or infection. In adults, the majority of partial status epilepticus is due to acute or remote focal brain lesion, especially stroke. Other common etiologies include remote symptomatic causes, metabolic disturbance, hypoxia, and low antiepileptic drug levels (4,20).The few population-based studies that report etiology data specifically for NCSE indicate that acute symptomatic causes are the most common. In the Minnesota study, partial status epilepticus included both SPSE and CPSE, and 48% were due to acute symptomatic causes, 21% were idiopathic, 21% remote symptomatic causes, and 9% progressive symptomatic causes. Four of the 6 ASE cases were idiopathic, whereas two were classified as acute symptomatic (30). In a series of 100 cases of NCSE identified in an EEG database, the majority (52%) were due to acute medical causes, 31% were attributable to epilepsy, and 17% were cryptogenic (32).

## MORTALITY DUE TO NONCONVULSIVE STATUS EPILEPTICUS

A major controversy in the study of status epilepticus concerns the influence of etiology on outcomes following status epilepticus. Using multivariate analysis, the independent predictors of mortality for status epilepticus (including all types) are etiology, age, and duration (33). Mortality is independently associated with anoxia as an etiology, with advancing age, and with status epilepticus duration exceeding 1 hour. In addition to the effect of etiology on outcome, there is evidence that status epilepticus itself can contribute to mortality. A study of acute stroke patients with and without status epilepticus found that those patients with both disorders had 3 times the short-term mortality of those with stroke alone (34).

## MORTALITY AND ETIOLOGY

Although population-based studies of status epilepticus have not included multivariate analyses of determinants of mortality that are specific to NCSE, case series suggest that etiology is an important contributor to NCSE outcome. In general, NCSE in the setting of epilepsy has a relatively benign prognosis, whereas acute symptomatic etiologies are associated with a higher mortality rate (32,35-38). The former patients are often ambulatory and confused, whereas the latter tend to have more severe changes in mental status, including coma, requiring an ICU setting.

In a study of 100 consecutive cases of NCSE from an EEG database, mortality during hospital admission was 18% and morbidity was 39% (32). The majority of cases had an acute medical etiology of NCSE, and mortality was 27% in this group. Complications were significantly more frequent in the acute medical group than in the other two groups: epilepsy and cryptogenic. Epilepsy was the etiology of 31% of the cases, with a mortality of 3%. Etiology was classified as cryptogenic in 17% of the sample, and this group had an 18% mortality rate. Compared with patients with mild impairment of mental status, those with severe changes in mental status were more likely to have complications and more likely to die (32).

## MORTALITY AND STATUS EPILEPTICUS TYPE

In studies combining all types of status epilepticus, seizure type is not an independent risk factor for short-term mortality (30,34). It is unclear whether NCSE type is independently associated with NCSE outcome, but it is recognized that some NCSE types have more-benign outcomes than others. For example, ASE is not associated with significant short-term mortality, whereas MSE, often occurring in the setting of anoxic encephalopathy, usually has a high short-term mortality rate of 50% to 86% (5,22,30). In these subsets of patients, etiology is a strong confounding variable that probably has a greater influence on outcome than does status epilepticus type.

Table 3.4 lists the proportion of each status epilepticus type that died within 30 days. The mortality rate for SPSE ranged from 16% to 25%, whereas CPSE was not associated with death in the Italian studies (5, 22). The Minnesota study combined SPSE and CPSE and found that a greater percentage of this group died than in either the generalized tonic-clonic or the secondarily generalized convulsive status epilepticus groups. When confounding influences were accounted for with multivariate analysis, the unconfounded relative risk for short-term mortality was 0.8 for partial status epilepticus, 2.3 for secondarily generalized convulsive status epilepticus, and 1 for generalized tonic-clonic status epilepticus (30).

The mortality rate for partial status epilepticus was 30.5%, whereas, for those with generalized tonic-clonic seizures, including secondarily generalized, the mortality rate was 20.7% (20). ASE was not associated with any significant mortality (5, 30). See also Chapters 21 and 22 for a review of prognosis in NCSE.

## NONCONVULSIVE STATUS EPILEPTICUS IN SELECTED POPULATIONS

Prospective studies of patients referred for EEG or retrospective analyses of EEG studies have selection bias because EEGs are requested when there is a clinical suspicion of seizures. Similarly, studies of NCSE in preselected cohorts of patients with epilepsy, altered mental status, coma, or ICU location may convey a falsely

**TABLE 3.4** PERCENT MORTALITY BY SE TYPE

| | NCSE % mortality by SE type | | | | Convulsive SE % Mortality | | |
|---|---|---|---|---|---|---|---|
| | SP | CP | Absence | Myoclonic | GTC | 2° Gen | Case Fatality – All Types SE |
| Minnesota, USA | 24[a] | See footnote[a] | 0 | 68 | 15 | 22 | 19% |
| Bologna, Italy | 25 | 0 | 0 | 86 | 0 | 44 | 39% |
| Rural Italy | 16.7 | 0 | N/A | 50 | 0 | 0 | 7% |

*[a]24% mortality for simple partial and complex partial SE combined*

high impression of the prevalence of NCSE in the general population.

## EPILEPSY

Several early case series found that the majority of patients with NCSE had a history of seizures (26,37,39,40). It was also recognized, however, that NCSE can be the initial manifestations of epilepsy and that it may be precipitated by a variety of metabolic, drug-related, and other factors (7,38,41). Population-based studies demonstrate a history of epilepsy in 18% to 50% of all status epilepticus cases (Table 3.2), but this parameter has not been reported for NCSE alone.

NCSE has been studied in various types of primary generalized epilepsy. A retrospective study of 69 patients with JME identified 3 patients with typical ASE, all women, with recurrence in 1. The authors estimated the prevalence of NCSE in JME at 5.8% and an incidence in JME patients of 1.2% annually (42). Another study identified 136 consecutive adult patients with idiopathic generalized epilepsies and found that 15.4% had experienced typical ASE. Typical ASE occurred only among those adults who continued to have typical absence seizures as one of their seizure types and included 6.7% of the patients with JME (43). The mean age of onset of ASE was 29 years, whereas the mean age of onset for absence seizures was 9 years. ASE was the first clinical manifestation of epilepsy in up to one third of patients and recurred, often numerous times, in up to 85% of patients (44). Based on these studies, ASE appears to occur more often in adults than in children and more often in women than in men.

## CHILDREN

The epidemiology of NCSE in children has not been fully described. In infants younger than one year of age, convulsive status epilepticus occurs far more frequently than does NCSE (3,20). SPSE is the most common type of NCSE in children (2). The age-specific incidence of partial status epilepticus (per 100,000 population) varies during childhood. In one study, it was shown to be 4.8 in babies younger than one year of age, 10.9 in children between ages 1 and 5 years, 5.1 between ages 5 and 10 years, and 1.1 between ages 10 and 15 years (3). In addition to the common types of partial and generalized status epilepticus, there are a number of severe childhood epileptic encephalopathies associated with continuous spike-wave on EEG, including Landau-Kleffner syndrome and electrical status epilepticus during slow sleep. These are rare forms of status epilepticus and are estimated to occur with a frequency less than 1 per 100,000 persons annually (9).

NCSE is a relatively common occurrence in children who are monitored with continuous EEG in an ICU. Of 117 children monitored during a 4-year period, NCSE occurred in 23%, and was purely nonconvulsive in 89% of these cases. The remainder had a combination of nonconvulsive and convulsive manifestations (45). The most common admitting diagnoses were epilepsy (26%), altered mental status (15%), congenital malformation (11%), and hypoxia or anoxia (11%) (45).

Few data are available regarding outcomes of NCSE in children, although the short-term mortality rate of all status epilepticus in children is very low, 3%, all occurring only with infectious etiologies (2,20).

## THE ELDERLY

Status epilepticus has a higher incidence in the elderly than in any other age group. In the Richmond study, the incidence of status epilepticus (all types) in the elderly was 86 per 100,000 annually, and localization-related NCSE occurred in 29% of the elderly cases (2,20). A review of all EEGs performed on elderly patients at an Irish hospital found that EEG abnormalities were common, but NCSE was identified on two of 300 records (0.65%) (47). Among the elderly, the age-specific annual incidence of partial status epilepticus per 100,000 increases with advancing age, ranging from 21.8 in those between 65 and 70 years of age to 64.1 in those between 85 and 90 years of age (3). Almost 0.4% of people surviving to age 75 will have experienced an episode of status epilepticus (3).

The mortality rate of status epilepticus in the elderly is 38% (2). It is likely that the increased occurrence of stroke, metabolic abnormalities, and degenerative disorders in the elderly increase their risk of status epilepticus and contribute to its high mortality rate. Although diverse etiologies contribute to status epilepticus in the elderly, cerebrovascular disease, either acute or remote, is the most common etiology (46). Among a series of 30 stroke patients with status epilepticus, NCSE was more common than convulsive status epilepticus, occurring in 73%. Onset of NCSE usually occurred within two weeks of stroke and was associated with a delay in time to treatment (48).

The prognosis in elderly patients with NCSE is poor, with reported short-term mortality rates ranging from 30% to 52% (49, 50). Given the high mortality rate among elderly patients with NCSE, the question arises as to whether NCSE contributes to mortality or is a manifestation of severe comorbid illnesses that lead to death. Several studies have demonstrated the dominant influence of etiology and comorbidities on outcome. A prospective series of 10 elderly NCSE patients with etiologies including epilepsy, electroconvulsive therapy, hyponatremia, tumor, head trauma, and hypoxia concluded that NCSE has a worse prognosis in the elderly than in younger patients, attributable to severity of underlying etiologies in the elderly (51). Hospital-acquired infection was frequent, occurring in 7 patients and leading to death in 3. Another series of 25 critically ill elderly patients with NCSE excluded cases with anoxic encephalopathy. Death was associated with the number of severe acute medical problems at presentation and occurred in more than half of the cases (49). In another series of 15 elderly patients with NCSE, 20% were alive 6 months after diagnosis, with most deaths occurring as the result of aspiration pneumonia or acute heart failure (52).

Elderly patients with NCSE have a higher morbidity rate and worse prognosis than those with altered mental status due to other causes (50). A case-control study investigated patients at least 75 years old who underwent EEG. Both groups had a variety of acute medical conditions, and many patients in each group had a history of dementia, stroke, or both. A history of epilepsy and tramadol use were significantly more frequent in the NCSE group, compared with controls. Compared with controls, those in the NCSE group were hospitalized longer and were more likely to have unfavorable outcomes. Mortality rate was 30% in the NCSE group and 5.9% in the control group. Within the NCSE group, unfavorable outcome was associated with a higher number of comorbidities and severely altered mental status at presentation (50).

Treatment of NCSE in the critically ill elderly is frequently ineffective and may contribute to death (49). Subtle status epilepticus in the elderly is also more refractory to treatment than is convulsive status epilepticus. The Veterans' Affairs Cooperative Study compared 4 treatments for generalized convulsive status epilepticus (53). Of the enrolled study patients older than 65 years of age, 71% had overt generalized convulsive status epilepticus, whereas 29% had subtle convulsive generalized status epilepticus, described as "the stage of generalized convulsive status when the patient is in continuous coma but only subtle motor convulsions are seen" (53). Although the groups did not differ in terms of recurrence rate, 30-day outcome, or adverse events, there was an important difference in response to treatment. Only 14.5% of the elderly patients with subtle status epilepticus responded to the first treatment, whereas 56.9% of those with overt convulsive status epilepticus responded to the first treatment (54).

Not all NCSE in the elderly has a dire prognosis. De novo ASE has been described in the elderly, presenting as ictal confusion, and associated with generalized spike-waves on EEG (19,38). Etiologies include drug toxicity and benzodiazepine withdrawal. The incidence of this entity is not known, but it is recognized to have a benign outcome.

## NONCONVULSIVE STATUS EPILEPTICUS IN SELECTED SETTINGS

### COMA

Early reports of NCSE tended to focus on status epilepticus in ambulatory patients. With the availability of continuous EEG monitoring in ICUs, it has become clear that patients with critical illnesses and acute brain injuries have a high incidence of NCSE. Because these clinical settings often cause altered level of consciousness, an additional causative diagnosis such as NCSE is not suspected and diagnosis does not occur until hours or days have passed (12,55,56).

Several studies have examined the occurrence of NCSE in comatose patients. NCSE is a frequent occurrence in patients with acute brain injuries who are in the neuro-ICU. In a series of 124 patients with admitting diagnoses including stroke, intracranial hemorrhage, metabolic coma, brain tumor, acute traumatic brain injury, and convulsive status epilepticus, 27% had NCSE, and an even higher proportion (34%) had nonconvulsive seizures that were not classifiable as status epilepticus (56). NCSE occurred with the highest incidence in those with metabolic derangements or following treated generalized convulsive status epilepticus (56).

In a study of patients evaluated with EEG for coma, NCSE was present in 8% of patients (28). The investigators studied 236 patients with unselected coma, aged one month to 87 years, specifically excluding those with overt seizures or clinical status epilepticus. Elderly patients (aged 60 or older) comprised 38% of the study group, and 51% of the patients were adults (aged 16-59 years). The most common precipitating etiology was hypoxia or anoxia, accounting for 42% of NCSE, followed by stroke (22%). See also Chapter 13 on NCSE in the ICU.

### FOLLOWING CONVULSIVE STATUS EPILEPTICUS

NCSE frequently occurs in the wake of convulsive status epilepticus and can be challenging to diagnose. When a patient has generalized convulsions that stop spontaneously or after treatment, it is frequently assumed that electrographic seizures have also ended, and a depressed level of consciousness is attributed to a postictal state. However, studies have documented that 12% to 53 % of convulsive status epilepticus "converts" to electrographic status epilepticus without clinical signs (46,53,57,58). This dissociation between obvious clinical signs and electrographic manifestations of status epilepticus has been termed "subtle status epilepticus" (53).

Several studies have investigated postconvulsive NCSE by investigating patients referred for EEG. Although this is a practical approach, selection bias is unavoidably present because a major reason for EEG referral is the suspicion of possible status epilepticus. Thus, these studies probably underestimate the actual frequency of postconvulsive NCSE. One study reviewed 198 prospectively identified patients in whom EEGs were ordered to evaluate altered consciousness or possible status epilepticus (29). Of the 48 patients who had altered consciousness preceded by tonic-clonic seizure, almost one third had NCSE on EEG (29). In a series of 19 pediatric patients with NCSE, 17 had convulsive seizures in the acute setting prior to diagnosis of NCSE (59). Convulsions were brief and isolated in 12 of these patients, and convulsive status epilepticus preceded NCSE in 5 (59).

In the Richmond, Virginia, study, 164 patients were prospectively evaluated with continuous EEG monitoring after clinical control of convulsive status epilepticus (60). Almost half, 48%, demonstrated ictal discharges after clinical status epilepticus had ended, and 14% had NCSE beginning within 30 minutes of convulsive status epilepticus. EEG patterns were heterogenous, but most patients had secondarily generalized or partial status epilepticus. Those with NCSE had the worst outcome, with a 51% mortality rate, compared with a 32%

mortality rate for those with delayed ictal discharges, and 13% for those without ictal discharges following convulsive status epilepticus. In addition to NCSE, advanced age and etiology were independent risk factors for poor outcome.

In the Veterans Affairs Status Epilepticus Cooperative Study, patients were treated with a series of intravenously administered antiepileptic medications until clinical seizure activity stopped (53). Of 518 convulsive patients, 26% demonstrated subtle status epilepticus, and this group of patients had a significantly higher 30-day mortality rate (65%), compared with those who had overt status epilepticus only (27%). Subtle status epilepticus in this study was also more refractory to treatment. Although 55% of patients with generalized convulsive status epilepticus responded to the first treatment, initial treatment succeeded in only 15% of patients with NCSE.

## IN THE INTENSIVE CARE UNIT

Two categories of patients with status epilepticus are found in the ICU: those who are admitted there because of status epilepticus and those who are being treated for severe surgical or medical illness and develop status epilepticus while in the ICU (61). The latter group presents the diagnostic challenge. The majority of these patients are not recognized as having NCSE prior to diagnostic EEG (55). Much of the ICU literature has focused on the importance of detecting nonconvulsive seizures in these critically ill patients, using continuous EEG. Nonconvulsive seizures and NCSE have been documented to occur frequently in severely affected neurologic populations, including those with traumatic brain injury, subarachnoid hemorrhage, and intracerebral hemorrhage (12,56,62-67). Continuous EEG monitoring significantly improves the detection of nonconvulsive seizures (68,69).

### *Mortality in the intensive care unit*

Although the incidence of NCSE in ICU populations with severe brain injury is unclear, there is evidence that outcomes differ between those with nonconvulsive seizures and those with NCSE (69).

In the ICU setting, NCSE is associated with a higher mortality rate than are nonconvulsive seizures alone, and the longer NCSE persists, the higher the mortality rate (12). In one study, continuous EEG monitoring in the ICU identified 49 cases of nonconvulsive seizures in 43 adult patients out of a total of 127 patients monitored over a 28-month interval (12). NCSE occurred in 47% of the cases, and nonconvulsive seizures without NCSE in the remainder. Although approximately one quarter of both groups became disabled, more than half (57%) of those with NCSE died, compared with 9% of those with nonconvulsive seizures (12). Those with acute symptomatic causes of seizures or NCSE had higher mortality rates, compared with the remote symptomatic group, but etiology was not an independent predictor of mortality because acute symptomatic seizures were associated with longer duration. With multivariate logistic regression, the only independent predictors of mortality associated with nonconvulsive seizures were delay to diagnosis and seizure duration (12).

NCSE in critically ill elderly patients has a high mortality rate. In a series of 25 cases of NCSE in elderly patients with critical illness due to multiple organ dysfunction syndrome or cancer, the mortality rate was 52% (49). Death was associated with the number of acute life-threatening medical problems on presentation, averaging 1.8 in survivors and 2.8 in those who died. Being treated with intravenously administered benzodiazepine increased the risk of death, and aggressive treatment of NCSE did not improve outcome. In this study, it was unclear whether NCSE independently affected patient outcome or was a manifestation of disease severity in predisposed patients (49).

## SUMMARY

NCSE comprises close to half of all status epilepticus, demonstrating subtle clinical signs and occurring in a variety of settings, including de novo, in patients with epilepsy, or in the setting of acute or remote symptomatic conditions. It is not uncommon for NCSE to be present after clinical manifestations of convulsive status epilepticus have stopped. Although the unadjusted annual incidence of NCSE per 100,000 ranges from 5 to 11, challenges in diagnosing and categorizing NCSE, particularly the need for EEG, make it likely that these incidences are underestimates. Epilepsy and acute symptomatic illnesses are common etiologies for NCSE. NCSE is associated with a significant mortality. In general, NCSE that occurs in patients with epilepsy has a relatively good prognosis, whereas NCSE that occurs in the setting of coma has a high mortality rate, which has been attributed to underlying etiology and comorbidities. A classification system that takes into account the heterogeneous clinical settings and manifestations of NCSE would allow more accurate epidemiologic assessment.

## REFERENCES


1. Coeytaux A, Jallon P, Galobardes B, Morabia A. Incidence of status epilepticus in French-speaking Switzerland: (EPISTAR). Neurology 2000;55:693-697.
2. DeLorenzo RJ, Pellock JM, Towne AR, Boggs JG. Epidemiology of status epilepticus. J Clin Neurophysiol 1995;12:316-325.
3. Hesdorffer DC, Logroscino G, Cascino G, Annegers JF, Hauser WA. Incidence of status epilepticus in Rochester, Minnesota, 1965-1984. Neurology 1998;50:735-741.
4. Knake S, Rosenow F, Vescovi M, Oertel WH, Mueller HH, Wirbatz A, Katsarou N, Hamer HM. Incidence of status epilepticus in adults in Germany: a prospective, population-based study. Epilepsia 2001;42:714-718.
5. Vignatelli L, Tonon C, D'Alessandro R. Incidence and short-term prognosis of status epilepticus in adults in Bologna, Italy. Epilepsia 2003;44:964-968.
6. Wu YW, Shek DW, Garcia PA, Zhao S, Johnston SC. Incidence and mortality of generalized convulsive status epilepticus in California. Neurology 2002;58:1070-1076.
7. Kaplan PW. Nonconvulsive status epilepticus. Semin Neurol 1996;16:33-40.
8. Shorvon S. Status epilepticus: its clinical features and treatment in children and adults. London, UK: Cambridge University Press; 1994:21-33.
9. Shorvon S. The definition, classification, and frequency of NCSE. Epileptic Disord 2005; 7:255-258.
10. Niedermeyer E, Ribeiro M. Considerations of nonconvulsive status epilepticus. Clinical Electroencephalogr 2000;31:192-195.
11. Brodtkorb E, Sand t, Kristiansen A, Torbergsen T. Nonconvulsive status epilepticus in the adult mentally retarded. Seizure 1993;2:115-123.
12. Young BG, Jordan KG, Doig GS. An assessment of nonconvulsive seizures in the intensive care unit using continuous EEG monitoring: an investigation of variables associated with mortality. Neurology 1996;47:83-89.
13. Kaplan PW. The clinical features, diagnosis, and prognosis of nonconvulsive status epilepticus. Neurologist 2005;11:348-361.
14. Chong DJ, Hirsch LJ. Which EEG patterns warrant treatment in the critically ill? Reviewing the evidence for treatment of periodic epileptiform discharges and related patterns. J Clin Neurophysiol 2005;22:79-91.
15. Kaplan PW. The EEG of status epilepticus. J Clin Neurophysiol 2006;23:221-229.
16. Kaplan PW. Prognosis in nonconvulsive status epilepticus. Epileptic Disord 2000;2:185-193.
17. Walker MC. Diagnosis and treatment of nonconvulsive status epilepticus. CNS Drugs 2001; 15:931-939.
18. DeLorenzo RJ, Garnett LK, Towne AR, Waterhouse EJ, Boggs JG, Morton L, Chouhry A, Barnes T, Ko D. Comparison of status epilepticus with prolonged seizure episodes lasting from 10 to 29 minutes. Epilepsia 1999;40:164-169.
19. Dunne JW, Summers QA, Stewart-Wynne EG. Non-convulsive status epilepticus: a prospective study in an adult general hospital. Q J Med 1987;62:117-126.
20. DeLorenzo RJ, Hauser WA, Towne AR, Boggs JG, Pellock JM, Penberthy, Garnett L, Fortner CA, Ko D. A prospective, population-based epidemiologic study of status epilepticus in Richmond, Virginia. Neurology 1996;46:1029-1035.
21. Waterhouse EJ. Epidemiology of status epilepticus. In: Drislane FW, ed. Status Epilepticus, a Clinical Perspective. Totowa, NJ: Humana Press; 2005:55-75.
22. Vignatelli L, Rinaldi R, Galeotti M, de CP, D'Alessandro R. Epidemiology of status epilepticus in a rural area of northern Italy: a 2-year popu-

lation-based study. Eur J Neurol 2005;12:897-902.
23. Gastaut H. Classification of status epilepticus. In: Delgado-Escueta AV, Wasterlain CG, Treiman DM, Porter RJ, eds. Status Epilepticus: Mechanisms of Brain Damage and Treatment. New York, NY; Raven Press; 1983:15-35.
24. Treiman DM, Degiorgio CMA, Salisbury SM, Wickboldt CL. Subtle generalized convulsive status epilepticus [abstract]. Epilepsia 1984; 25:653.
25. Krumholz A, Sung GY, Fisher RS, Barry E, Bergey GK, Grattan LM. Complex partial status epilepticus accompanied by serious morbidity and mortality. Neurology 1995;45:1499-1504.
26. Tomson T, Svanborg E, Wedlund JE. Nonconvulsive status epilepticus: high incidence of complex partial status. Epilepsia 1986;27:276-285.
27. Granner MA, Lee SI. Nonconvulsive status epilepticus: EEG analysis in a large series. Epilepsia 1994;35:42-47.
28. Towne AR, Waterhouse EJ, Boggs JG, Garnett LK, Brown AJ, Smith JR, DeLorenzo RJ, Smith JR Jr. Prevalence of nonconvulsive status epilepticus in comatose patients. Neurology 2000;54:340-345.
29. Privitera M, Hoffman M, Moore JL, Jester D. EEG detection of nontonic-clonic status epilepticus in patients with altered consciousness. Epilepsy Res 1994;18:155-166.
30. Logroscino G, Hesdorffer DC, Cascino G, Annegers JF, Hauser WA. Short-term mortality after a first episode of status epilepticus. Epilepsia 1997;38:1344-1349.
31. Haffey S, McKernan A, Pang K. Non-convulsive status epilepticus: a profile of patients diagnosed within a tertiary referral centre. J Neurol Neurosurg Psychiatry 2004;75:1043-1044.
32. Shneker BF, Fountain NB. Assessment of acute morbidity and mortality in nonconvulsive status epilepticus. Neurology 2003;61:1066-1073.
33. Towne AR, Pellock JM, Ko D, DeLorenzo RJ. Determinants of mortality in status epilepticus. Epilepsia 1994;35:27-34.
34. Waterhouse EJ, Vaughan JK, Barnes TY, Boggs JG, Towne AR, Kopec-Garnett L, DeLorenzo RJ. Synergistic effect of status epilepticus and ischemic brain injury on mortality. Epilepsy Res 1998;29:175-183.
35. Cockerell OC, Walker MC, Sander JW, Shorvon SD. Complex partial status epilepticus: a recurrent problem. J Neurol Neurosurg Psychiatry 1994;57:835-837.
36. Tomson T, Lindbom U, Nilsson BY. Nonconvulsive status epilepticus in adults: thirty-two consecutive patients from a general hospital population. Epilepsia 1992;33:829-835.
37. Guberman A, Cantu-Reyna G, Stuss D, Broughton R. Nonconvulsive generalized status epilepticus: clinical features, neuropsychological testing, and long-term follow-up. Neurology 1986;36:1284-1291.
38. Lee, S. Nonconvulsive status epilepticus: ictal confusion in later life. Arch Neurol 1985;42: 778-781.
39. Niedermeyer E, Khalifeh R. Petit mal status, an electroclinical appraisal. Epilepsia 1965;6:250-262.
40. Ballenger C, King D, Gallagher B. Partial complex status epilepticus. Neurology 1983;33: 1545-1552.
41. Jagoda A, Riggio S. Nonconvulsive status epilepticus in adults. Am J Emerg Med 1988;6:250-254.
42. Dziewas R, Kellinghaus C, Ludemann P. Nonconvulsive status epilepticus in patients with juvenile myoclonic epilepsy: types and frequencies. Seizure 2002;11:335-339.
43. Agathonikou A, Panayiotopoulos CP, Giannakodimos S, Koutroumanidis M. Typical absence status in adults: diagnostic and syndromic considerations. Epilepsia 1998;39:1265-1276.
44. Koutroumanidis M. Typical absence status epilepticus. In: Nonconvulsive Status Epilepticus: Epilepsy Research Foundation Workshop Reports. Epileptic Disord 2005;7:279-282.
45. Jette N, Claasen J, Emerson R, Hirsch L. Frequency and predictors of nonconvulsive seizures during continuous electroencephalographic monitoring in critically ill children. Arch Neurol 2006;63:1750-1755.
46. DeLorenzo RJ. Clinical and epidemiological study of status epilepticus in the elderly. In: Rowan AJ, Ramsey RE, eds. Seizures and Epilepsy in the Elderly. Newton, MA: Butterworth-Heinemann; 1997:191-205.
47. Widdess-Walsh P, Sweeney BJ, Galvin R, McNamara B. Utilization and yield of EEG in the elderly population. J Clin Neurophysiol 2005;22: 253-255.
48. Afsar N, Kaya D, Aktan S, Sykut-Bingol C. Stroke and status epilepticus: stroke type, type of status epilepticus, and prognosis. Seizure 2003;12:23-27.
49. Litt B, Wityk RJ, Hertz SH, Mullen PD, Weiss H, Ryan DD, Henry TR. Nonconvulsive status

epilepticus in the critically ill elderly. Epilepsia 1998;39:1194-1202.
50. Bottaro FJ, Martinez OA, Fernandez Pardal MM, Bruetman JE, Reisin RC. Nonconvulsive status epilepticus in the elderly: a case-control study. Epilepsia 2007;48:966-972.
51. Labar D, Barrera J, Solomon G, Harden C. Nonconvulsive status epilepticus in the elderly: a case series and review of the literature. J Epilepsy 1998;11:74-78.
52. Martin Y, Artaz MA, Bornand-Rousselot A. Nonconvulsive status epilepticus in the elderly. J Am Geriatr Soc 2004;52:476-477.
53. Treiman DM, Meyers PD, Walton NY, Collins JF, CollingC, Rowan AJ, Handforth A, Faught E, Calabrese A, Uthman BM, Ramsay RE, Mamdani MB. N Engl J Med 1998;339:792-798.
54. Treiman DM, Walker MC. Treatment of seizure emergencies: Convulsive and non-convulsive status epilepticus. Epilepsy Res 2006;68(Suppl 1):77-82.
55. Drislane FW, Blum AS, Schomer DL. Unsuspected electrographic status epilepticus in intensive care units. [abstract] Neurology 1998;50(Suppl 1):395-396.
56. Jordan KG. Nonconvulsive status epilepticus in acute brain injury. J Clin Neurophysiol 1999;16:332-340.
57. Drislane FR, Schomer DL. Clinical implications of generalized electrographic status epilepticus. Epilepsy Res 1994;19:111-121.
58. Jaitly R, Sgro JA, Towne AR, Ko D, DeLorenzo RJ. Prognostic value of EEG monitoring after status epilepticus: a prospective adult study. J Clin Neurophysiol 1997;14:326-334.
59. Tay SKH, Hirsch LJ, Leary L, Jette N, Wittman J, Akman CI. Nonconvulsive status epilepticus in children: Clinical and EEG characteristics. Epilepsia 2006;47:1504-1509.
60. DeLorenzo RJ, Waterhouse EJ, Towne AR, Boggs JG, Ko D, DeLorenzo GA, Brown A, Garnett L. Persistent nonconvulsive status epilepticus after the control of convulsive status epilepticus. Epilepsia 1998;39:833-840.
61. Walker MC. Status epilepticus on the intensive care unit. J Neurol 2003;250:401-406.
62. Grand'Maison F, Reiher J, Leduc CP. Retrospective inventory of EEG abnormalities in partial status epilepticus. Electroencephalogr Clin Neurophysiol 1991;79:264-270.
63. Scholtes FB, Renier WO, Meinardi H. Non-convulsive status epilepticus: causes, treatment, and outcome in 65 patients. J Neurol Neurosurg Psychiatry 1996;61:93-95.
64. Dennis LJ, Claassen J, Hirsch LJ, Emerson RG, Connolly ES, Mayer SA. Nonconvulsive status epilepticus after subarachnoid hemorrhage. Neurosurgery 2002;51:1136-1143.
65. Vespa PM, Nuwer MR, Nenov V, Ronne-Engstrom E, Hovda DA, Bergsneider M, Kelly DF, Martin NA, Becker DP. Increased incidence and impact of nonconvulsive and convulsive seizures after traumatic brain injury as detected by continuous EEG in the intensive care unit. J Neurosurg 1999;91:750-760.
66. Claassen J, Mayer SA, Kowalski BS, Emerson RG, Hirsch LJ. Detection of electrographic seizures with continuous EEG monitoring in critically ill patients. Neurology 2004;62:1743-1748.
67. Claassen J, Mayer SA, Hirsch LJ. Continuous EEG monitoring in patients with subarachnoid hemorrhage. J Clin Neurophysiol 2005;22:92-98.
68. Vespa PM, Nenov V, Nuwer MR. Continuous EEG monitoring in the intensive care unit: early findings and clinical efficacy. J Clin Neurophysiol 1999;16:1-13.
69. Vespa P. Continuous EEG monitoring for the detection of seizures in traumatic brain injury, infarction, and intracerebral hemorrhage: "to detect and protect." J Clin Neurophysiol 2005;22:99-106.
70. Logroscino G, Hesdorffer DC, Cascino GD, Annegers JF, Bagiella E, Hauser WA. Long-term mortality after a first episode of status epilepticus. Neurology 2002;58:537-541.
71. Waterhouse EJ, Towne AR. Seizures in the elderly: Nuances in presentation and treatment. Cleve Clin J Med 2005;72(Suppl 3):26-37.

CHAPTER 4

# THE ELECTROENCEPHALOGRAM OF NONCONVULSIVE STATUS EPILEPTICUS

SUSAN T. HERMAN

Nonconvulsive status epilepticus (NCSE) comprises a range of conditions in which prolonged (> 30 minutes) or recurrent electrographic seizure activity results in nonconvulsive clinical symptoms (1). There are as many types of NCSE as there are nonconvulsive epileptic seizures (Table 4.1) (2). NCSE has subtle and pleomorphic clinical manifestations—including impairment of consciousness (mild confusion to coma), automatisms, eye deviation or nystagmoid jerking, and subtle limb or facial twitching—and therefore may be difficult to distinguish from other disorders. To confirm NCSE, an electroencephalogram (EEG) must show electrographic seizure activity. This chapter will describe EEG criteria for the diagnosis of NCSE, common EEG patterns in the different types of NCSE, and the utility of EEG for the management of NCSE. The chapter will focus on the more "classic" examples of NCSE, as well as on the borderline areas of controversy; controversial patterns are fully discussed in Chapter 5.

## ELECTROENCEPHALOGRAPHIC CRITERIA FOR NONCONVULSIVE STATUS EPILEPTICUS AND COMMON PITFALLS IN DIAGNOSIS

There is no universally accepted classification of NCSE, and significant controversy exists regarding which EEG patterns are consistent with a diagnosis of NCSE. In addition to EEG findings, the patient's medical history, clinical state, and response to antiepileptic drugs (AEDs) may be required for accurate diagnosis. Several groups have proposed EEG criteria for NCSE (1,3-5), but the diagnosis remains subjective and somewhat arbitrary. A recent Epilepsy Research Foundation workshop report (1) proposed several "clear-cut patterns" of NCSE, but even these criteria engender some debate. The following findings, compared to those from a baseline EEG in patients with an epileptic encephalopathy, are usually considered to represent NCSE: frequent or continuous focal electrographic seizures that evolve in amplitude, frequency, and/or spatial distribution; frequent or continuous generalized spike-wave discharges at frequencies greater than 3 Hz; and more rapid generalized spike-wave discharges. Slower patterns are more controversial; repetitive discharges slower than 2.5 Hz are more likely to be ictal (ie, indicative of an epileptic seizure) if they evolve in frequency or follow the occurrence of clinical status epilepticus. Patterns that are generally agreed not to represent NCSE include periodic discharges in patients without prior seizures but with acute cerebral injuries and patients with epileptic encephalopathies in which the periodic generalized discharges are similar to those of the baseline EEG (1).

Figure 4.1 provides an algorithm for the EEG diagnosis of NCSE, focusing on several main features adapted from prior published criteria (3,5): (1) repetitive focal or generalized epileptiform activity (spikes, sharp waves, spike-and-wave, sharp-and-slow-wave complexes) or rhythmic waveforms faster than 2.5 Hz lasting longer than 10 seconds or (2) similar discharges slower than 2.5 Hz with any of the following features: (a) unequivocal evolution in frequency, morphology, or field; (b) focal clinical motor manifestations (eg, focal limb or face twitching); or (c) clear clinical and EEG improvement after intravenous administration of rapid-acting AEDs, typically benzodiazepines. To meet

TABLE 4.1 CLASSIFICATION OF NCSE

| NCSE Type | Clinical Characteristics | EEG characteristics |
|---|---|---|
| *Generalized NCSE* | | |
| Typical ASE | Impaired consciousness (usually mild), disorientation, staring, rhythmic blinking, in patients with primary generalized epilepsy | Continuous or recurrent generalized spike-and-wave or polyspike-and-wave at ≥ 3 Hz; normal interictal background |
| Atypical ASE | Increased confusion compared to baseline in patients with epileptic encephalopathy | Continuous or recurrent generalized spike-and-wave or polyspike-and-wave at < 3 Hz; diffuse slowing on interictal background |
| Late-onset ASE | Impaired consciousness, disorientation to stupor, staring, rhythmic blinking, in elderly patients with no history of epilepsy | Continuous or recurrent generalized spike-and-wave or polyspike-and-wave at 0.5-4 Hz; diffuse slowing on interictal background |
| SGCSE | Coma or obtundation; may show subtle limb jerking or nystagmoid eye movements | Generalized spike-and-wave or poly spike-and-wave 1-4 Hz, often on flat background |
| *Partial NCSE* | | |
| SPSE | Persistent sensory or autonomic phenomena which remain confined to one area of the body, no impairment of consciousness | Localized epileptiform activity (repetitive spikes or rhythmic waveforms) that remains confined; > 60% of foci may not be visible on surface EEG |
| CPSE | Impaired consciousness with confusion, bizarre behavior, automatisms | Focal rhythmic activity (usually involving temporal or frontal regions) with evolution in frequency, morphology, or field; may show diffuse pattern late in status epilepticus |
| Electrographic partial status epilepticus | Coma or obtundation; may show subtle limb jerking or nystagmoid eye movements | Focal rhythmic activity with evolution in frequency, morphology, or field; interictal EEG often shows PLEDs |
| *Age-related NCSE* | | |
| Neonatal status epilepticus | Clonic, tonic, myoclonic seizures | Focal activity in alpha, theta, delta band, sometimes with little evolution in frequency, morphology, or field |
| ESES | Progressive cognitive decline | Generalized spike-wave at 1.5-3.5 Hz occupying more than 85% of NREM sleep |
| Landau-Kleffner syndrome | Progressive receptive aphasia and behavioral disturbance | Unilateral or bilateral temporal spike-wave at 1.5-3.5 Hz during NREM sleep (< 85%) |
| Nonepileptic NCSE[a] | Unresponsiveness, staring, eyelid fluttering | Normal background |

NCSE refers to nonconvulsive status epilepticus; EEG, electroencephalographic; ASE, absence status epilepticus; ESES, Electrical status epilepticus during slow-wave sleep; Hz, Hertz, cycles per second; SGCSE, subtle or electrographic generalized convulsive status epilepticus; PLEDs, periodic lateralized epileptiform discharges; NREM, non-rapid eye movement sleep; SPSE, simple partial status epilepticus; CPSE, complex partial status epilepticus.

[a]*Psychogenic or pseudo-status epilepticus*

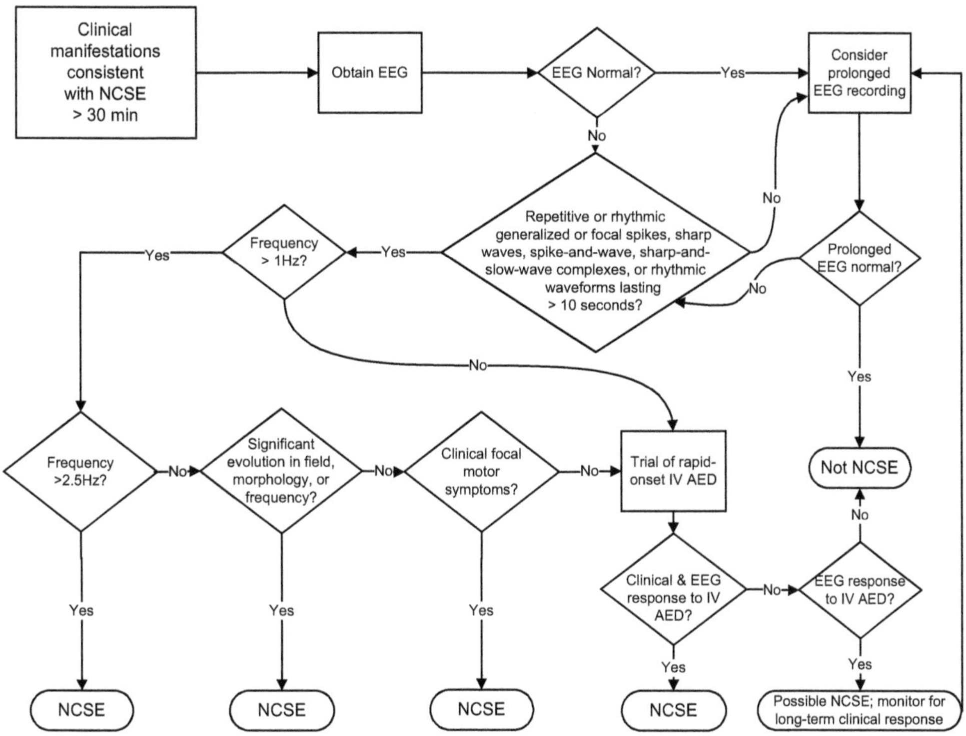


**Figure 4.1** Algorithm for electroencephalographic diagnosis of nonconvulsive status epilepticus (NCSE). See text for details.

criteria for evolution 2a, the electrographic discharges should show an increase or decrease in frequency by more than 1 Hz, significant change in waveform morphology, or spread to at least two adjacent EEG electrodes (5). A response to intravenously administered AEDs must include improvement in both the clinical state of the patient and the EEG or complete cessation of electrographic ictal activity with return of normal EEG background activity (6) (Figure 4.2). Figure 4.1 is merely a guide to diagnosis; many patterns cannot be definitely classified as ictal or nonictal even when all criteria are fulfilled.

## PARTIAL VERSUS GENERALIZED NONCONVULSIVE STATUS EPILEPTICUS

Classification of NCSE by the predominant EEG pattern yields 3 main groups: (1) patterns that are generalized at onset (Figure 4.2A); (2) patterns that begin focally, with or without secondary generalization (Figure 4.3); and (3) patterns that have both focal and generalized features or are otherwise poorly classified (7). Bihemispheric NCSE has features of both focal and generalized status epilepticus (8) and may show either a widespread field with focal predominance over one hemisphere (Figure 4.4) or shifting predominance between hemispheres. In a series of 85 episodes of NCSE in 78 patients, 69% showed a generalized pattern, 13% a focal pattern, and 18% a generalized pattern with focal predominance (7). In a study of NCSE in pediatric patients in the intensive care unit, focal or multifocal status epilepticus (65%) was shown to be more common than generalized status epilepticus (35%), often reflecting underlying focal acute structural brain lesions (9). It is important to remember that ictal activity may spread from focal areas to widespread brain regions, so an EEG recorded in established NCSE may not allow for a distinction to be made between focal and generalized status epilepticus.

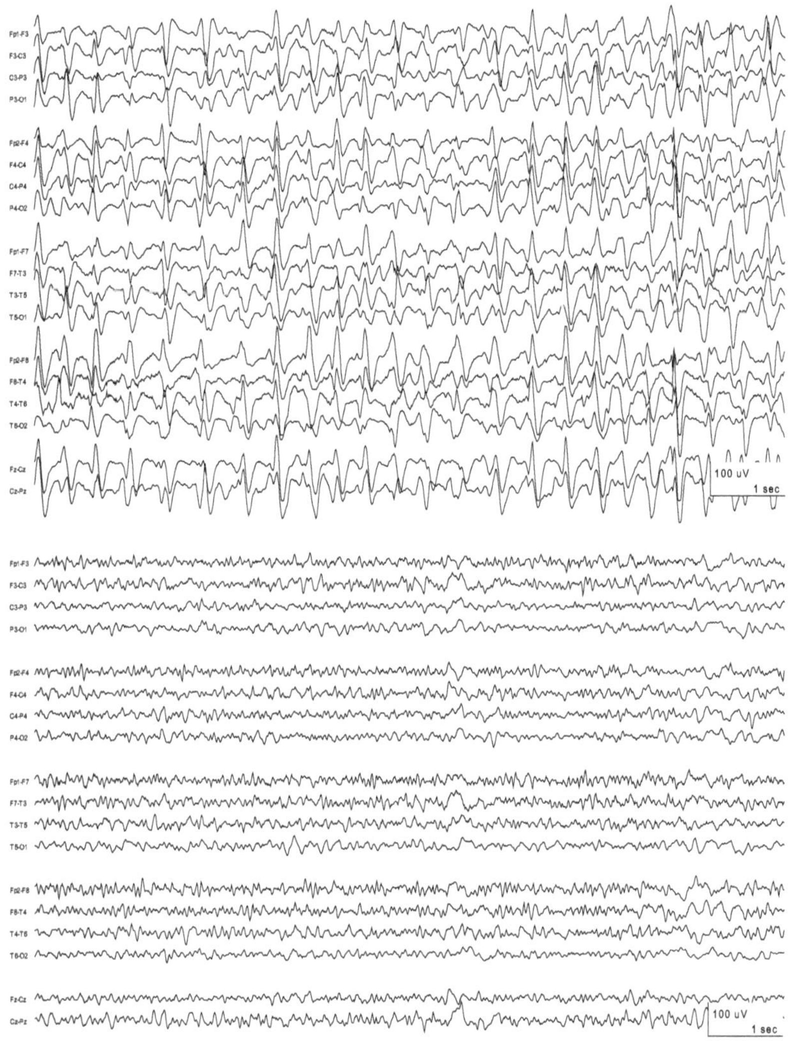


**Figure 4.2** (A) Generalized status epilepticus in a 75-year-old woman with a history of recent generalized tonic-clonic seizures, now confused and lethargic. The electroencephalogram (EEG) shows rhythmic, high-voltage, 3-Hz, sharp-and-slow-wave discharges, alternating with periods of diffuse delta activity and blunter epileptiform discharges. (B) Same patient as A. The EEG following intravenous administration of lorazepam shows complete cessation of ictal activity, with mild diffuse slowing and excess beta activity.

## ELECTROENCEPHALOGRAPHIC STAGES IN NONCONVULSIVE STATUS EPILEPTICUS

Treiman (10) proposed a stereotyped sequence of EEG changes in generalized convulsive status epilepticus: (1) discrete seizures, (2) merging seizures, (3) continuous ictal activity, (4) ictal activity with "flat" periods of background discontinuity, and finally (5) periodic epileptiform discharges (PEDs) on a flat background. These EEG changes are thought to represent progressive neuronal dysfunction secondary to metabolic exhaustion and parallel the diminution of clinical manifestations in generalized convulsive status epilepticus from convulsive motor movements to subtle limb twitching and eye movements. Stage 4 has subtle or no motor manifestations and is usually considered to represent NCSE. Stage 5, PEDs, is not accepted as ictal by most electroencephalographers.

This orderly temporal progression of EEG patterns does not often occur in NCSE (11,12). In a study of 40 patients (12), 53% had only discrete seizures without any other ictal patterns, 28% had discrete seizures with PEDs between seizures, and 8% had continuous ictal activity. Occurrence of continuous seizures, discrete seizures, or PEDs could occur at any time after SE, and no predictable pattern of evolu-

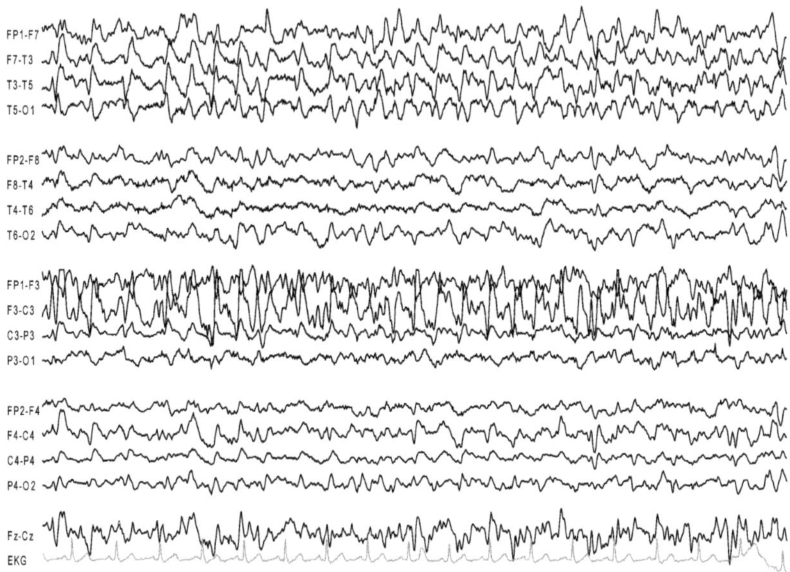


**Figure 4.3** Focal nonconvulsive status epilepticus (NCSE) in a 45-year-old man with a left frontal brain metastasis from testicular cancer. Clinically, he was confused and intermittently aphasic. The electroencephalogram shows rhythmic, 3- to 5-Hz, sharply contoured waveforms over the left hemisphere, maximal over the left frontal region.

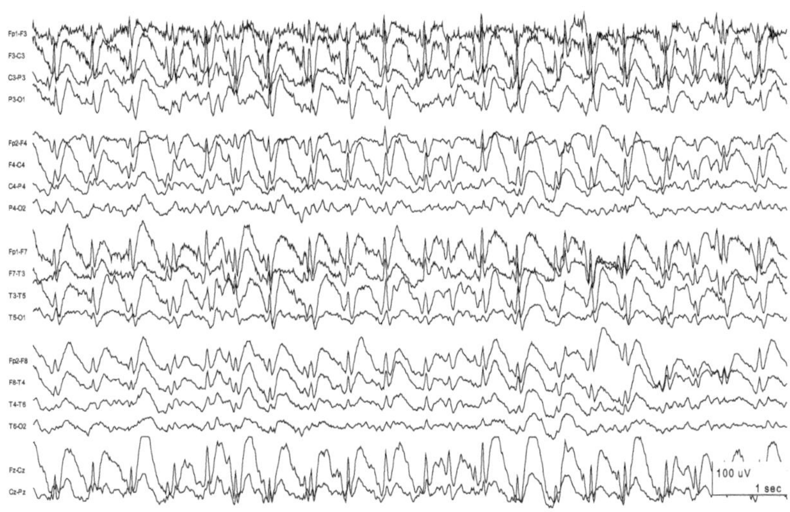


**Figure 4.4** Asymmetric nonconvulsive status epilepticus (NCSE). Broadly distributed, 2.5-Hz, spike-and-wave discharges, more prominent and higher amplitude over the left hemisphere, in a 62-year-old woman with a remote anterior cerebral artery infarct.

tion was identified. The evolution of the EEG depends on multiple factors: type of status epilepticus, baseline condition of the patient, etiology, duration of ictal activity, and type and duration of treatment. The variability in evolution adds to the controversy regarding which patterns are ictal.

## ICTAL PATTERNS VERSUS INTERICTAL PERIODIC PATTERNS

The borderland of NCSE is populated by a variety of PEDs with various morphologies and repetition rates, including periodic lateralized epileptiform discharges (PLEDs), bilateral independent periodic lateralized epileptiform discharges (BIPLEDs), generalized (GPEDs), and triphasic waves (TWs). These are fully discussed in Chapter 5. PEDs are seen in several clinical scenarios, including acute focal structural lesions and following convulsive seizures or status epilepticus. More than 75% of patients with periodic patterns may have clinical or electrographic seizures at some point in their course (13) (Figure 4.5). Periodic discharges are more likely to be "ictal" when they

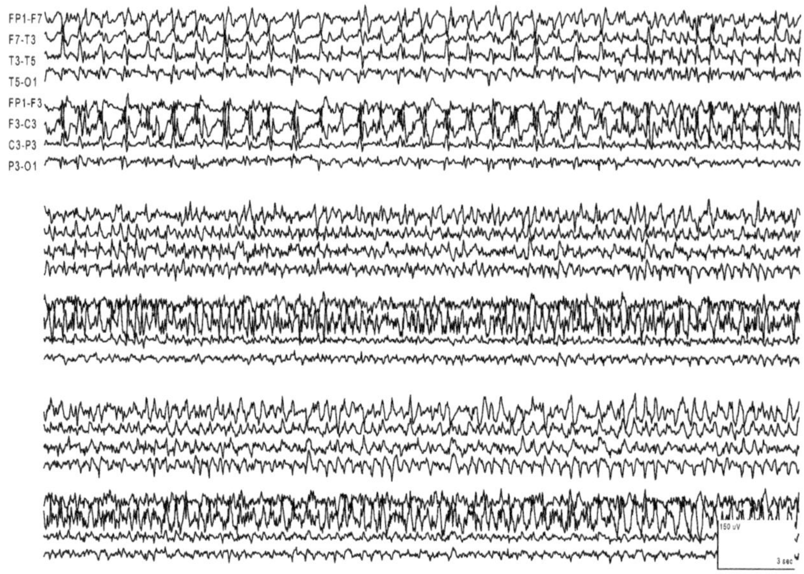


**Figure 4.5** Nonconvulsive status epilepticus (NCSE) evolving from left-hemisphere, periodic, lateralized, epileptiform discharges (PLEDs) in a 66-year-old man with a left frontal intracerebral hemorrhage. The electroencephalogram initially shows periodic discharges at 1.5 Hz, which are invariant for several minutes, then gradually increase in frequency and merge to electrographic theta activity over the entire left hemisphere. The pattern repeated every 5 to 10 minutes for several hours.

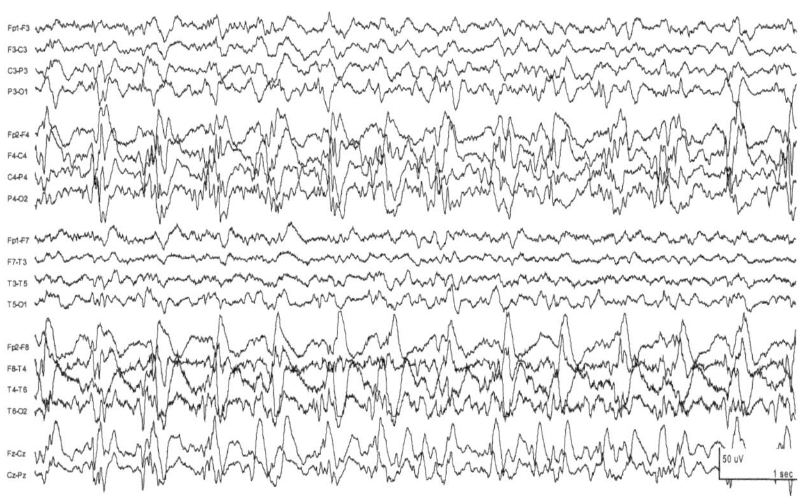


**Figure 4.6** Periodic, lateralized, epileptiform discharges (PLEDs)-plus in a 64-year-old woman with a right frontal astrocytoma. The electroencephalogram shows PLEDs at 1.5 Hz with intervening fast frequencies. PLEDs-plus is extremely likely to evolve into electrographic seizures; whether this pattern itself represents nonconvulsive status epilepticus is debated.

occur at rapid repetition rates (> 2 Hz) or show clear evolution in frequency (increase or decrease > 1 Hz), morphology, or field (14). Discharges with intervening fast components (PLEDs-plus) are more likely to be "ictal" than are bland isolated discharges (15) (Figure 4.6). Additional research will be needed to determine whether periodic discharges cause neuronal injury and whether aggressive treatment improves outcome (5). At the very least, the presence of PEDs should prompt consideration of continuous EEG monitoring for 24 hours to rule out frequent subclinical seizures. An American Clinical Neurophysiology Society subcommittee has proposed standardized terminology to describe rhythmic and periodic EEG patterns for research studies (16).

A particularly problematic area is the distinction between TWs and generalized NCSE (17). Although there are no absolute EEG criteria for diagnosis, epileptiform discharges in generalized NCSE typically show higher frequency (mean 2.4 versus 1.8 Hz), polyspikes, and sharper morphology than do TWs (18). A phase lag from anterior to posterior channels is often seen with TWs but not with NCSE. TWs are commonly state responsive and may be abolished by intravenous administration of AEDs (19).

## STIMULUS-INDUCED RHYTHMIC, PERIODIC, OR ICTAL DISCHARGES (SIRPIDS)

Focal or generalized periodic and quasi-periodic discharges can be elicited in stuporous or comatose patients by stimulation or occur with spontaneous arousal. Hirsch et al (20) termed these "stimulus-induced rhythmic, periodic, or ictal discharges" (Figure 4.7). The discharges abate when the patient lapses back into unresponsiveness. Whether these discharges represent seizures or an abnormal arousal process is debated; in general, discharges with repetition rates greater than 3 Hz or with clear evolution may be considered ictal, whereas invariant patterns slower than 3 Hz are less likely to be ictal.

## EFFECTS OF ANTIEPILEPTIC DRUGS ON THE ELECTROENCEPHALOGRAM IN NONCONVULSIVE STATUS EPILEPTICUS

A prompt clinical and EEG response to intravenous administration of AEDs is commonly used to determine if a particular EEG pattern represents NCSE. Lorazepam or midazolam may be given in small sequential doses while personnel monitor blood pressure, respiratory rate, and oxygenation. A "diagnostic response" is defined as marked improvement in both clinical status and EEG. EEG response alone is less helpful. Some nonictal EEG patterns, such as TWs of metabolic encephalopathy, may also improve after intravenous administration of benzodiazepines, likely because of state changes (19). Unfortunately, a rapid clinical response is uncommon in obtunded or comatose patients in NCSE (21); improvement in mental status after successful treatment of NCSE may take days (22,23). High doses of sedating benzodiazepines may also blunt the clinical response. In patients whose EEG improves but in whom no clinical change is evident, continuous EEG monitoring should be considered to look for recurrence of the ictal pattern.

## SPECIFIC ELECTROENCEPHALOGRAPHIC PATTERNS IN NONCONVULSIVE STATUS EPILEPTICUS

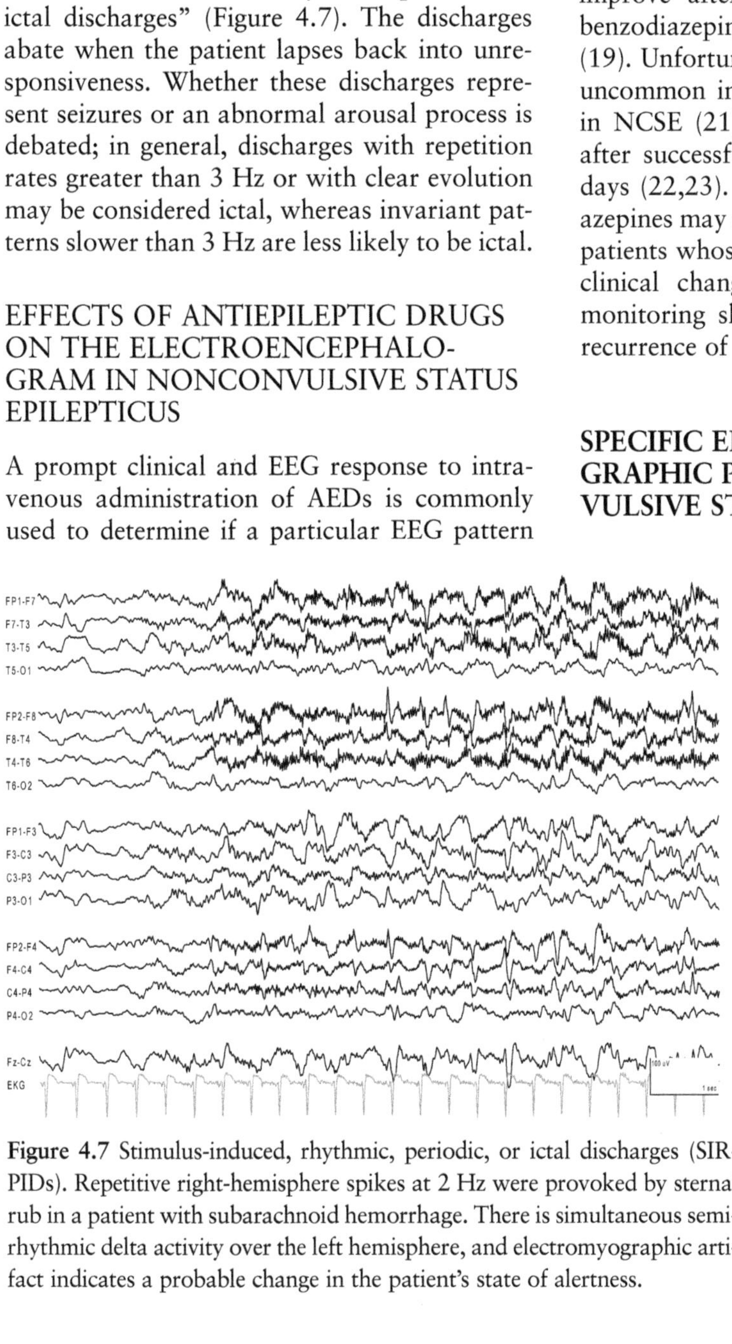


**Figure 4.7** Stimulus-induced, rhythmic, periodic, or ictal discharges (SIRPIDs). Repetitive right-hemisphere spikes at 2 Hz were provoked by sternal rub in a patient with subarachnoid hemorrhage. There is simultaneous semirhythmic delta activity over the left hemisphere, and electromyographic artifact indicates a probable change in the patient's state of alertness.

### GENERALIZED NONCONVULSIVE STATUS EPILEPTICUS

#### *Typical absence status epilepticus*

Typical absence status epilepticus (ASE) occurs most commonly in individuals who have primary generalized epilepsies and is characterized by impairment of consciousness, sometimes described as a "twilight state," with confusion, slowed thinking, repetitive blinking, or myoclonus (24). The EEG shows generalized 3-Hz spike-and-wave discharges or polyspike-and-wave discharges in frequent recurrent seizures (Figure 4.8) or prolonged seizures (Figure

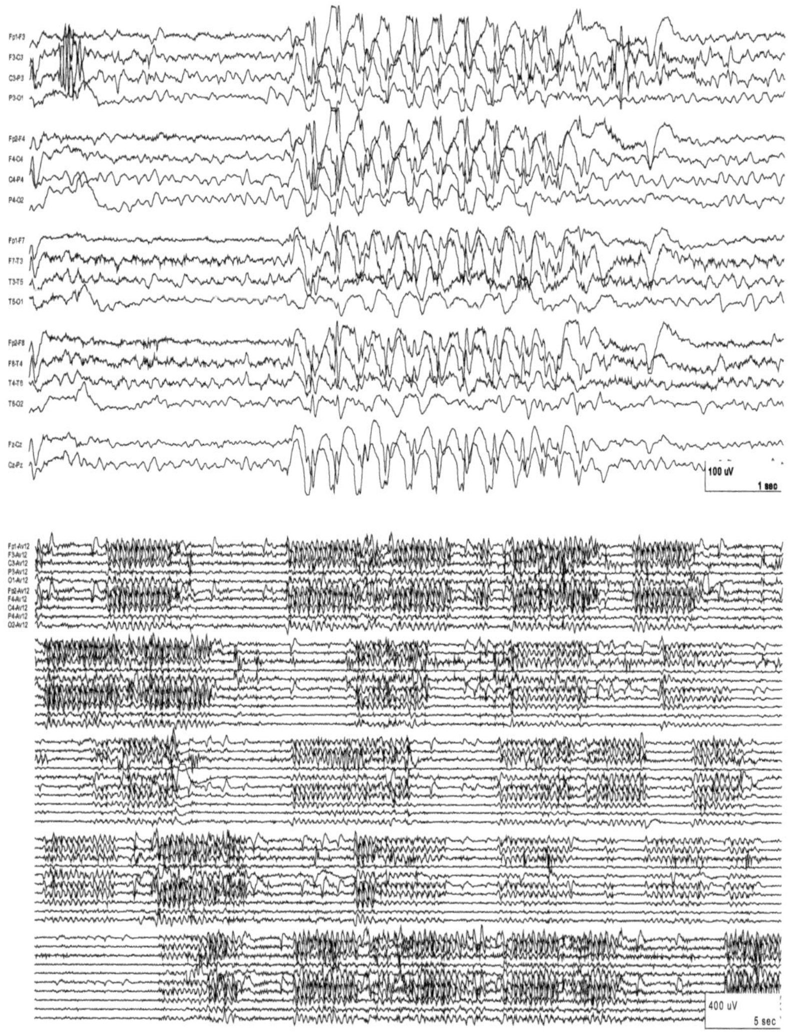


**Figure 4.8** Typical absence status epilepticus in a 17-year-old boy with juvenile absence epilepsy. A. Section of routine electroencephalogram (EEG) during hyperventilation shows a representative brief absence seizure with generalized, frontally maximal, spike-wave activity at 3 Hz. B. Longer section of EEG during an episode of absence status epilepticus precipitated by sleep deprivation. Frequent, 5- to 10-second, absence seizures recur every 5 to 10 seconds over 20 minutes until intravenous administration of lorazepam. Clinically, each absence seizure was accompanied by staring, unresponsiveness, eyelid fluttering, and subtle limb automatisms.

4.9) lasting more than 30 minutes (25,26). The epileptiform discharges are bilaterally synchronous and usually maximal over frontal or central head regions. Other EEG patterns include spike-and-wave activity at frequencies greater than 3 Hz, polyspike-and-wave discharges (Figure 4.10), generalized rhythmic slowing with intermixed spike-and-slow-wave complexes, irregular sharp-and-slow-wave discharges, or diffuse background slowing with superimposed bursts of fast activity (Figure 4.11) (24). If seizures are very prolonged, the spike-and-wave discharges may slow to less than 3 Hz (27). Typical ASE usually shows a prompt clinical and EEG response to intravenously administered AEDs.

*Atypical absence status epilepticus*

Atypical ASE is a rare type of status epilepticus seen in patients with epileptic encephalopathies such as the Lennox-Gastaut syndrome (28). To qualify as status epilepticus, there must be a clear change from baseline both clinically and electrographically (1). With atypical ASE, patients are more confused than they were at baseline and sometimes have subtle myoclonic, tonic, or atonic motor manifestations. The EEG shows either (1) generalized or asymmetric spike-wave activity at frequencies ranging from 1 to 2.5 Hz, which is more frequent or intense than baseline epileptiform activity and is superimposed on a diffusely slow background (Figure 4.12), or (2) low-voltage, generalized,

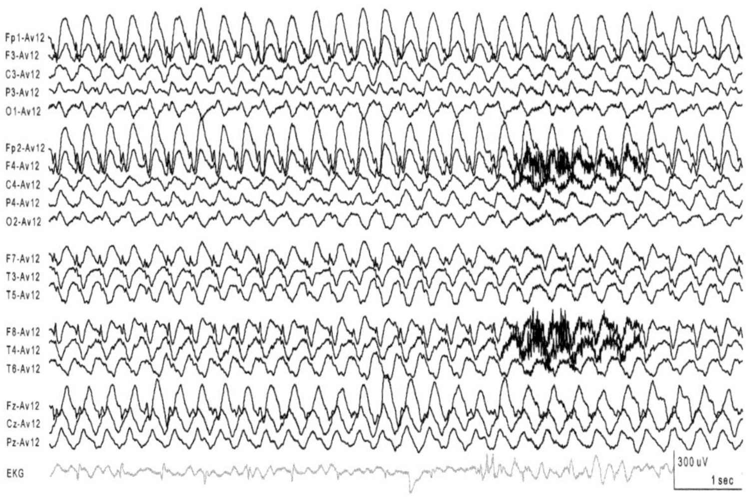


**Figure 4.9** Absence status epilepticus in a 42-year-old woman with juvenile myoclonic epilepsy, now with confusion, slowed responses, and "pauses in speech." The electroencephalogram shows a 3-Hz, generalized, spike-and- wave pattern.

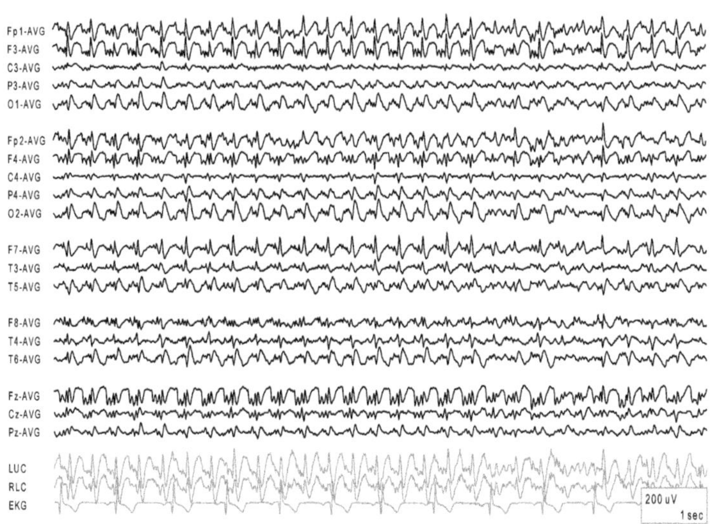


**Figure 4.10** Typical absence status epilepticus in a 35-year-old man presenting with mild confusion for 3 days. The electroencephalogram showed continuous polyspike-and-waves at 3 Hz.

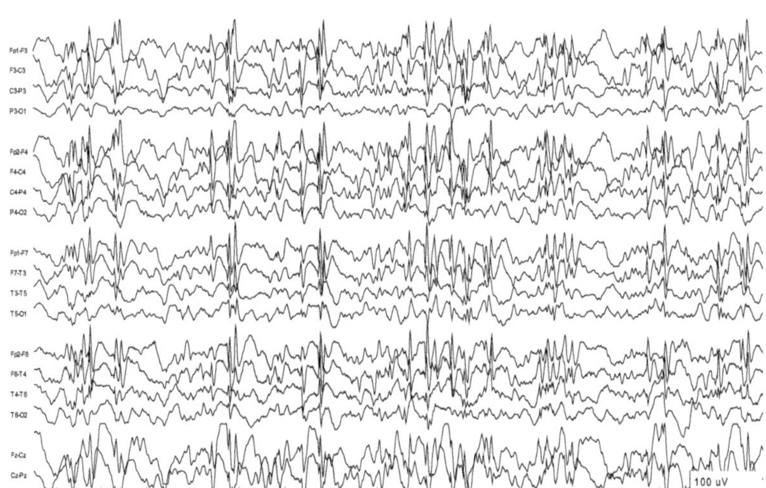


**Figure 4.11** Typical absence status epilepticus in a 54-year-old woman with juvenile myoclonic epilepsy. The electroencephalogram shows bursts of generalized, frontally maximal, irregular, polyspike-and-waves at 4-7 Hz, superimposed on a diffusely slow background.

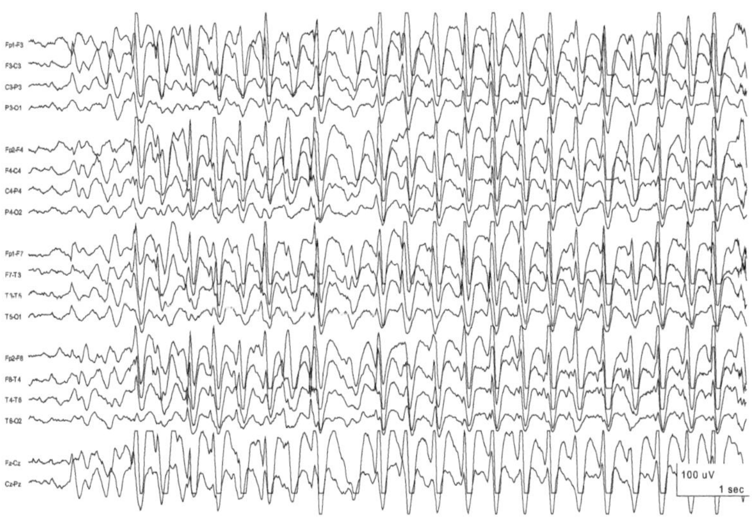


**Figure 4.12** Atypical absence status epilepticus in a 30-year-old woman with mild mental retardation and intractable epilepsy, presenting with lethargy and slurred speech after abrupt discontinuation of her antiepileptic drugs. The electroencephalogram shows generalized, frontally maximal, slow-spike-and-wave discharges at 2.5 Hz.

paroxysmal, fast activity (alpha or beta frequencies) (2,29).

*Late de novo absence status epilepticus*

Patterns of generalized NCSE can also be seen in older adults with no prior history of epilepsy, often in the setting of withdrawal from benzodiazepines, medication intoxication, systemic infection, or metabolic dysfunction (30). The EEG is highly variable, showing generalized spike-and-wave activity at frequencies from 0.5 to 4 Hz (31). The spike-and-wave component is often less prominent and more irregular than in typical ASE (Figure 4.2) but does show a similar frontally or centrally maximal distribution (7).

*Subtle or electrographic generalized convulsive status epilepticus*

Subtle or electrographic generalized convulsive status epilepticus occurs as the late stages of generalized convulsive status epilepticus (ie, stages 4 and 5, as described by Treiman) (10). Patients are typically comatose, with minimal or no motor manifestations. The EEG shows repetitive, generalized, periodic, epileptiform discharges or bursts of polyspikes, with frequencies from 0.5 to 4 Hz (Figure 4.13) (10,32). Similar discharges can be seen in patients with severe encephalopathy (eg, uremic or postanoxic) but no history of seizures (33).

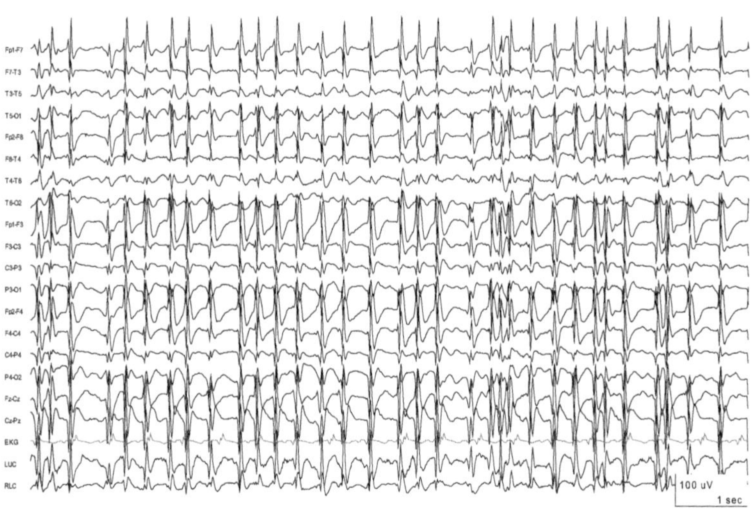


**Figure 4.13** Subtle generalized convulsive status epilepticus (SGCSE). A 68-year-old man with renal failure remained unresponsive following treatment for generalized convulsive status epilepticus with lorazepam, phenytoin, and phenobarbital. Exam showed nystagmoid eye movements and fine twitching of fingers. The electroencephalogram shows a discontinuous pattern of spikes and polyspikes at 2-3 Hz with brief periods of diffuse background attenuation.

## FOCAL NONCONVULSIVE STATUS EPILEPTICUS

### *Simple partial status epilepticus*

Clinical manifestations of simple partial status epilepticus reflect ictal involvement of discrete brain regions, such as motor, sensory, special sensory, psychic, or autonomic symptoms, without impairment of consciousness (34,35). Because only a small volume of brain tissue is involved, only 20% to 35% of simple partial seizures have an ictal correlate detectable with scalp EEG (36); the EEG is often normal or shows nonspecific changes such as focal slowing (37). A variety of ictal patterns may occur, such as focal fast-frequency discharges, rhythmic waveforms with evolving morphology, and repetitive epileptiform discharges (37-39). Ictal activity may be either continuous or discontinuous, with discrete seizures showing evolving frequencies of 3 to 6 Hz lasting 30 to 60 seconds (39). Epilepsia partialis continua is a specific form of simple partial status epilepticus characterized by continuous clonic or myoclonic motor seizures involving part or all of one side of the body. Focal epileptiform discharges such as irregular spikes and sharp waves or PLEDs may be seen in 22% to 71% of patients with epilepsia partialis continua (40,41).

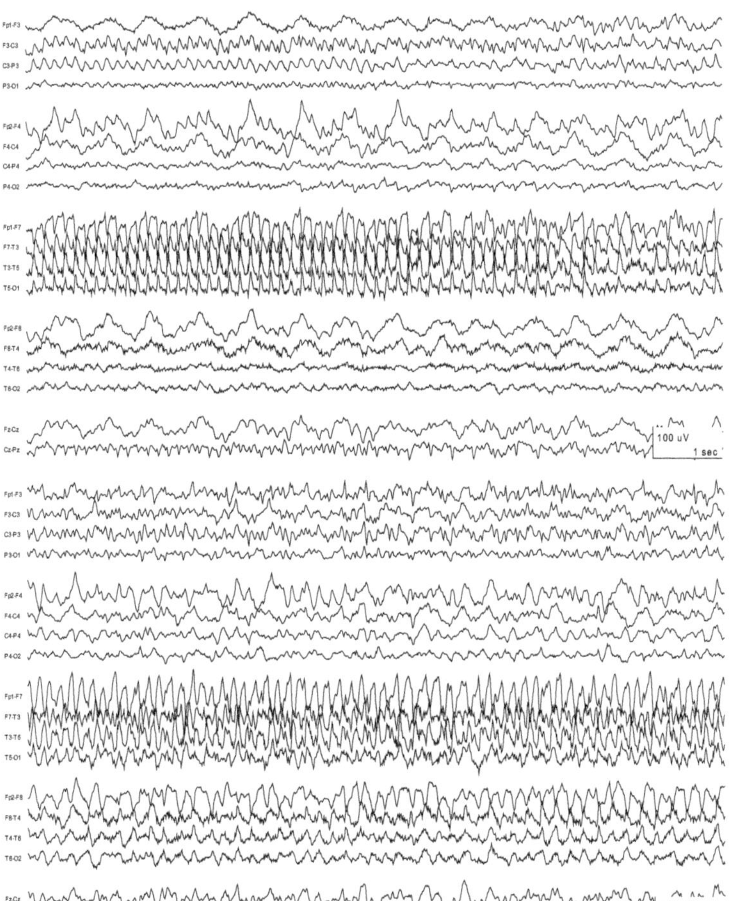


**Figure 4.14** Progression of focal nonconvulsive status epilepticus (NCSE) in a 21-year year-old with intractable temporal lobe epilepsy. A. Initial well-localized, 7-Hz, sharply contoured, ictal activity over the left temporal region, with some spread to the left. B. Later epoch from same patient as A. Ictal activity has now spread to right frontal region, with some spread to the left parasagittal region.

### *Complex partial status epilepticus*

EEG findings are essential to distinguish complex partial status epilepticus (CPSE) from other causes of altered mental status. CPSE nearly always shows discernable ictal patterns on scalp EEG, but EEG during frontal or parietal CPSE may be normal or obscured by artifact (42,43). CPSE may arise from any brain region, most commonly frontal or temporal (44). The EEG patterns of CPSE are highly variable, reflecting differences in ictal onset zones and propagation pathways (45). Morphologies include repetitive spikes, spike-and-slow-wave discharges, and rhythmic waveforms in the theta, delta, or alpha frequency range. Early EEG manifestations are usually focal or lateralized, but spread of ictal activity results in diffuse or generalized patterns difficult to distinguish from ASE (Figure 4.14) (7,46,47). CPSE may show recurrent seizures, each showing focal onset with evolution in field, morphology, amplitude, or frequency (Figure 4.15) or continuous ictal discharges (Figure 4.16) (2,48-50). Background activity between discrete seizures shows focal slowing, focal epileptiform discharges, or periodic lateralized epileptiform discharges. As CPSE progresses, seizures may become fragmentary, with periods of background attenuation between seizures (Figure 4.17).

### *Focal nonconvulsive status epilepticus in critically ill obtunded or comatose patients*

The diagnosis of NCSE in coma is problematic. EEG patterns are not pathognomonic; similar changes can be seen in NCSE, acute focal structural lesions, and encephalopathies. NCSE has been reported to occur in 8% of patients with coma but no other clinical signs of seizures (51) and 16% of pediatric patients in the intensive care unit with unexplained alteration in consciousness (52). Some authors consider subtle or electrographic status to be present only if the patient has previously experienced clinical seizures or status epilepticus (11).

Electrographic partial status epilepticus is seen in stuporous or comatose patients with no clear clinical signs of seizure activity (5). Seizures may be either continuous or repetitive, and EEG patterns are similar to those in simple partial status epilepticus and CPSE (Figure 4.18). Such partial status epilepticus is frequently seen after strokes or other acute brain injuries and should be suspected when conditions do not stabilize or improve as expected

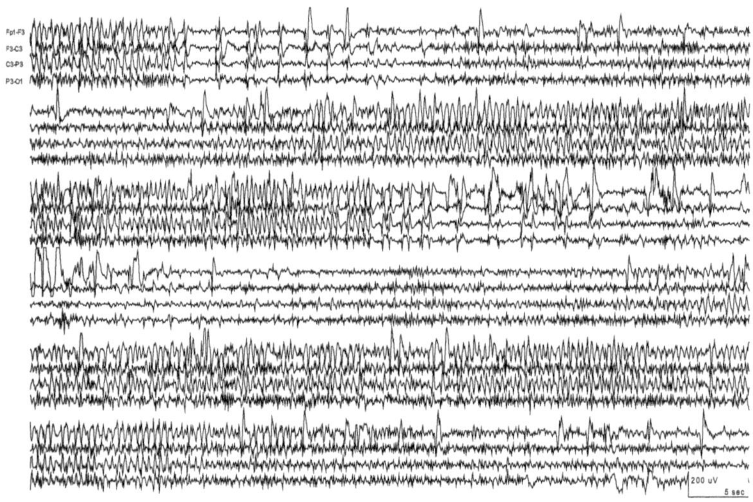


**Figure 4.15** Focal nonconvulsive status epilepticus (NCSE). Frequent recurrent seizures in a patient with parietal epilepsy and NCSE. Seizures arise from the left hemisphere, gradually increase in frequency and amplitude, then stop abruptly, followed by diffuse slowing for approximately one minute before the next seizure begins. Each group of 4 electroencephalographic channels follows the 4 channels above sequentially.

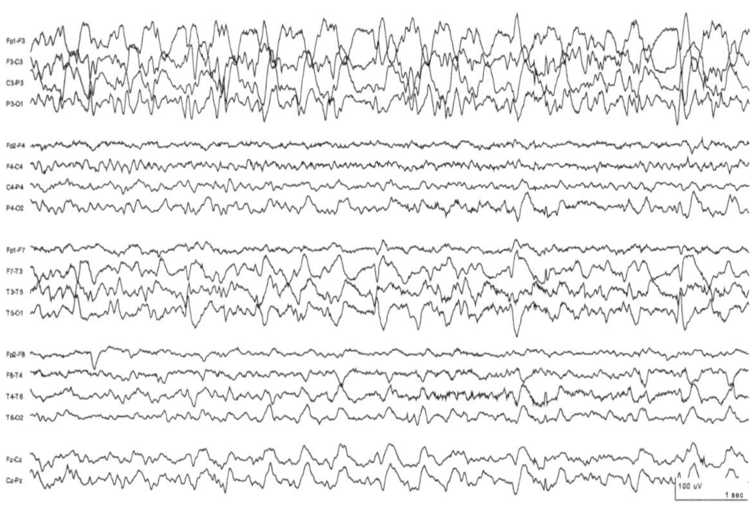


**Figure 4.16** Focal nonconvulsive status epilepticus (NCSE). Continuous focal ictal activity in the left hemisphere in a 54-year-old man with central nervous system vasculitis.

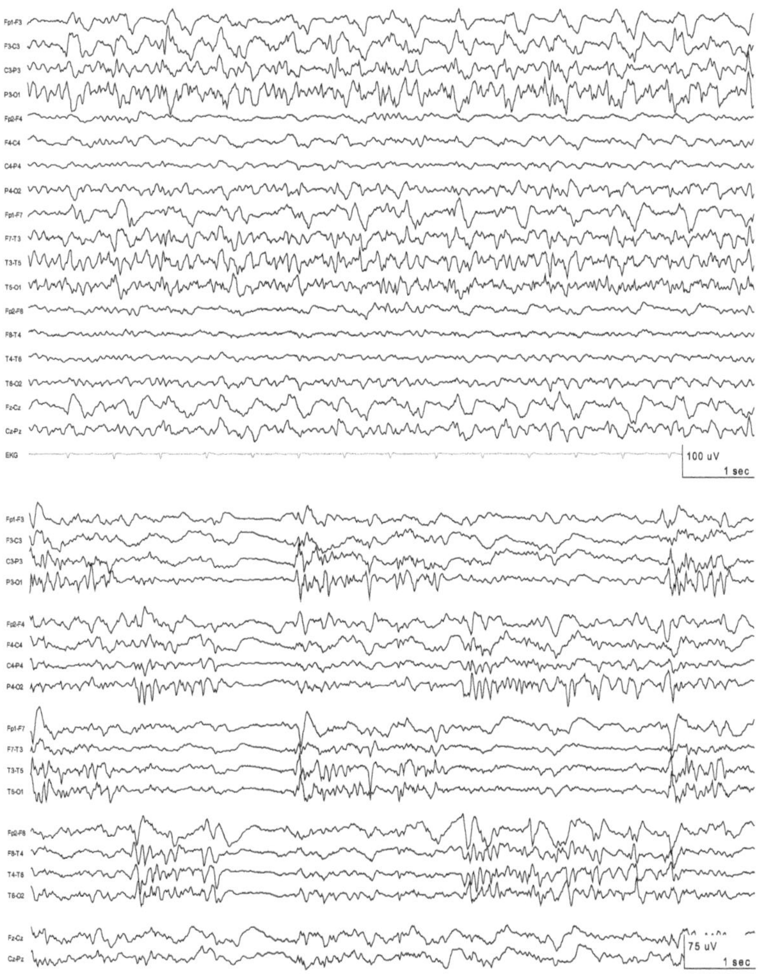


**Figure 4.17** A. Continuous focal ictal activity (rhythmic theta and delta with intermixed spikes) in a 68-year-old woman with herpes encephalitis. B. Later electroencephalogram (EEG) in same patient as A. At the time of this EEG, she was comatose. EEG shows discontinuous ictal activity independently from the right and left hemispheres.

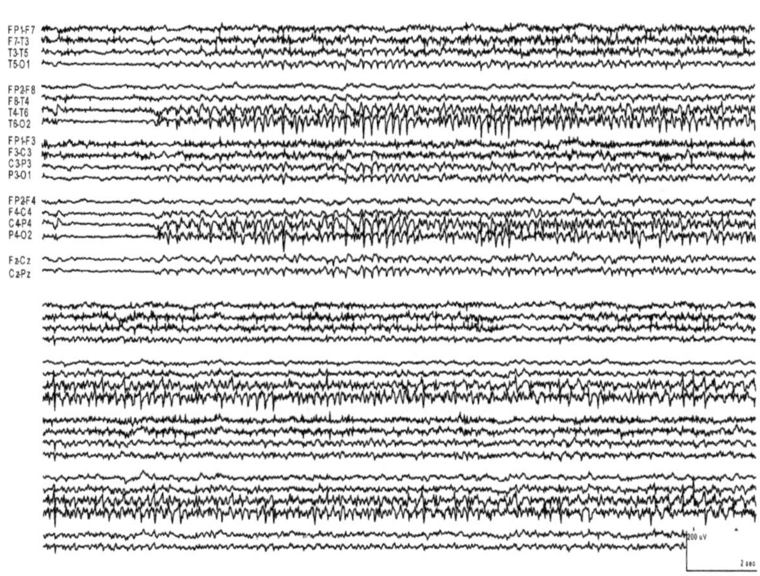


**Figure 4.18** Electrographic status epilepticus in a 54 year old woman with reversible posterior leukoencephalopathy syndrome. EEG showed recurrent electrographic seizures arising from the right occipital region, with clinical correlate of eye deviation and nystagmoid jerking to the right. The EEG tracing on the lower half of the figure is a continuation of that above.

(45). In some NCSE in critically ill patients, seizures occur cyclically, with brief electrographic seizures occurring every 5 to 10 minutes over several hours, possibly representing a "wearing off" of the factor responsible for stopping the electrographic seizure (53).

## AGE-RELATED NONCONVULSIVE STATUS EPILEPTICUS

### *Neonatal status epilepticus*

Continuous video-EEG monitoring is an essential tool for optimal diagnosis and management of neonatal status epilepticus (54). As in critically ill adults, neonates with severe brain injury, prior treatment with AEDs, and pharmacologic paralysis may have few or no clinical manifestations of seizure (55), resulting in underdiagnosis of status epilepticus if EEG is not monitored (56). EEG can also avoid inappropriately aggressive treatment of nonepileptic abnormal movements, such as swimming, pedaling, rowing, myoclonic jerks, jitteriness, and stimulus-sensitive clonus or myoclonus.

Ictal discharges in neonates are usually focal and localized to relatively small brain areas, likely secondary to incomplete myelination and neuronal migration (57). Seizures arise most frequently in midtemporal areas of one hemisphere, followed by the central and occipital regions (54). Multifocal seizures (more than 3 foci in both hemispheres) are common. Some seizures show evolution in frequency, amplitude, morphology, or spatial distribution, but many show little or no evolution (Figure 4.19) (57). Morphologies include sharply contoured, sinusoidal, or rounded waveforms in the alpha, theta, and delta frequency range. Because of the unusual patterns in neonatal SE, particular attention must be paid to exclude artifact mimicking electrographic seizures. Most neonatal seizures last 2 to 3 minutes but recur frequently; prolonged continuous seizures are less frequently seen (58). Brief ictal rhythmic discharges (BIRDS) have characteristics similar to those of seizures but last less than 10 seconds (59).

### *Electrical status epilepticus during slow-wave sleep (ESES) or continuous spikes and waves during sleep (CSWS)*

Electrical status epilepticus during slow-wave sleep is a childhood-onset disorder characterized by seizures, continuous generalized spike-and-wave discharges during slow-wave sleep, and progressive cognitive decline (60). EEG during wakefulness and rapid eye movement sleep shows only rare focal or generalized epileptiform discharges. As soon as patients fall asleep, non-rapid eye movement sleep demonstrates continuous generalized or bilaterally synchronous spike-and-wave complexes at 1.5 to 3.5 Hz, occupying at least 85% of slow-wave sleep (Figure 4.20) (61,62). The spike component is most prominent. The typical EEG pattern is usually first seen between ages 5 and 15 years and then often disappears.

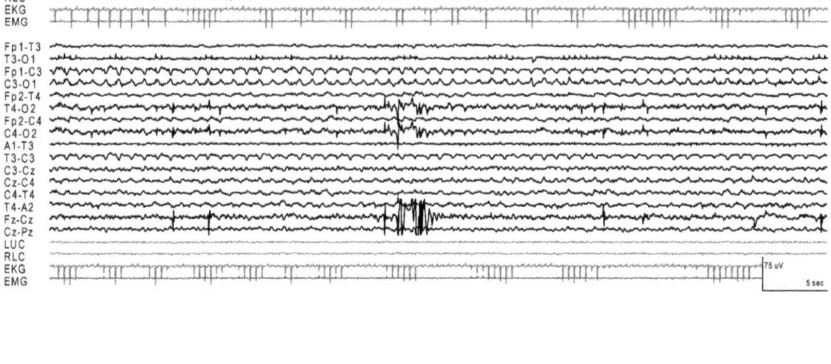


**Figure 4.19** Neonatal status epilepticus in a 36-week-conceptional- age neonate with left periventricular hemorrhage. The electroencephalogram shows onset with intermixed alpha and delta activity in the left occipital region, which shifts to the left central parasagittal region and continues as monomorphic, low-amplitude, delta activity for 15 minutes. Seizures recurred frequently but were multifocal.

*Landau-Kleffner syndrome*

The Landau-Kleffner syndrome is an epileptic encephalopathy characterized by an acquired receptive aphasia, seizures, and a behavior disorder (63). EEG findings are variable. As in electrical status epilepticus during slow-wave sleep, waking EEG may be normal or may show unilateral or bilateral temporal spike-and-wave discharges. Bursts of focal or bilateral spike-and-wave discharges at 1.5 to 3.5 Hz are present in less than 85% of slow-wave sleep (64). Epileptiform discharges are usually seen over the anterior or midtemporal regions, but also in the temporo-parieto-occipital regions, and may have a very broad, nearly generalized field (Figure 4.21) (62,65). A vertical dipole is often present in the intraperisylvian region (66). The EEG manifestations usually appear between the ages of 3 and 5 years and resolve after approximately 15 years of age.

## NONEPILEPTIC NONCONVULSIVE STATUS EPILEPTICUS

Misdiagnosis of nonepileptic NCSE (psychogenic or pseudo-status epilepticus) can result in inappropriately aggressive treatment (67,68), so EEG should be performed for any patient with suspected status epilepticus

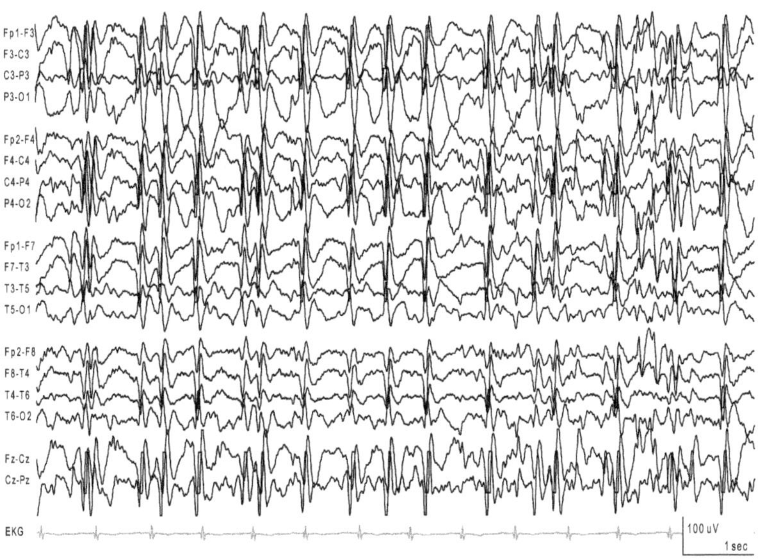


**Figure 4.20** Electrical status epilepticus in sleep (ESES) in a 12-year-old girl. She presented with a single generalized tonic-clonic seizure, several falls, and deterioration in school performance. The electroencephalogram in sleep showed continuous, high-voltage, bilaterally symmetric, sharp-and-slow-wave discharges at 1-3 Hz.

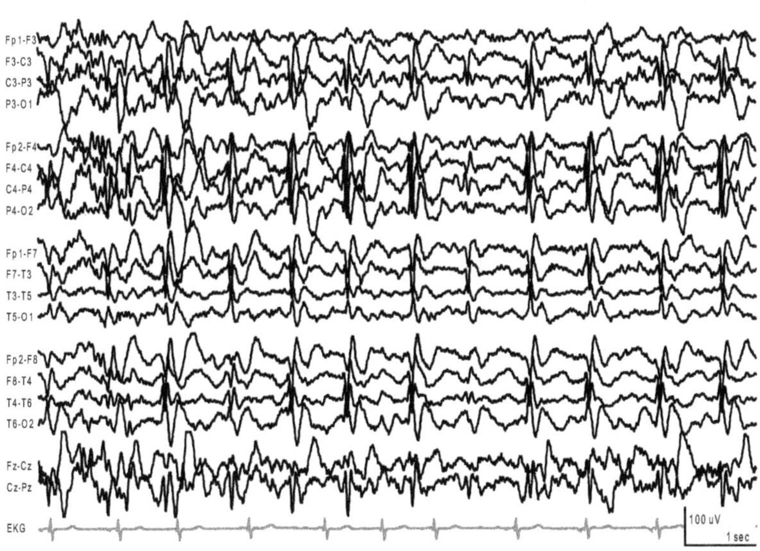


**Figure 4.21** Landau-Kleffner syndrome in a 4-year-old boy with a history of language regression. The electroencephalogram shows high-voltage, sharp-and-slow-wave discharges over the right centrotemporal region, with less prominent synchronous spikes over the left centrotemporal region.

who does not respond to initial treatment. Nonepileptic psychogenic seizures can mimic NCSE, with prolonged staring, eye blinking, and unresponsiveness. The EEG shows normal background activity or artifact from muscle or eye movements (69). Alpha rhythm can be elicited by passive eye opening and closure.

## USE OF EEG IN DIAGNOSIS AND MANAGEMENT OF NCSE

### *Indicators for electroencephalography for diagnosis*

The diagnosis of NCSE is often delayed for more than 24 hours or missed entirely if EEG is not performed (3,23,39). An EEG should therefore be obtained in all patients with (1) unexplained acute changes in mental status or personality, especially in patients with a history of epilepsy or remote neurologic injuries (70); (2) alterations in consciousness out of proportion to an acute neurologic injury (71); (3) persistent unresponsiveness following convulsive status epilepticus or clinically evident seizures (72); or (4) subtle limb twitching or nystagmoid eye movements (70,73). Critically ill patients in the intensive care unit have high rates of nonconvulsive seizures (18%) and NCSE (10%) (74), including those with intracerebral hemorrhage (18%-28%) (75,76), severe traumatic brain injury (28%) (77), central nervous system infection (26%) (78), brain tumor (23%) (78), and subarachnoid hemorrhage (8%) (79). In obtunded or comatose patients, continuous EEG monitoring for 24 to 48 hours may be necessary to detect NCSE (78). Unfortunately, emergency EEG is not available in all hospitals and may take 1 to 24 hours to obtain and interpret (80). Additional research is necessary to determine the utility and cost effectiveness of providing continuous availability for emergency EEG (81).

### *Monitoring of treatment efficacy*

Because clinical signs of NCSE are nonspecific, subtle, or nonexistent, continuous EEG monitoring is often necessary to assess the response to therapy and to exclude recurrent seizures. Once NCSE is diagnosed, EEG should be reviewed continuously until seizures are stopped or a burst-suppression pattern is induced with continuous intravenous administration of AEDs. Continuous EEG should be maintained until the patient returns to normal consciousness or electrographic seizures are controlled for 24 hours after initial therapy or after continuous intravenous administration of AEDs is withdrawn.

NCSE persists in 14% to 20% of patients after medical treatment and cessation of clinically evident motor activity (21,72). Patients requiring continuous intravenous administration of AEDs for the management of NCSE should have continuous EEG monitoring or, at a minimum, periodic EEGs during therapy. Typical endpoints are suppression of all electrographic seizures (82,83), a burst-suppression EEG pattern with interburst intervals of 2 to 30 seconds (84-86), or complete suppression pattern (87), but there are no controlled trials of outcome of status epilepticus based on depth and duration of EEG suppression. Breakthrough seizures during continuous intravenous administration of AED treatment are common (56%) and often subclinical (89%) (88), and relapse rates are high (18%-68%) (83).

### *Technical aspects of electroencephalography in nonconvulsive status epilepticus*

The emergency room and intensive care unit environments in which NCSE is usually diagnosed present significant technical challenges to obtaining good-quality EEGs; these challenges may include artifacts from patient movement, nursing care, 60-Hz line noise, and equipment, such as respirators and vibrating beds. Simultaneous video recording can help to determine the etiology of some artifacts (20).

Large quantities of continuous EEG data must be reviewed to ensure that breakthrough or recurrent seizures have not occurred. Computer analysis can aid in data compression but, at this point, cannot replace expert electroencephalographer review. Automatic spike-and-seizure-detection algorithms developed for patients in the epilepsy monitoring unit (89,90)

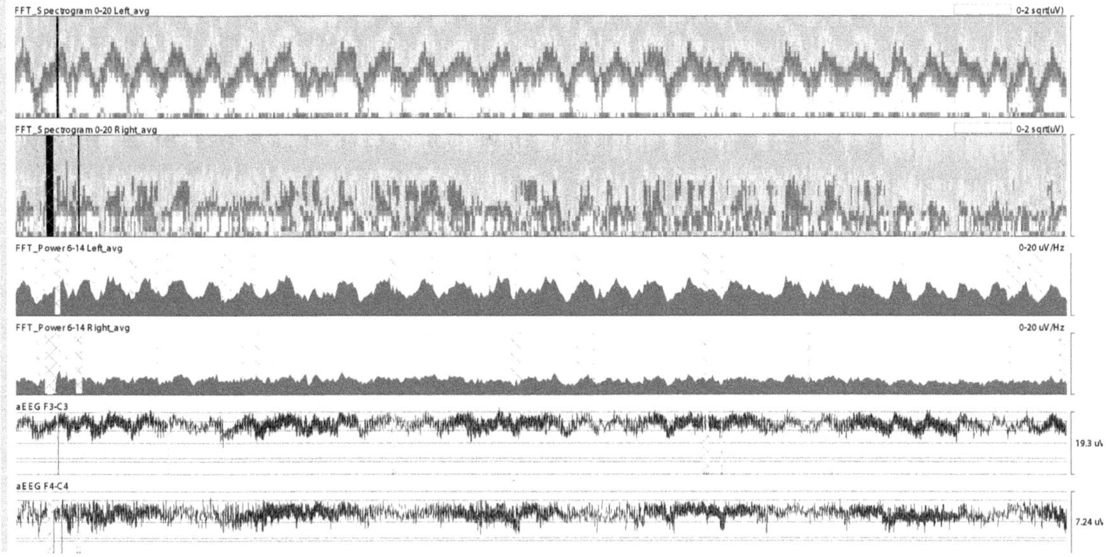


**Figure 4.22** Cyclic seizures over a 2-hour period in a 29-year-old woman with focal status epilepticus causing confusion and aphasia. Spectrogram shows recurrent increases in delta power (white color in row 1) over the left hemisphere. Power in the 6- to 14-Hz band (row 3) shows the same cyclic increases.

are inadequate for detection of ictal patterns in NCSE, especially in patients with acute brain injuries. Quantitative analysis techniques display EEG activity as a graph versus time. Color spectrograms, compressed spectral arrays, displays of total power in certain EEG frequency bins, ratios of power in certain bands to total EEG power, amplitude integrated EEG, and spectral edge displays can be displayed for single-channel or groups of channels to detect electrographic seizures (Figures 4.22 and 4.23) (91). The sensitivity and specificity of these techniques for NCSE has not been explored. Raw EEG traces must be immediately available to exclude artifacts (Figure 4.24) and state changes causing changes in quantitative EEG

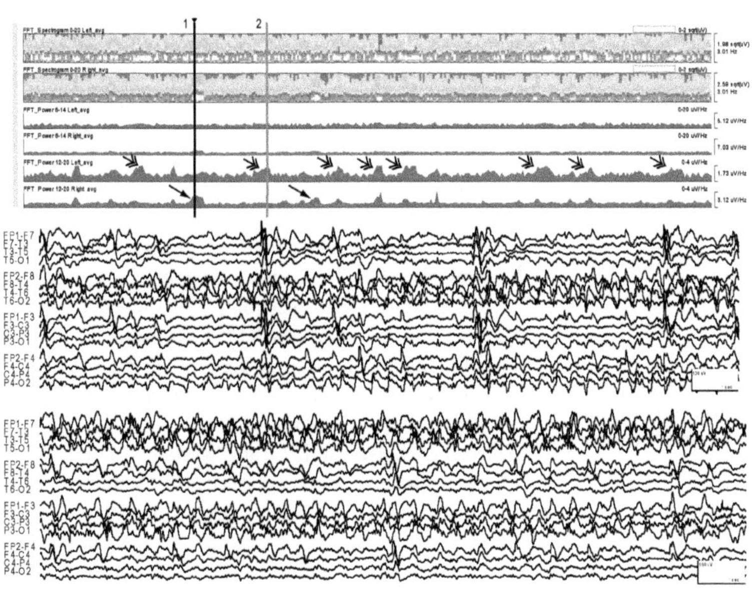


**Figure 4.23** Quantitative electroencephalogram (EEG) can distinguish between left and right hemisphere seizures. Single arrowheads show increases in beta power corresponding to electrographic seizures from the right hemisphere, as shown in the first EEG trace. The double arrowheads show increases in theta power in the left hemisphere, corresponding to the electrographic seizures in the lower EEG trace.

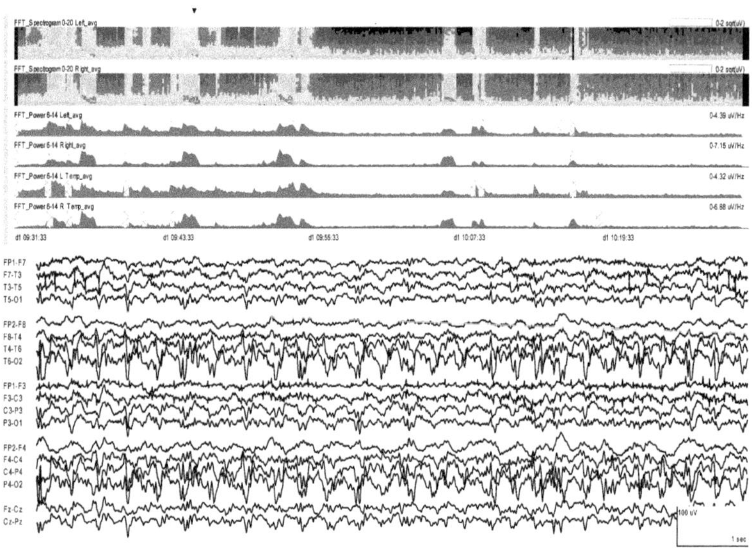

**Figure 4.24** Quantitative electroencephalogram (EEG) shows increases in power in the right hemisphere (line at arrowhead), corresponding to right occipital electrographic seizures. Assessment of activity in the left hemisphere is limited by continuous muscle artifact on the left. Artifacts from a variety of sources can limit the utility of quantitative EEG displays, either by obscuring ictal changes or by producing changes in quantitative trends that mimic those caused by seizures. Quantitative EEG should therefore always be performed as an adjunct to review of the raw EEG tracing.

and to confirm that electrographic seizures are not missed.

## REFERENCES

1. Walker M, Cross H, Smith S, Young C, Aicardi J, Appleton R, Aylett S, Besag F, Cock H, DeLorenzo R, Drislane F, Duncan J, Ferrie C, Fujikawa D, Gray W, Kaplan P, Koutroumanidis M, O'Regan M, Plouin P, Sander J, Scott R, Shorvon S, Treiman D, Wasterlain C, Wieshmann U. Nonconvulsive status epilepticus: Epilepsy Research Foundation workshop reports. Epileptic Disord 2005;7:253-296.
2. Gastaut H. Classification of status epilepticus. Adv Neurol 1983;34:15-35.
3. Young GB, Jordan KG, Doig GS. An assessment of nonconvulsive seizures in the intensive care unit using continuous EEG monitoring: an investigation of variables associated with mortality. Neurology 1996;47:83-89.
4. Jordan KG. Continuous EEG and evoked potential monitoring in the neuroscience intensive care unit. J Clin Neurophysiol 1993;10:445-475.
5. Chong DJ, Hirsch LJ. Which EEG patterns warrant treatment in the critically ill? Reviewing the evidence for treatment of periodic epileptiform discharges and related patterns. J Clin Neurophysiol 2005;22:79-91.
6. Kaplan PW. The EEG of status epilepticus. J Clin Neurophysiol 2006;23:221-229.
7. Granner MA, Lee SI. Nonconvulsive status epilepticus: EEG analysis in a large series. Epilepsia 1994;35:42-47.
8. Litt B, Wityk RJ, Hertz SH, Mullen PD, Weiss H, Ryan DD, Henry TR. Nonconvulsive status epilepticus in the critically ill elderly. Epilepsia 1998;39:1194-1202.
9. Abend NS, Dlugos DJ. Nonconvulsive status epilepticus in a pediatric intensive care unit. Pediatr Neurol 2007;37:165-170.
10. Treiman DM, Walton NY, Kendrick C. A progressive sequence of electroencephalographic changes during generalized convulsive status epilepticus. Epilepsy Res 1990;5:49-60.
11. Lowenstein D, Aminoff M. Clinical and EEG features of status epilepticus in comatose patients. Neurology 1992;42:100-104.
12. Nei M, Lee JM, Shanker VL, Sperling MR. The EEG and prognosis in status epilepticus. Epilepsia 1999;40:157-163.
13. Snodgrass SM, Tsuburaya K, Ajmone-Marsan C. Clinical significance of periodic lateralized epileptiform discharges: relationship with status epilepticus. J Clin Neurophysiol 1989;6:159-172.
14. Garzon E, Fernandes RM, Sakamoto AC. Serial EEG during human status epilepticus: evidence for PLED as an ictal pattern. Neurology 2001;57:1175-1183.
15. Reiher J, Rivest J, Grand'Maison F, Leduc CP. Periodic lateralized epileptiform discharges with transitional rhythmic discharges: association with seizures. Electroencephalogr Clin Neurophysiol 1991;78:12-17.

16. Hirsch LJ, Brenner RP, Drislane FW, So E, Kaplan PW, Jordan KG, Herman ST, LaRoche SM, Young B, Bleck TP, Scheuer ML, Emerson RG. The ACNS subcommittee on research terminology for continuous EEG monitoring: proposed standardized terminology for rhythmic and periodic EEG patterns encountered in critically ill patients. J Clin Neurophysiol 2005; 22:128-135.
17. Brenner RP. EEG in convulsive and nonconvulsive status epilepticus. J Clin Neurophysiol 2004;21:319-331.
18. Boulanger JM, Deacon C, Lecuyer D, Gosselin S, Reiher J. Triphasic waves versus nonconvulsive status epilepticus: EEG distinction. Can J Neurol Sci 2006;33:175-180.
19. Fountain NB, Waldman WA. Effects of benzodiazepines on triphasic waves: implications for nonconvulsive status epilepticus. J Clin Neurophysiol 2001;18:345-352.
20. Hirsch LJ. Continuous EEG monitoring in the intensive care unit: an overview. J Clin Neurophysiol 2004;21:332-340.
21. Treiman DM, Meyers PD, Walton NY, Collins JF, Colling C, Rowan AJ, Handforth A, Faught E, Calabrese VP, Uthman BM, Ramsay RE, Mamdani MB. A comparison of four treatments for generalized convulsive status epilepticus. Veterans Affairs Status Epilepticus Cooperative Study Group. N Engl J Med 1998;339:792-798.
22. Fagan K, Lee S. Prolonged confusion following convulsions due to generalized nonconvulsive status epilepticus. Neurology 1990;40:1689-1694.
23. Kaplan PW. Nonconvulsive status epilepticus in the emergency room. Epilepsia 1996;37:643-650.
24. Andermann F, Robb JP. Absence status: a reappraisal following review of thirty-eight patients. Epilepsia 1972;13:177-187.
25. Baykan B, Gokyigit A, Gurses C, Eraksoy M. Recurrent absence status epilepticus: clinical and EEG characteristics. Seizure 2002;11:310-319.
26. Berkovic SF, Bladin PF. Absence status in adults. Clin Exp Neurol 1983;19:198-207.
27. Treiman DM. Electroclinical features of status epilepticus. J Clin Neurophysiol 1995;12:343-362.
28. Proposal for revised clinical and electroencephalographic classification of epileptic seizures. From the Commission on Classification and Terminology of the International League Against Epilepsy. Epilepsia 1981;22:489-501.
29. Roger J, Lob H, Tassinari C. Status epilepticus. In: Finken P, Bruyn G, eds. The Epilepsies. New York, NY: American Elsevier; 1974:145-188.
30. Fernandez-Torre JL. De novo absence status of late onset following withdrawal of lorazepam: a case report. Seizure 2001;10:433-437.
31. D'Agostino MD, Andermann F, Dubeau F, Fedi M, Bastos A. Exceptionally long absence status: multifactorial etiology, drug interactions and complications. Epileptic Disord 1999;1:229-232.
32. Drislane FW, Schomer DL. Clinical implications of generalized electrographic status epilepticus. Epilepsy Res 1994;19:111-121.
33. Husain AM, Mebust KA, Radtke RA. Generalized periodic epileptiform discharges: etiologies, relationship to status epilepticus, and prognosis. J Clin Neurophysiol 1999;16:51-58.
34. Delgado-Escueta AV, Fong CY. Status epilepticus: recent trends and prospects. Neurologia 1997;12:62-73.
35. Ferrie CD, Caraballo R, Covanis A, Demirbilek V, Dervent A, Fejerman N, Fusco L, Grunewald RA, Kanazawa O, Koutroumanidis M, Lada C, Livingston JH, Nicotra A, Oguni H, Martinovic Z, Nordli DR, Parisi P, Scott RC, Specchio N, Verrotti A, Vegevano F, Walker MC, Watanabe K, Yoshinaga H, Panayiotopoulos CP. Autonomic status epilepticus in Panayiotopoulos syndrome and other childhood and adult epilepsies: a consensus view. Epilepsia 2007;48:1165-1172.
36. Devinsky O, Kelley K, Porter RJ, Theodore WH. Clinical and electroencephalographic features of simple partial seizures. Neurology 1988;38:1347-1352.
37. Schomer DL. Focal status epilepticus and epilepsia partialis continua in adults and children. Epilepsia 1993;34(Suppl 1):S29-S36.
38. Grand'Maison F, Reiher J, Leduc CP. Retrospective inventory of EEG abnormalities in partial status epilepticus. Electroencephalogr Clin Neurophysiol 1991;79:264-270.
39. Drislane FW, Blum AS, Schomer DL. Focal status epilepticus: clinical features and significance of different EEG patterns. Epilepsia 1999;40:1254-1260.
40. Thomas JE, Reagan TJ, Klass DW. Epilepsia partialis continua. A review of 32 cases. Arch Neurol 1977;34:266-275.
41. Chatrian GE, Shaw CM, Plum F. Focal Periodic Slow Transients in epilepsia partialis continua: clinical and pathological correlations in two cases. Electroencephalogr Clin Neurophysiol 1964;16:387-393.

42. Salanova V, Morris HH, Van Ness P, Kotagal P, Wyllie E, Luders H. Frontal lobe seizures: electroclinical syndromes. Epilepsia 1995;36:16-24.
43. Williamson PD, Spencer DD, Spencer SS, Novelly RA, Mattson RH. Complex partial seizures of frontal lobe origin. Ann Neurol 1985; 18:497-504.
44. Williamson PD, Spencer DD, Spencer SS, Novelly RA, Mattson RH. Complex partial status epilepticus: a depth-electrode study. Ann Neurol 1985;18:647-654.
45. Drislane FW. Presentation, evaluation, and treatment of nonconvulsive status epilepticus. Epilepsy Behav 2000;1:301-314.
46. Tomson T, Lindbom U, Nilsson BY. Nonconvulsive status epilepticus in adults: thirty-two consecutive patients from a general hospital population. Epilepsia 1992;33:829-835.
47. Tomson T, Svanborg E, Wedlund JE. Nonconvulsive status epilepticus: high incidence of complex partial status. Epilepsia 1986;27:276-285.
48. Ballenger C 3d, King D, Gallagher B. Partial complex status epilepticus. Neurology 1983;33:1545-1552.
49. Markand ON, Wheeler GL, Pollack SL. Complex partial status epilepticus (psychomotor status). Neurology 1978;28:189-196.
50. Mayeux R, Lueders H. Complex partial status epilepticus: case report and proposal for diagnostic criteria. Neurology 1978;28:957-961.
51. Towne AR, Waterhouse EJ, Boggs JG, Garnett LK, Brown AJ, Smith JR, DeLorenzo RJ. Prevalence of nonconvulsive status epilepticus in comatose patients. Neurology 2000;54:340-345.
52. Saengpattrachai M, Sharma R, Hunjan A, Shroff M, Ochi A, Otsubo H, Cortez MA, Carter Snead O. Nonconvulsive seizures in the pediatric intensive care unit: etiology, EEG, and brain imaging findings. Epilepsia 2006;47:1510-1518.
53. Friedman DE, Schevon C, Emerson RG, Hirsch LJ. Cyclic electrographic seizures in critically ill patients. Epilepsia 2008;49:281-287.
54. Clancy RR. The contribution of EEG to the understanding of neonatal seizures. Epilepsia 1996;37:S52-59.
55. Mizrahi EM, Kellaway P. Characterization and classification of neonatal seizures. Neurology 1987;37:1837-1844.
56. Olmos-Garcia de Alba G, Udaeta Mora E, Malagon Valdez J, Villaneuva Garcia D, Valarezo Crespo F. Neonatal status epilepticus II: Electroencephalographic aspects. Clin Electroencephalogr 1984;15:197-201.
57. Scher MS. Controversies regarding neonatal seizure recognition. Epileptic Disord 2002;4:139-158.
58. Clancy RR, Legido A. The exact ictal and interictal duration of electroencephalographic neonatal seizures. Epilepsia 1987;28:537-541.
59. Shewmon DA. What is a neonatal seizure? Problems in definition and quantification for investigative and clinical purposes. J Clin Neurophysiol 1990;7:315-368.
60. Patry G, Lyagoubi S, Tassinari CA. Subclinical "electrical status epilepticus" induced by sleep in children. A clinical and electroencephalographic study of six cases. Arch Neurol 1971;24:242-252.
61. Tassinari CA, Rubboli G, Volpi L, Meletti S, d'Orsi G, Franca M, Sabetta AR, Riguzzi P, Gardella E, Zaniboni A, Michelucci R. Encephalopathy with electrical status epilepticus during slow sleep or ESES syndrome including the acquired aphasia. Clin Neurophysiol 2000;111(Suppl 2):S94-S102.
62. De Negri M. Electrical status epilepticus during sleep (ESES). Different clinical syndromes: towards a unifying view? Brain Dev 1997; 19:447-451.
63. Engel J, Jr. A proposed diagnostic scheme for people with epileptic seizures and with epilepsy: report of the ILAE Task Force on Classification and Terminology. Epilepsia 2001;42:796-803.
64. McVicar KA, Shinnar S. Landau-Kleffner syndrome, electrical status epilepticus in slow wave sleep, and language regression in children. Ment Retard Dev Disabil Res Rev 2004;10:144-149.
65. Van Hirtum-Das M, Licht EA, Koh S, Wu JY, Shields WD, Sankar R. Children with ESES: variability in the syndrome. Epilepsy Res 2006;70(Suppl 1):S248-S258.
66. Morrell F, Whisler WW, Smith MC, Hoeppner TJ, de Toledo-Morrell L, Pierre-Louis SJC, Kanner AM, Buelow JM, Ristanovic R, Bergen D, Chez M, Hasegawa H. Landau-Kleffner syndrome. Treatment with subpial intracortical transection. Brain 1995;118(Pt 6):1529-1546.
67. Wilner AN, Bream PR. Status epilepticus and pseudostatus epilepticus. Seizure 1993;2:257-260.
68. Walker M. Status epilepticus: an evidence based guide. Bmj 2005;331:673-677.
69. Holtkamp M, Othman J, Buchheim K, Meierkord H. Diagnosis of psychogenic

nonepileptic status epilepticus in the emergency setting. Neurology 2006;66:1727-1729.
70. Husain AM, Horn GJ, Jacobson MP. Non-convulsive status epilepticus: usefulness of clinical features in selecting patients for urgent EEG. J Neurol Neurosurg Psychiatry 2003;74:189-191.
71. Privitera M, Hoffman M, Moore JL, Jester D. EEG detection of nontonic-clonic status epilepticus in patients with altered consciousness. Epilepsy Res 1994;18:155-166.
72. DeLorenzo RJ, Waterhouse EJ, Towne AR, Boggs JG, Ko D, DeLorenzo GA, Brown A, Garnett L. Persistent nonconvulsive status epilepticus after the control of convulsive status epilepticus. Epilepsia 1998;39:833-840.
73. Praline J, Grujic J, Corcia P, Lucas B, Hommett C, Autret A, de Toffol B. Emergent EEG in clinical practice. Clin Neurophysiol 2007;118: 2149-2155.
74. Jirsch J, Hirsch LJ. Nonconvulsive seizures: developing a rational approach to the diagnosis and management in the critically ill population. Clin Neurophysiol 2007;118:1660-1670.
75. Claassen J, Jette N, Chum F, Green R, Schmidt M, Choi H, Jirsch J, Frontera JA, Connolly ES, Emerson RG, Mayer SA, Hirsch LJ. Electrographic seizures and periodic discharges after intracerebral hemorrhage. Neurology 2007;69: 1356-1365.
76. Vespa PM, O'Phelan K, Shah M, Mirabelli J, Starkman S, Kidwell C, Saver J, Nuwer MR, Frazee JG, McArthur DA, Martin NA. Acute seizures after intracerebral hemorrhage: A factor in progressive midline shift and outcome. Neurology 2003;60:1441-1446.
77. Vespa PM, Nuwer MR, Nenov V, Ronne-Engstrom E, Hovda DA, Bergsneider M, Kelly DF, Martin NA, Becker DP. Increased incidence and impact of nonconvulsive and convulsive seizures after traumatic brain injury as detected by continuous electroencephalographic monitoring. J Neurosurg 1999;91:750-760.
78. Claassen J, Mayer SA, Kowalski RG, Emerson RG, Hirsch LJ. Detection of electrographic seizures with continuous EEG monitoring in critically ill patients. Neurology 2004;62:1743-1748.
79. Dennis LJ, Claassen J, Hirsch LJ, Emerson RG, Connolly ES, Mayer SA. Nonconvulsive status epilepticus after subarachnoid hemorrhage. Neurosurgery 2002;51:1136-1144.
80. Quigg M, Shneker B, Domer P. Current practice in administration and clinical criteria of emergent EEG. J Clin Neurophysiol 2001;18:162-165.
81. Bautista RE, Godwin S, Caro D. Incorporating abbreviated EEGs in the initial workup of patients who present to the emergency room with mental status changes of unknown etiology. J Clin Neurophysiol 2007;24:16-21.
82. Walker MC. Diagnosis and treatment of nonconvulsive status epilepticus. CNS Drugs 2001;15:931-939.
83. Claassen J, Hirsch LJ, Emerson RG, Mayer SA. Treatment of refractory status epilepticus with pentobarbital, propofol, or midazolam: a systematic review. Epilepsia 2002;43:146-153.
84. Van Ness PC. Pentobarbital and EEG burst suppression in treatment of status epilepticus refractory to benzodiazepines and phenytoin. Epilepsia 1990;31:61-67.
85. Rashkin MC, Youngs C, Penovich P. Pentobarbital treatment of refractory status epilepticus. Neurology 1987;37:500-503.
86. Lowenstein DH, Aminoff MJ, Simon RP. Barbiturate anesthesia in the treatment of status epilepticus: clinical experience with 14 patients. Neurology 1988;38:395-400.
87. Krishnamurthy KB, Drislane FW. Depth of EEG suppression and outcome in barbiturate anesthetic treatment for refractory status epilepticus. Epilepsia 1999;40:759-762.
88. Claassen J, Hirsch LJ, Emerson RG, Bates JE, Thompson TB, Mayer SA. Continuous EEG monitoring and midazolam infusion for refractory nonconvulsive status epilepticus. Neurology 2001;57:1036-1042.
89. Wilson SB. A neural network method for automatic and incremental learning applied to patient-dependent seizure detection. Clin Neurophysiol 2005;116:1785-1795.
90. Gotman J. Automatic detection of seizures and spikes. J Clin Neurophysiol 1999;16:130-140.
91. Scheuer ML, Wilson SB. Data analysis for continuous EEG monitoring in the ICU: seeing the forest and the trees. J Clin Neurophysiol 2004;21:353-378.

CHAPTER 5

# CONTROVERSIAL ELECTROENCEPHALOGRAPHIC PATTERNS AND NONCONVULSIVE STATUS EPILEPTICUS

Richard P. Brenner

Because of the spectrum of electroencephalogram (EEG)-ictal patterns and the diversity of clinical presentations, "Is it nonconvulsive status epilepticus (NCSE)?" is often a difficult question for an electroencephalographer to answer, particularly in an intensive care unit setting. Diagnostic criteria for NCSE are controversial, and there are no agreed-upon criteria to diagnose NCSE in obtunded or comatose patients. Young and colleagues proposed primary and secondary criteria (1), subsequently modified (2), for an electrographic or nonconvulsive seizure, which, in turn, help define NCSE.

NCSE consists of EEG-ictal episodes, which are continuous or recurrent for 30 minutes or greater without improvement in clinical state or return to the pre-ictal EEG pattern between seizures. It is relatively easy to diagnose NCSE when there are frequent focal electrographic seizures in which there is a change in frequency, field, voltage, and morphology of the discharge. The problem is greater with periodic generalized or lateralized spikes, sharp waves, spike-and-wave, and sharp-and-slow-wave complexes (SSWC) that occur less frequently than 3 per second. The latter should not be invariant; that is, they should show evolution. If not, then a secondary criterion is required. This involves response to anticonvulsant medications such as benzodiazepines. Clearly marked clinical improvement following administration is the preferred response. Although this often occurs in absence status (also referred to as petit mal status or spike-wave stupor [3]) in ambulatory but confused patients ("the walking wounded"), it is rare in obtunded or comatose patients in NCSE (the ictally comatose) (4,5). Improvement of the EEG alone, without clinical improvement, requires resolution of the discharges and the appearance of previously normal EEG patterns to satisfy secondary criteria for NCSE when discharges are fewer than 3 per second (2).

A test dose of lorazepam may complicate matters because many EEG patterns, including triphasic waves (TWs) due to a metabolic encephalopathy, may resolve if the patient is given an adequate dose (6). Sometimes this can be shown to be due to a state change, as the pattern recurs after painful stimulation. After treatment, the presence of diffuse slowing on the EEG only, without clinical improvement, does not prove that the discharges were ictal and were responsible for the patient's decreased responsiveness. Furthermore, if the patient is in a coma following a subarachnoid hemorrhage or due to a central nervous system infection and is also in NCSE, treatment with anticonvulsant medications might improve the EEG, but the patient might not awaken due to the underlying brain disorder.

There are a number of EEG patterns described as being associated with NCSE that are controversial, particularly as to whether or not they are ictal. These include periodic patterns, such as periodic lateralized epileptiform discharges (PLEDs); bilateral independent PLEDs (BIPLEDs); and periodic epileptiform discharges (PEDs), which can be either lateralized (PLEDs) or generalized (GPEDs); and generalized TWs. All may become prominent following stimulation and, as such, can be considered stimulus-induced, rhythmic, periodic, or ictal discharges (SIRPIDs) (7).

## PERIODIC LATERALIZED EPILEPTIFORM DISCHARGES

A pattern often seen with acute or subacute unilateral lesions is PLEDs. Chatrian and colleagues (8) described PLEDs as consisting of lateralized complexes usually recurring every one to two seconds (Figure 5.1A). The complexes often consist of sharp waves or spikes that may be followed by a slow wave. Reiher and colleagues (9) proposed a classification of PLEDs that included PLEDs-plus and PLEDs-proper. PLEDs-plus consist of brief, low-amplitude, focal, rhythmic, activity that occurs in association with PLEDs, whereas PLEDs-proper consist of repetitive and stereotyped PLEDs without the low-amplitude, focal, rhythmic discharges. PLEDs-plus is more likely to be associated with clinical seizures and seizure discharges than is PLEDs-proper.

PLEDs occur in a variety of disorders, most often infarcts or tumors. They may also be seen in patients with chronic seizure disorders or old static lesions, especially when associated with recent seizures, alcohol withdrawal, or a toxic-metabolic disorder (10). In a literature review of 586 cases (11), etiologies were found to be stroke (35%), mass lesion (26%), infection (6%), hypoxia (2%), and other (22%). The clinical picture associated with PLEDs is usually obtundation, focal seizures, and focal neurologic signs.

Regardless of etiology, PLEDs are usually a transient phenomenon. With time, the discharges usually decrease in amplitude, the repetition rate decreases, and ultimately the discharges cease. An exception to this is the report by Westmoreland and colleagues of 6 patients with epilepsy who had persistent PLEDs, ranging from 30 months to 20.5 years, in their interictal EEGs (12). These they termed chronic PLEDs.

The majority of patients with PLEDs will have seizures during the acute stage of illness. During the recording of the EEG, PLEDs usually will be transiently replaced by a new pattern if a seizure occurs, often consisting of faster rhythmic activity (Figure 5.1B). For this reason, PLEDs are usually considered an interictal pattern, although not all agree (13-15). In several studies of NCSE, PLEDs alone were not considered an ictal pat-

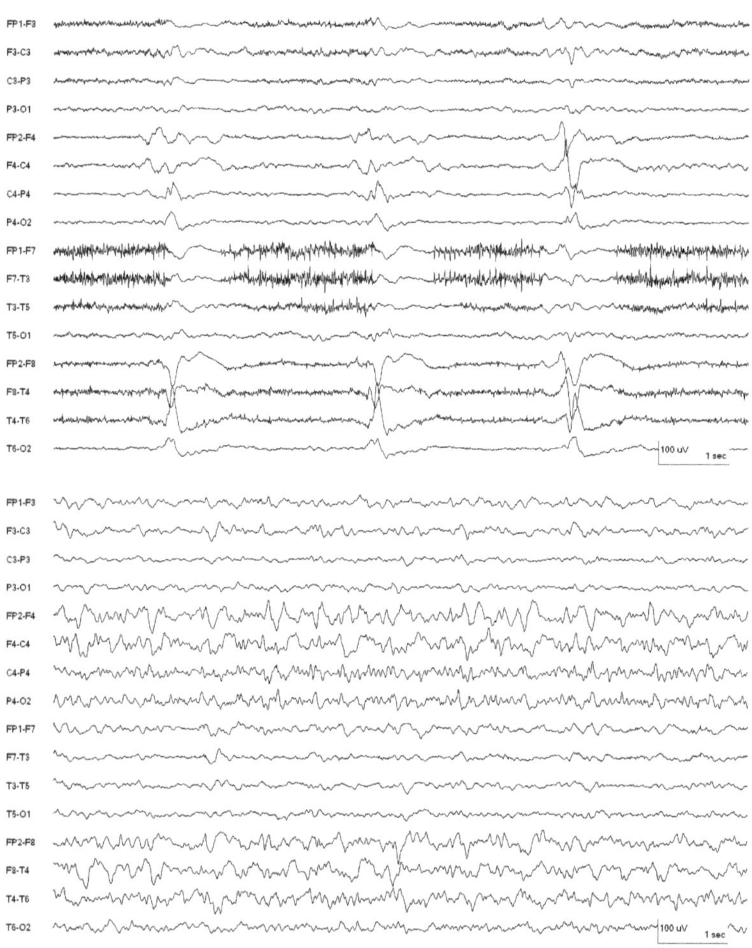


**Figure 5.1** (A) Periodic lateralized epileptiform discharges (PLEDs) in an 87-year-old-woman with herpes simplex encephalitis. (B) Right-sided electrographic seizure in the same patient.

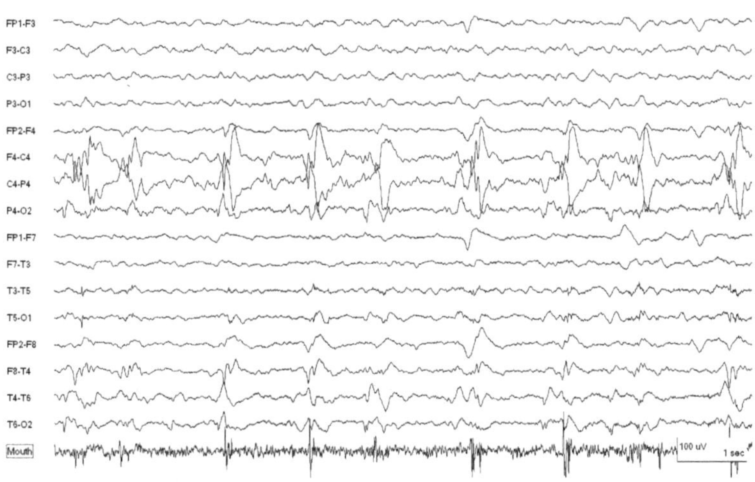


**Figure 5.2** Ictal periodic lateralized epileptiform discharges (PLEDs) in a 79-year-old man. There is left-sided facial twitching associated with right-sided PLEDs.

tern (16-18). Pohlmann-Eden and colleagues (19) viewed PLEDs as an electrographic signature of a dynamic pathophysiologic state in which unstable neurobiologic processes create an ictal-interictal continuum.

Clearly there are times when PLEDs are ictal. For example, they may be associated with repetitive jerks of the contralateral extremity, ie, epilepsia partialis continua (Figure 5.2). In addition, Terzano and colleagues (20) reported data from 7 patients over the age of 60 who suffered from recurrent and prolonged episodes of a confusional state associated with psychic and neurologic manifestations. All episodes were accompanied by PLEDs on the EEG, which became normal when the ictal episodes subsided, either spontaneously or following the intravenous administration of diazepam.

## BILATERAL INDEPENDENT PLEDS

PLEDs are lateralized, but they are often reflected synchronously to a lesser degree over homologous areas in the contralateral hemisphere. In contrast, in patients with BIPLEDs, the complexes are asynchronous, usually differing in morphology, amplitude, rate of repetition, and site of maximal involvement (Figure 5.3). De la Paz and Brenner (21) reported clinical findings in 18 patients whose EEGs showed this pattern. The most common causes of BIPLEDs were hypoxic encephalopathy (5), central nervous system infection (encephalitis or meningitis) (5), and chronic seizure disorders (4). When compared with patients with PLEDs, those with BIPLEDs were more likely to be comatose (72% vs 24%) and had a higher mortality rate (61% vs 29%), but focal neurologic deficits and focal seizures were less common. BIPLEDs are much less common than PLEDs, with few other patient series having been reported. Like PLEDs, the complexes are often replaced by a lateralized rhythmic pattern during a seizure.

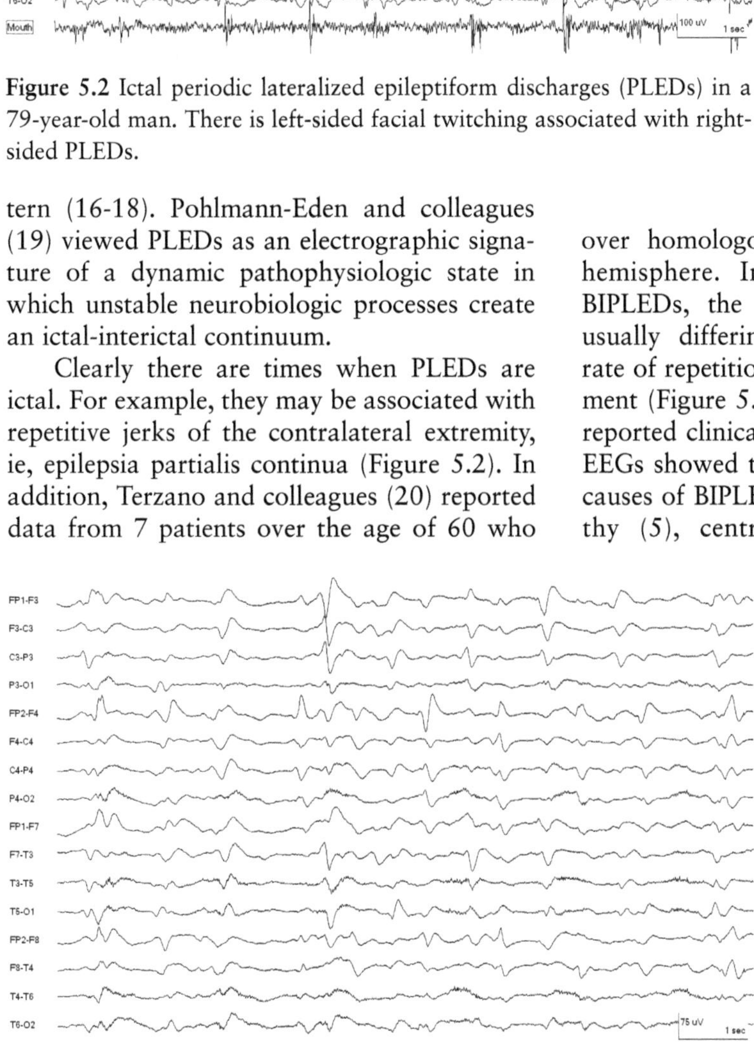


**Figure 5.3** Bilateral independent periodic lateralized epileptiform discharges (BIPLEDs) in an 82-year-old man.

## PERIODIC EPILEPTIFORM DISCHARGES

Treiman and colleagues (22) described 5 identifiable EEG patterns that they felt occurred in a predictable sequence during the course of secondarily generalized convulsive status epilepticus. These were

1. EEG changes of discrete seizures with interictal slowing
2. Merging seizures with waxing and waning ictal discharge
3. Continuous ictal discharges
4. Continuous ictal discharges with "flat" periods
5. PEDs on a "flat" background. When these complexes are lateralized, the term PLEDs is used; when generalized, then *GPEDs* is employed.

Others, however, have not found this sequence of EEG changes (14,23-25). Whether the final pattern of this proposed sequence, particularly GPEDs with a "flat" background (Figure 5.4), should be considered ictal is debatable (14,25-27). Some feel that GPEDs may represent NCSE; others view it as an epileptic encephalopathy in which spikes and sharp waves may not impair clinical function but, rather, reflect damage from severe brain injury (28,29).

As in patients with PLEDs or BIPLEDs, a longer recording (1 hour instead of 25 minutes) may demonstrate discrete seizures. How to define GPEDs with continuous EEG monitoring, however, has become more difficult; in prolonged recordings, patients with GPEDs may also have periods of PLEDs and BIPLEDs.

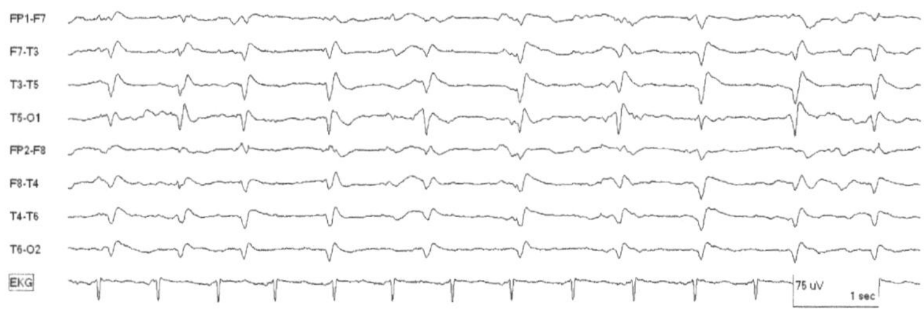


**Figure 5.4** Generalized periodic epileptiform discharges (GPEDs) in a 45-year-old-man.

## TRIPHASIC WAVES

Foley and colleagues (30) have described blunt spike-and-slow-wave complexes in patients with hepatic coma and have felt that, at times, these could not be distinguished from the electrical activity frequently associated with petit mal epilepsy. Distinguishing these complexes from epileptiform abnormalities has remained a problem (31). Recommendations to differentiate these entities have been provided by several investigators (32-34).

These waveforms were subsequently termed *TWs* (35) and consist of bursts of moderate-to high-amplitude (100- to-300-uV) activity, usually of 1.5 to 2.5 Hz, often occurring in clusters (Figure 5.5). Although frequently predominant in the frontal regions, they are occasionally maximal posteriorly. A fronto-occipital lag may be present. The initial negative component is the sharpest, whereas the following positive portion of the complex is the largest and is subsequently followed by another negative wave. TWs may increase with stimulation (31). They are bisynchronous but can show shifting asymmetries. A persistent asymmetry (not related to technical factors or a skull defect) suggests an underlying structural lesion on the side of the lower amplitude.

TWs were initially believed to be highly specific for hepatic dysfunction. In a study of 50 patients whose EEGs showed TWs (36), however, etiologies were hepatic (28), azotemia (10), hypoxia (9), hyperosmolarity (2), and hypoglycemia (1). Bahamon-Dussan and col-

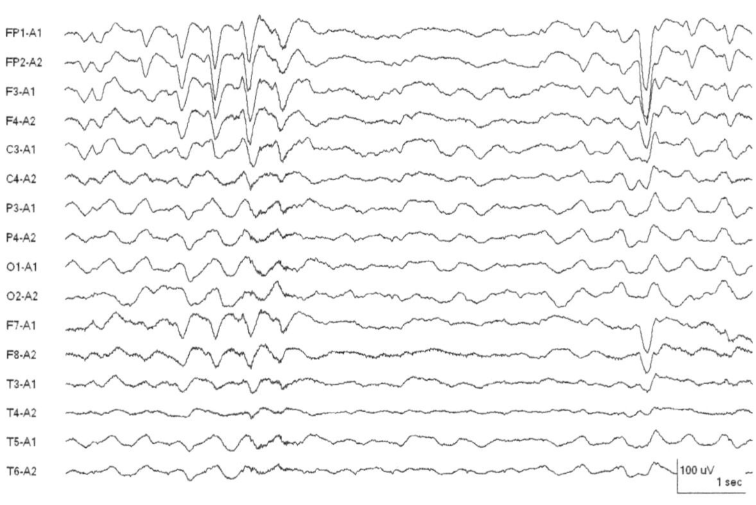


**Figure 5.5** Triphasic waves in a 51-year-old man with hepatic failure.

leagues (37) found multiple metabolic derangements to be the most common cause of TWs, present in 12 of 30 patients. Patients were either very lethargic or comatose, and the mortality rate was 77%. Sundaram and Blume (38) found that the etiology of TWs was more closely related to the level of consciousness at the time of recording than they were to any morphologic or distribution features or nature of EEG background activity. Awake but confused patients all had nonmetabolic encephalopathies, particularly Alzheimer disease, whereas all unarousable patients had metabolic encephalopathies. In general, patients with absence status, however, are confused but arousable, whereas those with NCSE are obtunded or comatose, particularly if patients in the intensive care unit are included. Periodic sharp complexes, most often triphasic or biphasic and occurring approximately every second, can also be seen in patients with degenerative disorders, such as Creutzfeldt-Jakob disease (39) (Figure 5.6). Clearly, the causes of TWs depend on the patient population at the institution where the study is performed.

Rae-Grant and colleagues (40) found TWs in 15 of 268 EEG studies (6%) done in patients with Alzheimer disease but did not comment on the distribution of the TWs. TWs were always associated with other severe EEG disturbances, such as excessive delta activity. Sundaram and Blume (38) found that TWs were maximal anteriorly in the majority of patients with Alzheimer disease. Others (41,42) have found the discharges usually maximal posteriorly.

In a study of the diagnostic specificity of TWs, those occurring in hepatic encephalopathy were more likely to be associated with severe EEG background slowing than in other encephalopathies with these waveforms (43). None of the morphologic features of TWs (longitudinal topography, phase lag, symmetry, or longitudinal, bipolar, phase-reversal sites) reliably distinguished hepatic encephalopathy from other forms of metabolic encephalopathy. Our concern, however, is not distinguishing between the various

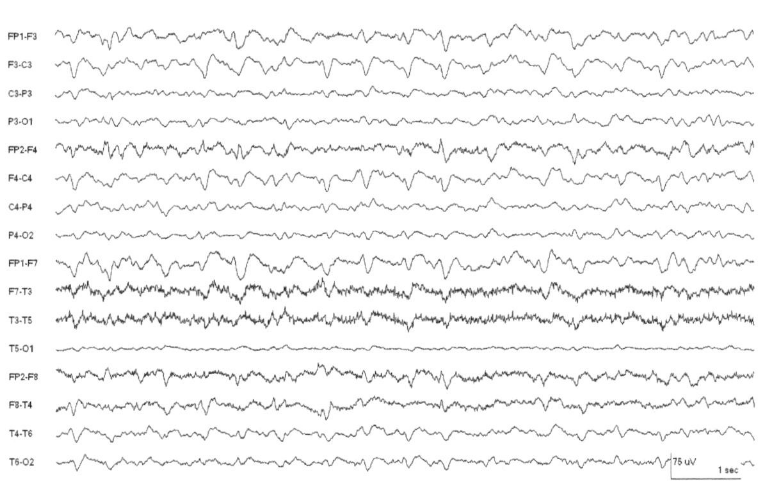


**Figure 5.6** Generalized periodic complexes in a 62-year-old-woman with Creutzfeldt-Jakob disease.

metabolic encephalopathies associated with TWs but, rather, whether these waveforms are more consistent with a metabolic encephalopathy or with NCSE.

When electroencephalographers use the term *TWs*, they are usually implying a pattern seen with a variety of encephalopathies, particularly hepatic or renal dysfunction, or following hypoxia. The term triphasic, however, can also be used to describe the morphology of the waveform because SSWC or spike-and-wave discharges usually have 3 phases; hence they are TWs. Difficulties in distinguishing TWs from generalized epileptiform abnormalities were initially noted by Foley and colleagues (30) and subsequently by others (44-46). Sundaram and Blume (38) indicated that TWs and SSWC, also often called slow-spike-and-wave, share many morphologic features. They also searched for TWs in another 100 EEGs in which the main finding was SSWC to compare the morphology with that of the TWs present in the 63 consecutive patients in whom TWs were the major finding. They found similarities, including 3 components (spike, trough and slow wave), bilaterally synchronous complexes with frontal predominance, and occurrence in groups or runs on a slow background. The relative durations of the 3 components of some TWs were similar to those of SSWC (ie, first component shortest and the third component longest). Of 100 EEGs containing SSWC, 40 had sporadic TWs. The major differences were the relative amplitudes of the waveforms of TWs occurring in EEGs with SSWC compared with most TWs seen in other conditions, including toxic-metabolic disorders. Waves 2 and 3 were the largest waveforms, or all 3 were equally large, in 37 of 40 EEGs with SSWC and sporadic TWs. In contrast, in the patients with and without metabolic disorders, wave 2 was usually the largest, followed in incidence by equally prominent waves 1 and 2. Equal prominence of components 2 and 3 was infrequent, whereas equal amplitude of all 3 waves rarely occurred. The authors used a referential montage to ipsilateral ears for these measurements, as have others (31).

TWs and generalized spike-wave discharges in generalized nonconvulsive status epilepticus (GNCSE) or absence status can also closely resemble one another. Kaplan (47) felt that TWs may straddle the border between epilepsy and encephalopathy and that the distinction between GNCSE and encephalopathy can be difficult to identify, whereas Litt and colleague (48) felt that monorhythmic TWs could be distinguished from ictal patterns. Clearly, there are times when this distinction can be difficult to make; hence the terms *triphasic-like waves* and *nonepileptiform true TWs* (27).

EEG features that help differentiate TWs from epileptiform discharges seen in GNCSE include wave 1 is of shorter duration and the frequency of the complexes is higher in GNCSE (mean = 2.4 Hz vs 1.8 Hz); in addition, there are often extra spikes preceding wave 1 and less background slowing in patients with NCSE (31). In patients with TWs due to metabolic encephalopathies, phase 2 is maximal, exceeding all other wave forms by at least 50%. In the study by Boulanger and colleagues (31), this did not occur in the group with GNCSE. There was usually a lag of phase 2 in the encephalopathy group only, which more commonly was anterior to posterior but could be posterior to anterior. TWs increased in a large percentage of cases following stimulation, whereas stimulation had no effect on the discharges in GNCSE. The morphologic features and response to stimulation, however, although helpful in distinguishing TWs from GNCSE, were not always present. As noted by Young (49), the study had limitations. It was retrospective and used traditional differentiating EEG criteria that have never been subjected to pathophysiologic investigations for confirmation. Thus, the study was almost tautologic in its approach.

Generalized, bisynchronous sharp complexes, at times periodic and often with a triphasic configuration, can occur following hypoxia-ischemia (26,50), in metabolic encephalopathies (51), in Creutzfeldt-Jakob disease (39), during or following status epilepticus (22), and in a variety of drug-related disorders. One such example is with cefepime, a

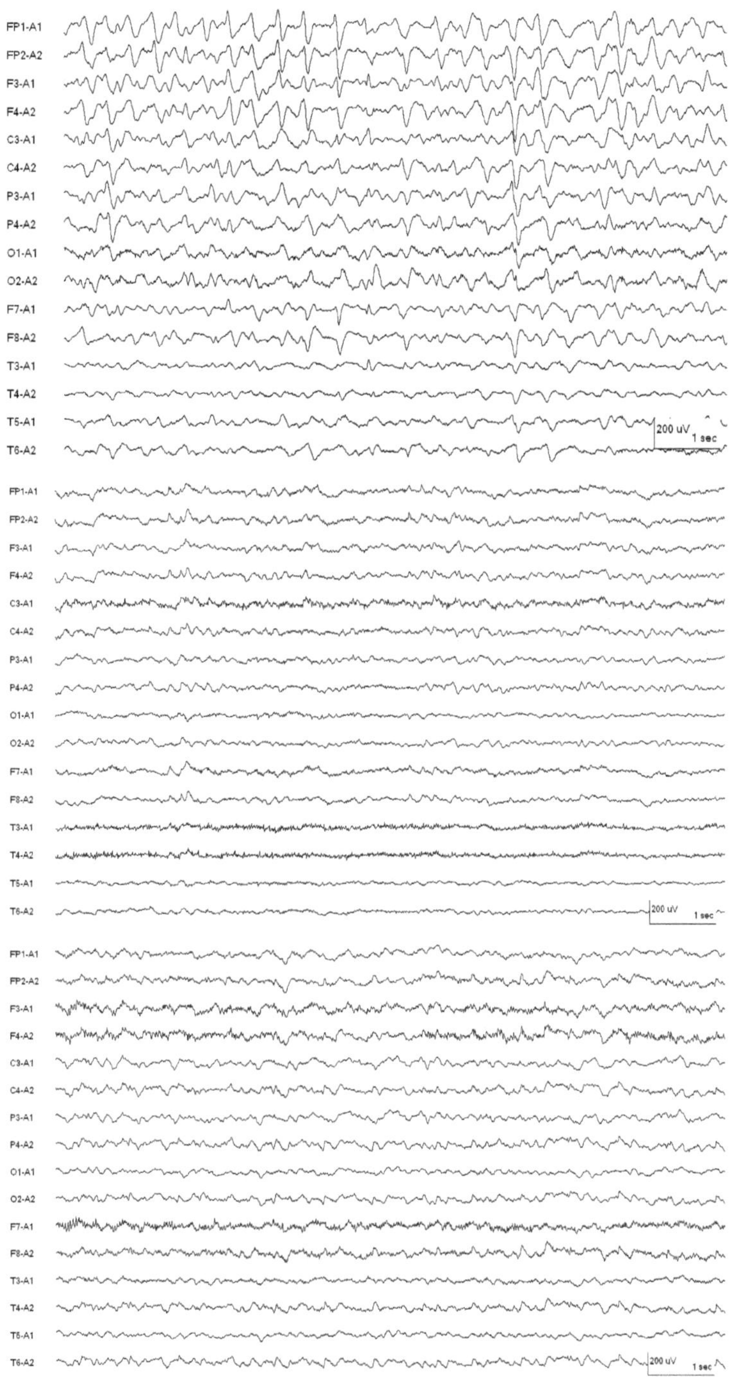

**Figure 5.7** (A) The initial electroencephalogram (EEG) in a 61-year-old-man in renal failure receiving cefepime. (B) Although the EEG improved following the administration of lorazepam, the patient remained unresponsive. (C) Cefepime was stopped, and the patient was treated with intravenously administered phenytoin. Both the EEG and the patient's condition improved the following day.

fourth-generation cephalosporin. Patients with renal failure receiving this antibiotic have become unresponsive, and the EEG often shows triphasic activity (52-56) (Figure 5.7A- C). Whether this is due to renal failure (although it has recently been reported in a patient with normal renal function (57)), an encephalopathy due to the drug, or NCSE (an epileptic mechanism caused by the drug) is uncertain. As has been emphasized, the diagnosis is often difficult to make. Should it require strict morphologic EEG criteria or should the clinical and EEG response be required? Finally, there are cases in which the morphologic EEG criteria are more suggestive of an encephalopathy, but treatment results in both a good clinical and EEG response.

Other drugs associated with generalized periodic patterns include baclofen (46,58,59), levodopa (60), lithium (61,62), ifosfamide (63-65), metrizamide (66-70), and tiagabine (71,72). Some have felt that these patterns represent NCSE, whereas others view them as encephalopathies that resolve when the offending agent is discontinued. As noted previously, the use of medications such as benzodiazepines may not resolve the issue, and a test dose of lorazepam may complicate matters because TWs due to a metabolic encephalopathy can regress without clinical improvement if the patient is given an adequate dose (6).

TWs may increase with stimulation (31). This is also true of PLEDs, BIPLEDs, GPEDs, and frontal rhythmic delta activity (7) (Figure 5.8A and B). One of the reasons that SIRPIDs have been recognized with greater frequency is that, due to recent technologic advances, it is now feasible and practical to record 24-hour, continuous, digital EEG with simultaneous digital video. Using these techniques, Hirsch and colleagues (7) noted striking EEG changes when stuporous or comatose patients were stimulated. In their study of 150 critically ill patients undergoing continuous EEG monitoring (with or without video), 33 patients exhibited SIRPIDs. No significant difference was found in the incidence of clinical seizures in patients with SIRPIDs (30%), compared with those without (45%), nor did the authors find any particular correlation between subtypes of SIRPIDs and clinical findings. The authors concluded that further research was necessary to determine the pathophysiologic, prognostic, and therapeutic significance of SIRPIDs. As with the other patterns described in this chapter, there are no easy answers.

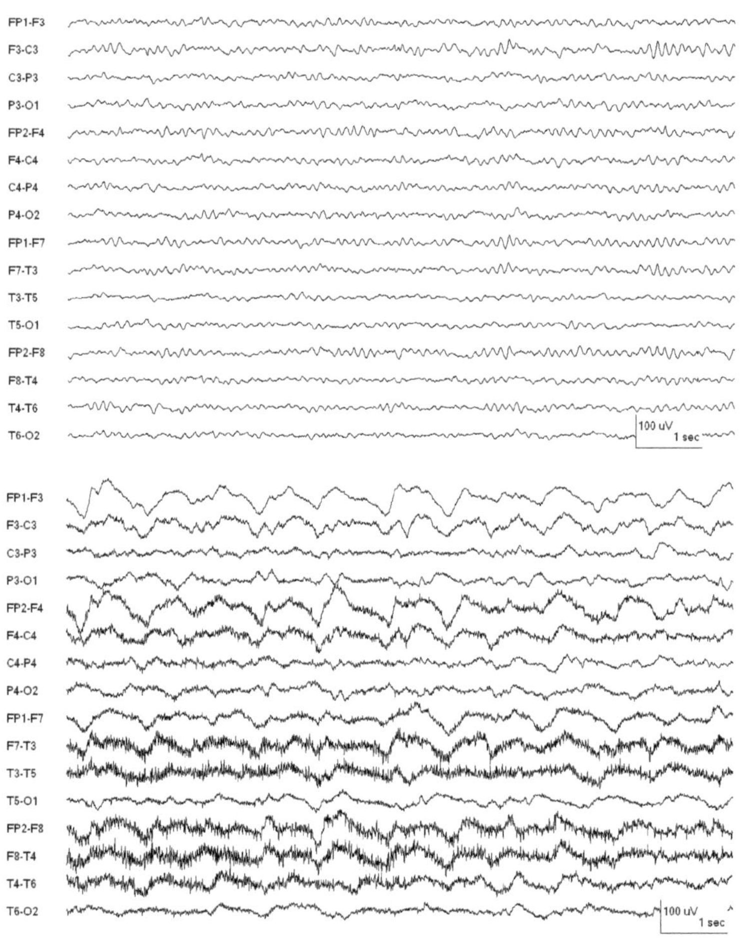


**Figure 5.8** (A) The electroencephalogram in a comatose 71-year-old man. (B) Following stimulation, stimulus-induced, rhythmic, periodic, or ictal discharges, consisting of frontal rhythmic delta activity, are present.

## REFERENCES

1. Young GB, Jordan KG, Doig GS. An assessment of nonconvulsive seizures in the intensive care unit using continuous EEG monitoring: an investigation of variables associated with mortality. Neurology 1996;47:83-89.
2. Chong DJ, Hirsch LJ. Which EEG patterns warrant treatment in the critically ill? Reviewing the evidence for treatment of periodic epileptiform discharges and related patterns. J Clin Neurophysiol 2005;22:79-91.
3. Niedermeyer E, Khalifeh R. Petit mal status ("spike-wave stupor"). An electro-clinical appraisal. Epilepsia 1965;6: 250-262.
4. Treiman DM, Meyers PD, Walton NY, Collins JF, Colling C, Rowan AJ, Handforth A, Faught E, Calabrese VP, Uthman BM, Ramsay RE, Mamdani MB. A comparison of four treatments for generalized convulsive status epilepticus. Veterans Affairs Status Epilepticus Cooperative Study Group. N Engl J Med 1998;339:792-798.
5. Walker M, Cross H, Smith S. Nonconvulsive status epilep-

ticus: Epilepsy Research Foundation Workshop Reports. Epileptic Disord 2005;7:253-296.
6. Fountain NB, Waldman WA. Effects of benzodiazepines on triphasic waves: implications for nonconvulsive status epilepticus. J Clin Neurophysiol 2001;18:345-352.
7. Hirsch LJ, Claassen J, Mayer SA, Emerson RG. Stimulus-induced rhythmic, periodic, or ictal discharges (SIRPIDs): a common EEG phenomenon in the critically ill. Epilepsia 2004;45:109-123.
8. Chatrian GE, Shaw CM, Leffman H. The significance of periodic lateralized epileptiform discharges in EEG: an electrographic, clinical and pathological study. Electroencephalogr Clin Neurophysiol 1964;17:177-193.
9. Reiher J, Rivest J, Grand'Maison F, Leduc CP. Periodic lateralized epileptiform discharges with transitional rhythmic discharges: association with seizures. Electroencephalogr Clin Neurophysiol 1991;78:12-17.
10. Garcia-Morales I, Garcia MT, Galan-Davila L, Gomez-Escalonilla C, Saiz-Diaz R, martinez-Salio A, de la Pena P, Tejerina JA. Periodic lateralized epileptiform discharges: etiology, clinical aspects, seizures, and evolution in 130 patients. J Clin Neurophysiol 2002;19:172-177.
11. Snodgrass SM, Tsuburaya K, Ajmone-Marsan C. Clinical significance of periodic lateralized epileptiform discharges: relationship with status epilepticus. J Clin Neurophysiol 1989;6:159-172.
12. Westmoreland BF, Klass DW, Sharbrough FW. Chronic periodic lateralized epileptiform dicharges. Arch Neurol 1986;43:494-496.
13. Handforth A, Cheng JT, Mandelkern MA, Treiman DM. Markedly increased mesiotemporal lobe metabolism in a case with PLEDs: further evidence that PLEDs are a manifestation of partial status epilepticus. Epilepsia 1994;35:876-881.
14. Garzon E, Fernandes RM, Sakamoto AC. Serial EEG during human status epilepticus: evidence for PLED as an ictal pattern. Neurology 2001;57:1175-1183.
15. Assal F, Papazyan JP, Slosman DO, Jallon P, Goerres BW. SPECT in periodic lateralized epileptiform discharges (PLEDs): a form of partial status epilepticus? Seizure 2001;10:260-265.
16. Claassen J, Hirsch LJ, Emerson RG, Bates JE, Thompson TB, Mayer SA. Continuous EEG monitoring and midazolam infusion for refractory nonconvulsive status epilepticus. Neurology 2001;57:1036-1042.
17. Jordan KG. Nonconvulsive status epilepticus in acute brain injury. J Clin Neurophysiol 1999;16:332-340; discussion 353.
18. Jaitly R, Sgro JA, Towne AR, Ko D, DeLorenzo RJ. Prognostic value of EEG monitoring after status epilepticus: a prospective adult study. J Clin Neurophysiol 1997;14:326-334.
19. Pohlmann-Eden B, Hoch DB, Cochius JI, Chiappa KH. Periodic lateralized epileptiform discharges—a critical review. J Clin Neurophysiol 1996;13:519-530.
20. Terzano MG, Parrino L, Mazzucchi A, Moretti G. Confusional states with periodic lateralized epileptiform discharges (PLEDs): a peculiar epileptic syndrome in the elderly. Epilepsia 1986;27:446-457.
21. de la Paz D, Brenner RP. Bilateral independent periodic lateralized epileptiform discharges. Clinical significance. Arch Neurol 1981;38:713-715.
22. Treiman DM, Walton NY, Kendrick C. A progressive sequence of electroencephalographic changes during generalized convulsive status epilepticus. Epilepsy Res 1990;5:49-60.
23. Lowenstein DH, Aminoff MJ. Clinical and EEG features of status epilepticus in comatose patients. Neurology 1992;42:100-104.
24. So E, Ruggles KH, Ahmann PA, Trudeau SK, Weatherford KJ, Trenerry MR. Clinical significance and outcome of subclinical status epilepticus in adults. Epilepsy 1995;8:11-15.
25. Nei M, Lee JM, Shanker VL, Sperling MR. The EEG and prognosis in status epilepticus. Epilepsia 1999;40:157-163.
26. Brenner RP, Schaul N. Periodic EEG patterns: classification, clinical correlation, and pathophysiology. J Clin Neurophysiol 1990;7:249-267.
27. Husain AM, Mebust KA, Radtke RA. Generalized periodic epileptiform discharges: etiologies, relationship to status epilepticus, and prognosis. J Clin Neurophysiol 1999;16:51-58.
28. Krumholz A. Epidemiology and evidence for morbidity of nonconvulsive status epilepticus. J Clin Neurophysiol 1999;16:314-322; discussion 353.
29. Niedermeyer E, Ribeiro M. Considerations of nonconvulsive status epilepticus. Clin Electroencephalogr 2000;31:192-195.
30. Foley JM, Watson CW, Adams RD. Significance of the electroencephalographic changes in hepatic coma. Trans Am Neurol Assoc 1950;75:161-164.

31. Boulanger JM, Deacon C, Lecuyer D, Gosselin S, Reiher J. Triphasic waves versus nonconvulsive status epilepticus: EEG distinction. Can J Neurol Sci 2006;33:175-180.
32. Klass DW. Principles in the differentiation of atypical spike-waves and triphasic waves. Am J EEG Technol 1990;30:313-314.
33. Hughes J. Principles in the differentiation of atypical spike-waves and triphasic waves. Am J EEG Technol 1990;30:309-312.
34. Ghigo J. Principles in the differentiation of atypical spike-waves and triphasic waves: a tecnologist's view. Am J EEG Technol 1990;30: 315-316.
35. Bickford RG, Butt HR. Hepatic coma: the electroencephalographic pattern. J Clin Invest 1955;34:790-799.
36. Karnaze DS, Bickford RG. Triphasic waves: a reassessment of their significance. Electroencephalogr Clin Neurophysiol 1984;57:193-198.
37. Bahamon-Dussan JE, Celesia GG, Grigg-Damberger MM. Prognostic significance of EEG triphasic waves in patients with altered state of consciousness. J Clin Neurophysiol 1989;6:313-319.
38. Sundaram MB, Blume WT. Triphasic waves: clinical correlates and morphology. Can J Neurol Sci 1987;14:136-140.
39. Wieser HG, Schindler K, Zumsteg D. EEG in Creutzfeldt-Jakob disease. Clin Neurophysiol 2006;117:935-951.
40. Rae-Grant A, Blume W, Lau C, Hachinski VC, Fisman M, Merskey H. The electroencephalogram in Alzheimer-type dementia. A sequential study correlating the electroencephalogram with psychometric and quantitative pathologic data. Arch Neurol 1987;44:50-54.
41. Muller HF, Kral VA. The electroencephalogram in advanced senile dementia. J Am Geriatr Soc 1967;15:415-426.
42. Blatt I, Brenner RP. Triphasic waves in a psychiatric population: a retrospective study. J Clin Neurophysiol 1996;13:324-329.
43. Fisch BJ, Klass DW. The diagnostic specificity of triphasic wave patterns. Electroencephalogr Clin Neurophysiol 1988;70:1-8.
44. Yamamoto M, Hosokawa K. Triphasic spike-wave stupor in portal-systemic encephalopathy: a case report. J Neurol Neurosurg Psychiatry 1985;48:386-387.
45. Sheridan PH, Sato S. Triphasic waves of metabolic encephalopathy versus spike-wave stupor. J Neurol Neurosurg Psychiatry 1986;49:108-109.
46. Nowack WJ, King JA. Triphasic waves and spike wave stupor. Clin Electroencephalogr 1992;23:100-104.
47. Kaplan PW. Assessing the outcomes in patients with nonconvulsive status epilepticus: nonconvulsive status epilepticus is underdiagnosed, potentially overtreated, and confounded by comorbidity. J Clin Neurophysiol 1999;16:341-352.
48. Litt B, Wityk RJ, Hertz SH, Mullen PD, Weiss H, Ryan DD, Henry TR. Nonconvulsive status epilepticus in the critically ill elderly. Epilepsia 1998;39:1194-1202.
49. Young GB. Those troublesome but never tiresome triphasic waves. Can J Neurol Sci 2006;33:125.
50. Yamashita S, Morinaga T, Ohgo S, Sakamoto T, Kaku N, Sugimoto S, Matsukura S. Prognostic value of electroencephalogram (EEG) in anoxic encephalopathy after cardiopulmonary resuscitation: relationship among anoxic period, EEG grading and outcome. Intern Med 1995;34:71-76.
51. Yemisci M, Gurer G, Saygi S, Ciger A. Generalised periodic epileptiform discharges: clinical features, neuroradiological evaluation and prognosis in 37 adult patients. Seizure 2003;12:465-472.
52. Martinez-Rodriguez JE, Barriga FJ, Santamaria J, Iranzo A, Pareja JA, Revilla M, de la Rosa CR. Nonconvulsive status epilepticus associated with cephalosporins in patients with renal failure. Am J Med 2001;111:115-119.
53. Dixit S, Kurle P, Buyan-Dent L, Sheth RD. Status epilepticus associated with cefepime. Neurology 2000;54:2153-2155.
54. Primavera A, Cocito L, Audenino D. Nonconvulsive status epilepticus during cephalosporin therapy. Neuropsychobiology 2004;49:218-222.
55. Jallon P, Fankhauser L, Du Pasquier R, Coeytaux A, Picard F, Hefft S, Assal F. Severe but reversible encephalopathy associated with cefepime. Neurophysiol Clin 2000;30:383-386.
56. Fernandez-Torre JL, Martinez-Martinez M, Gonzalez-Rato J, Maestro I, et al. Cephalosporin-induced nonconvulsive status epilepticus: clinical and electroencephalographic features. Epilepsia 2005;46:1550-1552.
57. Capparelli FJ, Diaz MF, Hlavnika A, Wainsztein NA, Leiguarda R, Del Castillo ME. Cefepime-

and cefixime-induced encephalopathy in a patient with normal renal function. Neurology 2005;65:1840.
58. Hormes JT, Benarroch EE, Rodriguez M, Klass DW. Periodic sharp waves in baclofen-induced encephalopathy. Arch Neurol 1988;45:814-815.
59. Zak R, Solomon G, Petito F, Labar D. Baclofen-induced generalized nonconvulsive status epilepticus. Ann Neurol 1994;36:113-114.
60. Neufeld MY. Periodic triphasic waves in levodopa-induced encephalopathy. Neurology 1992;42:444-446.
61. Roccatagliata L, Audenino D, Primavera A, Cocito L. Nonconvulsive status epilepticus from accidental lithium ingestion. Am J Emerg Med 2002;20:570-572.
62. Kaplan PW, Birbeck G. Lithium-induced confusional states: nonconvulsive status epilepticus or triphasic encephalopathy? Epilepsia 2006;47:2071-2074.
63. Simonian NA, Gilliam FG, Chiappa KH. Ifosfamide causes a diazepam-sensitive encephalopathy. Neurology 1993;43:2700-2702.
64. Wengs WJ, Talwar D, Bernard J. Ifosfamide-induced nonconvulsive status epilepticus. Arch Neurol 1993;50:1104-1105.
65. Primavera A, Audenino D, Cocito L. Ifosfamide encephalopathy and nonconvulsive status epilepticus. Can J Neurol Sci 2002;29:180-183.
66. Drake ME, Erwin CW. Triphasic EEG discharges in metrizamide encephalopathy. J Neurol Neurosurg Psychiatry 1984;47:324-325.
67. Elian M, Fenwick P. Metrizamide and the EEG: three case reports and a review. J Neurol 1985;232:341-345.
68. Levin R, Lee SI. Nonconvulsive status epilepticus following metrizamide myelogram. Ann Neurol 1985;17:518-519.
69. Obeid T, Yaqub B, Panayiotopoulos C, al-Jasser S, Shabaan A, Hawass NE. Absence status epilepticus with computed tomographic brain changes following metrizamide myelography. Ann Neurol 1988;24:582-584.
70. Potts K. Seizures and encephalopathies following metrizamide myelography and cisternography. Am J EEG Technol 1990;30:45-57.
71. de Borchgrave V, Lienard F, Willemart T, van Rijckevorsel K. Clinical and EEG findings in six patients with altered mental status receiving tiagabine therapy. Epilepsy Behav 2003;4:326-337.
72. Ettinger AB, Bernal OG, Andriola MR, Bagchi S, Flores P, Just C, Pitocco C, Rooney T, Tuominen J, Devinsky O. Two cases of nonconvulsive status epilepticus in association with tiagabine therapy. Epilepsia 1999;40:1159-1162.

CHAPTER 6

# IMAGING IN NONCONVULSIVE STATUS EPILEPTICUS

JONATHAN C. EDWARDS AND DIANA GOMEZ-HASSAN

Tremendous progress has been made in the field of epileptology over the last few decades, and this has been true nowhere more so than in the neuroimaging of epilepsy. Modern neuroimaging has made it possible to demonstrate gross and subtle structural etiologies for seizures that would previously have been considered "cryptogenic," while nuclear imaging can demonstrate metabolic and functional changes that occur ictally, interictally, or postictally.

The imaging of status epilepticus has certain practical limitations. Status epilepticus is typically an emergency, and detailed imaging takes considerable time. A second challenge arises from the availability of several different types of imaging and many potential imaging sequences for each modality. Practical, financial, and safety constraints make it necessary to choose the most appropriate imaging modality for a particular clinical situation.

## PRACTICAL ASPECTS OF IMAGING IN NONCONVULSIVE STATUS EPILEPTICUS

Often, the only imaging that has been obtained at the time of diagnosis of status epilepticus is a screening computed tomography (CT) scan. Once a diagnosis of status epilepticus has been established by clinical or electrocephalographic (EEG) means or both, the focus of care turns to the termination of seizures as quickly as possible. Further imaging with other modalities often becomes a secondary concern that must wait until the status epilepticus has been controlled successfully.

Additionally, because of seizure activity or because of the medications used to suppress seizures, intubation and mechanical ventilation are often necessary. Patients undergoing treatment for status epilepticus may also have hemodynamic instability and require close monitoring, creating further challenges in obtaining detailed or multimodal imaging. For a variety of reasons, the medical literature on imaging during nonconvulsive status epilepticus (NCSE) is limited, and large controlled series are not available. Nevertheless, modern imaging facilities include protocols for CT scanning, magnetic resonance imaging (MRI), positron emission tomography (PET), and single-photon emission computerized tomography (SPECT) in critically ill patients, including those who require mechanical ventilation.

Most patients in the intensive care unit who have external monitors, lines, and devices, including ventilatory equipment, can safely undergo CT or SPECT studies. Depending on the location of these devices, certain metallic equipment on or near the head may cause streak artifacts on CT images or appear as defects on SPECT images and may have to be moved or repositioned to avoid these artifacts. If contrast-enhanced CT imaging is needed, patients must be evaluated for potential reactions to intravenously administered contrast agents. Although uncommon, a severe reaction can be life threatening. Such studies should be performed when physicians are present and available to treat any untoward reaction that might occur.

For MRI studies, it must be determined whether the patient can safely undergo the study. Metallic implants, stimulators, and other devices are absolute contraindications to MRI scanning. Patients with some invasive blood pressure-measuring devices, pacer wires, and infusion pumps are also unable to undergo MRI studies. For critically ill patients, nonferromagnetic supportive equipment, including dedicated MRI-compatible ventilators, are necessary. In addition to the MRI technologist, adequately trained critical care personnel must accompany the patient from the intensive care unit, and anesthesia personnel are needed to prepare a patient for imaging. Preparation is time consuming but essential for patient safety. Although most university or tertiary care centers have the trained staff and compatible equipment and accessories, some may not be able to perform these studies in critically ill patients.

## COMPUTED TOMOGRAPHY

CT is an important diagnostic tool in screening for intracranial injury such as hemorrhage or mass lesions, especially acutely, but CT is of limited value in evaluating the brain parenchyma. It is easy to screen patients presenting in status epilepticus using a noncontrast or even contrast-enhanced head CT, but the diagnostic yield is low in patients with a history of long-standing epilepsy.

The advantages of CT include its availability in most institutions and the short time needed to scan. Currently, a state-of-the-art, 64-slice, helical CT scanner can perform a head CT in less than 10 seconds in a cooperative nonmoving patient. Additional time is needed to position the patient and obtain the appropriate scout images prior to full imaging. This can take up to 10 or 15 minutes. Contrast-enhanced CT imaging generally adds another 10 to 15 minutes for the administration of contrast material. Contrary to the case with MRI, osseous structures, surgical clips, and hemorrhages are seen better on CT. Epilepsy patients with intracranial and extracranial electrodes are often imaged to assess the position of the leads. A CT scan of the head is much less expensive than MRI.

A disadvantage of CT is the use of radiation, but multidector, multislice, high-speed scanners have been optimized to reduce the amount of radiation exposure. The greatest disadvantage of CT as an imaging tool, however, is its low sensitivity in the detection of abnormalities in patients with refractory epilepsy, as compared with MRI. Although CT has a role in identifying acute abnormalities or large structural lesions in patients presenting in status epilepticus, it has no diagnostic role in evaluating more subtle cortical malformations or parenchymal signal abnormalities in these patients.

CT findings reported in patients presenting with NCSE are usually nonspecific. In a case report, transient CT changes included focal cortical swelling in the acute phase, with the results confirmed with MRI (1). These changes, including narrow sulci and a hypodensity in the right frontal lobe, resolved after cessation of the seizures. In another report, a CT study performed on a patient with a known left frontal abscess (previously treated, both medically and surgically) did not have any new changes when presenting in NCSE; the subtle parenchymal distortion in the left frontal region (from the earlier abscess) was seen again (Figure 6-1). Kutluay and colleagues showed localizing CT changes in 1 of 3 patients presenting with NCSE (2). Subtle ischemic changes were detected in this patient and confirmed on MRI. Overall, the sensitivity for detecting any CT abnormality in epilepsy patients ranges from 30% to 40%, and the specificity is much lower.

## MAGNETIC RESONANCE IMAGING

MRI is an essential tool for the evaluation of patients with epilepsy. It provides far greater resolution of brain structures than do other imaging methods. MRI technology (including equipment, field strength, and software) is continuously being improved for better resolution. Rather than radiation, MRI uses radiofrequency pulses and magnetic fields to temporarily change atomic spins to generate images. Although the lack of ionizing radiation is beneficial, the magnetic fields of MRI scanners can be dangerous in patients with internal pacer wires, stimulators, or ferromagnetic foreign bodies or devices. Although 1- to 1.5-Tesla unit

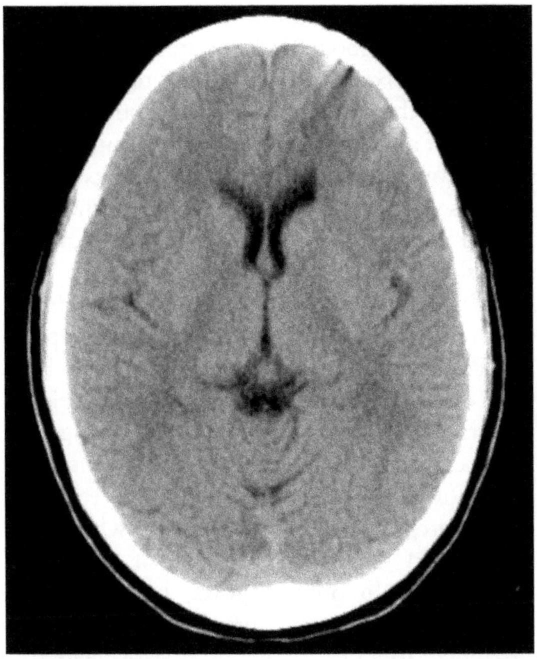

**Figure 6.1** A 16-year-old girl with a history of surgically treated pansinusitis and a left frontal cerebritis and abscess, who had nonconvulsive status epilepticus 4 months later.

MRIs have become available at many imaging centers and hospitals, higher field-strength equipment and the latest software and technology are generally available only in tertiary care facilities. Dedicated high-resolution protocols for epilepsy imaging may be available only in multidisciplinary epilepsy centers. The excellent resolution of detail in these images and the multiplanar capabilities of MRI provide a significant advantage in evaluating patients with epilepsy. With these technologies, tumors, infection, and inflammatory lesions are often readily seen, as are the extent of surrounding edema and mass effect. Developmental or structural disorders are best detected with MRI. Structural deformities such as schizencephaly and lissencephaly can be seen, as can more subtle heterotopias or cortical malformations.

A disadvantage of MRI is that a routine screening study of the brain may take from 30 to 60 minutes—and 60 to 90 minutes for a high-resolution epilepsy-focused MRI. Immobilizing the patient is essential to provide adequate resolution. Even subtle movement such as swallowing or eye blinking can compromise the quality of the images. Because multiple sequences in different planes are needed, the procedure lasts a long time. The sequences used in more focused epilepsy protocols can take as long as 9 to 11 minutes each; those used in screening studies range from 2 to 4 minutes each. MRI-compatible surgical clips, coils, shunts, and other hardware can also distort images. Patients with epilepsy who need ventilatory support require MRI-compatible ventilators and monitors. MRI studies are considerably more costly than CT, and many patients with epilepsy require multiple studies during their evaluations. Patients in NCSE may have an initial MRI to evaluate acute changes, followed by a separate study to assess resolution of abnormalities.

To evaluate more subtle pathology in patients with epilepsy, high-resolution MRI with 3-D thin-section spoiled gradient T1-weighted images in the coronal plane are often helpful. This sequence is ideal in evaluating the cortical morphology and gray-white matter interface and provides the anatomic detail necessary to calculate the volume of individual structures. Atrophy of mesial temporal structures associated with hippocampal sclerosis is now easily detected with this sequence.

Many epileptic lesions are detected by changes in signal intensities. Fluid-attenuated inversion recovery (FLAIR) and T2-weighted images improve detection of the hyperintensities associated with hippocampal sclerosis or cortical malformations. At least 1 post–contrast-imaging sequence is obtained to detect contrast-enhancing lesions. Diffusion-weighted imaging provides information regarding the microstructure of the brain and diffusion of water in the local environment. Acute changes in the brain can be detected best with diffusion-weighted-imaging sequences.

Many patients in NCSE require EEG monitoring, and imaging is typically performed prior to or after monitoring. Occasionally, patients with surface electrodes may require urgent imaging, and the MRI compatibility of the electrodes must be confirmed prior to imaging. Patients requiring invasive monitoring often undergo imaging; their electrodes are typically made of titanium and are MRI compatible.

As with CT, MRI changes in patients with NCSE are often nonspecific. Bauer and colleagues reported T1-weighted changes and edema in the right frontal lobe of a patient who had been in NCSE for 5 days (1). Reversible diffusion and FLAIR-weighted cortical changes have been noted in several other NCSE patients (3). Patients with hippocampal sclerosis can also present with NCSE (Figure 6-2A and B). In a patient who presented in hypoglycemic coma with persistent seizures despite metabolic correction, NCSE was confirmed by EEG, and MRI demonstrated multiple areas of signal hyperintensities throughout the supratentorial and infratentorial compartments (4). After seizures resolved, only atrophy was noted in some of those areas.

## POSITRON EMISSION TOMOGRAPHY

PET, typically using 2-deoxy-2-($^{18}$F) fluoro-D-glucose (FDG), is usually performed in the interictal state to demonstrate hypometabolic areas in the epileptogenic regions. Although PET lacks the anatomic resolution of MRI, it can be more sensitive in detecting potential epileptogenic foci. Still, the availability of PET is limited, and it is costly. It is possible, and often helpful, to record an EEG throughout a PET scan. The PET scan takes approximately an hour to complete, including the time for the administration and uptake of a contrast agent. PET scanning is ventilator compatible. Although the study itself does not pose a risk to patients in NCSE, trained personnel must be present to monitor the patient's vital signs during the procedure.

Extensive published data on PET scanning during NCSE are not available. Most reports on PET during status epilepticus have been with convulsive status and have shown regional hypermetabolism (5,6). FDG-PET changes in case reports during NCSE have been inconsistent. One report demonstrated focal, regional, or multiregional hypermetabolism, which may correspond to the localization of EEG ictal activity (7). In other reports, however, focal hypometabolism seen during NCSE has been attributed to a destructive process (8). The role of PET in the diagnosis and treatment of NCSE has not been defined.

## SINGLE-PHOTON EMISSION COMPUTERIZED TOMOGRAPHY

SPECT shows blood flow to the brain. A radioactive tracer, typically 99Tc, is injected

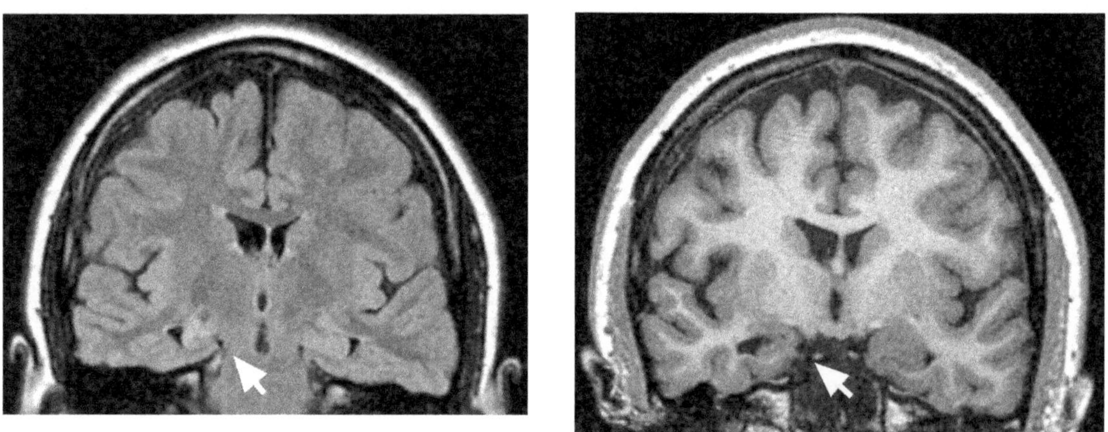

**Figure 6.2** (A) An 18-year-old woman with a history of seizures presented with nonconvulsive status epilepticus. Coronal FLAIR (fluid-attenuated inversion recovery)-weighted images show an increased signal in the right hippocampus (left side of image). (B). Coronal spoiled gradient recall acquisition and steady state (SPGR)-weighted images show atrophy of the right anterior hippocampus (left side of image).

intravenously and then detected using a dual-headed scintillation camera and high-resolution collimator. Ictal and interictal images are often obtained, and the images are then subtracted from one another to identify areas of hyperperfusion. Imaging can usually be obtained within 15 to 30 minutes of injection, but it can be delayed for several hours if necessary. Scan time is 15 to 25 minutes, and SPECT is ventilator compatible. EEG may be obtained concomitantly, but there is a risk for attenuation artifact on the SPECT images, depending on the protocol used. As is the case for PET, ictal SPECT imaging itself does not pose a particular risk to the patient, but trained medical personnel must monitor the patient's medical and neurologic stability in cases of status epilepticus.

There are several published reports of the utility of ictal SPECT in status epilepticus. Most are isolated case reports (5,9,10), and almost all describe changes during convulsive status. In 3 studies with multiple patients, however, SPECT imaging has shown increased focal or regional ictal perfusion during NCSE (2,11,12).

Tatum and colleagues reported 7 cases of patients with status epilepticus who underwent SPECT scans reviewed by an experienced nuclear medicine physician (11). Six were obtained during NCSE and demonstrated areas of definite focal hyperperfusion. One had stopped having seizures 24 hours before the SPECT, and the scan showed focal hypoperfusion. In contrast, there were 6 patients in whom a clinical suspicion of status was considered initially but later disproved, and none showed focal changes on SPECT.

Another report evaluated the diagnostic and localizing value of ictal SPECT in 3 patients with NCSE (2). All had ictal scans that were later subtracted digitally from interictal scans. The 3 patients each displayed different EEG patterns associated with NCSE, as well as different localizations. All demonstrated a well-localized increase in cerebral perfusion on ictal SPECT.

Another 5 patients with NCSE of frontal origin underwent ictal SPECT (12). NCSE was caused by a wide range of etiologies. Injection was performed 10 seconds after ictal onset, and status epilepticus was treated with benzodiazepines 10 minutes later. SPECT scans obtained 45 to 60 minutes after the termination of status epilepticus showed regional hyperperfusion.

Through these 3 series and 2 other single-patient case reports, 17 cases have shown consistent results for SPECT scanning during NCSE(13). Sixteen scans were obtained with injection during NCSE, and all 16 showed EEG-congruent focal or regional hyperperfusion; 1 injection performed postictally showed focal hypoperfusion. Because of the variability of clinical features and EEG patterns that are associated with NCSE, ictal SPECT may be a useful adjunctive tool for the diagnosis of NCSE. In several cases, the use of ictal SPECT assisted with localization, surgical planning, or both.

## REFERENCES

1. Bauer J, Stefan H, Huk WJ, Feistel H, Hilz MJ, Brinkmann HG, Druschky KF, Neundorfer B. CT, MRI and SPECT neuroimaging in status epilepticus with simple partial and complex partial seizures: case report. J Neurol 1989;236: 296-299.
2. Kutluay E, Beattie J, Passaro EA, Edwards JC, Minecan D, Milling C, Selwa L, Beydoun A. Diagnostic and localizing value of ictal SPECT in patients with nonconvulsive status epilepticus. Epilepsy Behav 2005;6:212-217.
3. Lansberg MG, O'Brien MW, Norbash AM, Moseley ME, Morrell M, Albers GW. MRI abnormalities associated with partial status epilepticus. Neurology 1999;52:1021-1027.
4. Kawai N, Miyake K, Kuroda Y, Yamashita S, Nishiyama Y, Monden T, Sasakawa Y, Nagao S. Magnetic resonance imaging and positron emission tomography findings in status epilepticus following severe hypoglycemia. Ann Nucl Med 2006;20:371-376.
5. Doherty CP, Cole AJ, Grant PE, Fischman A, Dooling E, Hoch DB, White TE, Cosgrove R. Multimodal longitudinal imaging of focal status epilepticus. Can J Neurol Sci 2004;31:276-281.
6. Tatum WO, Stecker MM. Serial FDG-PET scans in a patient with partial status epilepticus. Epilepsia 1995;36:214-215.

7. Maeda Y, Oguni H, Saitou Y, Mutoh A, Imai K, Osawa M, Fukuyama Y, Hori T, Yamane F, Kubo O, Ishii K, Ishiwata K. Rasmussen syndrome: multifocal spread of inflammation suggested from MRI and PET findings. Epilepsia 2003;44:1118-1121.
8. Kim J, Park JH, Ryu YH, Lee KY. Tc-99m ECD SPECT and FDG PET in partial status epilepticus resulting from cerebral sparganosis. Clin Nucl Med 2006;31:307-309.
9. Juhász C, Scheidl E, Szmirmai I. Reversible focal MRI abnormalities due to status epilepticus. An EEG, single photon emission computed tomography, transcranial Doppler follow-up study. Electroencephalogr Clin Neurophsiol 1998;107: 402-407.
10. Ali I, Pirzada N, Vaughn B. Periodic lateralized epileptiform discharges after complex partial status epilepticus associated with increased focal cerebral blood flow. J Clin Neurophysiol 2001;18:565-569.
11. TatumWO, Alavi A, Stecker MM. Technetium-99m-HMPAO SPECT in partial status epilpepticus. J Nucl Med 1994;35:1087-1094.
12. Thomas P, Zifkin B, Migneco O, Lebrun C, Darcourt J, Andermann F. Nonconvulsive status epilepticus of frontal origin. Neurology 1999;52:1174-1183.
13. Kaplan PW. Neurophysiological localization of epileptic nystagmus. Am J END Technol 1999;39:77-83.

# CHAPTER 7

# PATHOPHYSIOLOGY OF NONCONVULSIVE STATUS EPILEPTICUS

Jaideep Kapur

Broadly, nonconvulsive status epilepticus (NCSE) refers to prolonged electrographic seizure activity that results in nonconvulsive clinical symptoms. There are several clinical conditions associated with NCSE. Among these are prolonged complex partial seizures of temporal lobe or extratemporal lobe origin and prolonged typical or atypical absence seizures. There are other types of NCSE in which it is not possible to classify the seizures into complex partial or absence, such as NCSE in comatose patients, electrical status epilepticus of sleep, etc. This chapter discusses the extant literature on various types of status epilepticus, specifically focusing on gaps in our knowledge that need to be addressed in carefully designed studies.

## COMPLEX PARTIAL STATUS EPILEPTICUS ORIGINATING IN EXTRATEMPORAL NEOCORTEX

Nonconvulsive, complex, partial status epilepticus can arise from limbic structures (including in the temporal lobe) or from extratemporal neocortical structures. Status epilepticus of neocortical onset has not been studied extensively, except for epilepsia partialis continua (EPC), a form of partial status epilepticus with simple motor manifestations, typically clonic activity of a group of muscles, lasting hours to months. Although EPC is not strictly "nonconvulsive," this entity is instructive when trying to understand the pathophysiology of simple and complex partial status epilepticus arising from the extratemporal neocortex. A large body of evidence suggests that seizures in EPC arise from the neocortex and remain confined to it without involving limbic circuits. Injury to the neocortex caused by neoplasms, stroke, inflammation (especially Rasmussen encephalitis), and cortical malformations result in EPC. Positron emission tomography (PET) imaging studies demonstrate cortical hypermetabolism in patients with EPC (1-3). Resection of neocortical foci, especially in patients with Rasmussen encephalitis, leads to resolution of EPC. There are few reports detailing the site of origin of seizures of nonmotor complex partial status epilepticus.

The pathophysiology of status epilepticus of extratemporal neocortical origin remains poorly understood for several reasons. There is a paucity of animal models of neocortical extratemporal status epilepticus. Also, inherited and acquired cortical malformations in experimental animals lead to isolated seizures or interictal spikes. Similarly, vascular lesions of the cortex in experimental animals lead to discrete seizures.

In contrast to these models, focal application of tetanus toxin to neocortex causes prolonged neocortical seizures that may persist as EPC (4), and, following infusion of tetanus toxin into cat cerebral cortex, prolonged seizures occur (5). Seizures begin shortly after intracortical infusion of the toxin and may continue for at least 6 hours (4-6). There are few detailed descriptions of seizures that follow the toxin infusion.

Electroencephalographic (EEG) findings during toxin-induced status epilepticus have not been described in detail. Previous studies have focused on chronic, recurrent, spontaneous seizures (4,6). A detailed study of tetanus–toxin-induced neocortical status epilepticus would be useful for comparing it with well-described changes in electrographic seizures during temporal lobe (or limbic)-onset status epilepticus (see subsequent text).

The functional anatomy of tetanus–toxin-induced neocortical status epilepticus has not been described well, but there were early studies describing the functional anatomy of neocortical-onset focal motor seizures using 2-deoxyglucose techniques (7). Within the focus, a columnar pattern of activation is present, and activation of lamina V is particularly evident. The cortical focus is surrounded by an area of hypometabolism. Seizures spread laterally, activating columns. There is transcallosal spread of activity to the contralateral cortex. Finally, activity spreads to the thalamus, thus engaging thalamocortical circuits. These studies refer to brief seizures caused by acute application of penicillin, but the circuits sustaining neocortical status epilepticus have not been delineated. Furthermore, it is unclear whether there are specific circuits or structures that are necessary for sustaining neocortical status epilepticus. Recent advances in small-animal imaging, such as high-strength magnetic resonance imaging and positron emission tomography scanning could address these questions.

Once microcircuits and large-scale circuits within the neocortex that can generate and sustain status epilepticus have been defined, cellular, molecular, and synaptic dysfunction associated with status epilepticus originating in a small neocortical island can be studied. The tetanus-toxin model offers an opportunity to approach these problems. Current evidence indicates that tetanus toxin blocks the release of the inhibitory neurotransmitter -amino butyric acid (GABA) from presynaptic terminals (8). Cellular, synaptic, and molecular mechanisms sustaining extratemporal neocortical status epilepticus, however, remain unknown.

## COMPLEX PARTIAL STATUS EPILEPTICUS OF TEMPORAL LOBE OR LIMBIC ORIGIN

Perhaps the best understood form of status epilepticus is complex partial status epilepticus of the temporal lobe, or status epilepticus of limbic origin. It is important to note that, in animal models, status epilepticus of limbic origin is associated with both convulsive and nonconvulsive seizures, and published reviews on generalized convulsive status epilepticus and NCSE refer to these animal models (9-13). The pathophysiology of limbic-onset status epilepticus has been described extensively in primary literature and in reviews.

## ANIMALS MODELS OF LIMBIC STATUS EPILEPTICUS

Several animal models have been developed to study various facets of status epilepticus. They can be divided into 2 major categories: chemical convulsant-induced and electrogenic models. A progression of behavior and EEG changes similar to those described in humans has also been demonstrated in both the chemical convulsant model and the electrogenic model of status epilepticus in experimental animals, thus validating their use in understanding the pathophysiology of status epilepticus (10). The chemical convulsant-induced models can be classified into antagonism of GABAergic inhibition (14), excitatory amino-acid activation (15), cholinergic stimulation (16), and other models (17).

Chemical convulsant models of status epilepticus have been useful in determining the systemic effects of generalized convulsive status epilepticus, elucidating the functional anatomy of status epilepticus, and comparing the efficacy of antiepileptic drugs in treatment. In addition, they are very convenient to use. Experimental studies of status epilepticus based on chemical convulsant-induced seizures have the inherent difficulty that the effects of the convulsant drug must be separated from the effects of seizures.

Electrical stimulation models of status epilepticus are useful to study the effect of prolonged and recurrent seizures in a controlled fashion. Electrogenic models are derived from kindling protocols and involve prolonged electrical stimulation of limbic structures (9,18). Prolonged electrographic seizures have been induced by electrical stimulation of hippocampal slices from young animals with a combination of electrical stimulation and manipulation of extracellular magnesium concentrations (19,20).

Key anatomic structures involved in sustaining limbic status epilepticus have been delineated by means of 2-deoxyglucose mapping studies performed on the electrical stimulation and lithium-pilocarpine models. Limbic status epilepticus is maintained by an interconnected circuit consisting of entorhinal cortex, dentate gyrus, areas CA1 and CA3, subiculum, and parasubiculum (21-26). Combined entrorhinal cortex and hippocampal slices from young animals can maintain prolonged electrographic discharges (19,27).

## GABA-MEDIATED INHIBITION DURING STATUS EPILEPTICUS

GABA-mediated inhibition in the CA1 region of hippocampus has been studied by the paired-pulse method in several models of status epilepticus (28,29). CA1 pyramidal neurons are inhibited by interneurons activated by both feedforward and feedback inhibition. Feedforward inhibition results from Schaffer collaterals from CA3 pyramidal neurons simultaneously activating inhibitory basket cells and CA1 pyramidal neurons. The activated basket cells inhibit the CA1 pyramidal neurons activated by Schaffer collaterals. Feedback inhibition consists of 2 steps: (a) a pyramidal cell excites a local GABAergic interneuron and (b) the inhibitory interneuron in turn inhibits the same pyramidal cell. The connection between pyramidal and inhibitory cells is strong. The inhibitory postsynaptic potentials (IPSP) generated in pyramidal cells prevent recruitment of intrinsic bursts in individual pyramidal cells. Extensive divergence of projections of interneurons onto pyramidal neurons reduces the spread of bursts of action potentials downstream from an initially excited pyramidal neuron (30). Epileptiform discharges can be experimentally produced in the hippocampal CA1 pyramidal layer with $GABA_A$ receptor antagonists such as penicillin, bicuculline, and picrotoxin. The paired-pulse method primarily measures feedback inhibition of CA1 pyramidal neurons. Briefly, it involves placement of a stimulating electrode in the CA1/CA3 region of 1 hippocampus and a recording electrode in the homotopic contralateral CA1 hippocampus to record extracellular field potentials in response to the stimuli. When 2 pulses are delivered close to each other at low stimulus intensities, the inhibition of the response to the second stimulus depends both on the interpulse interval and on the stimulus intensity. At higher stimulus intensity, the inhibition is dependent on the interpulse interval alone. Paired-pulse inhibition in the 20- to 70-millisecond interpulse interval range is enhanced by benzodiazepines and diminished by bicuculline.

The relationship of GABA-mediated paired-pulse inhibition in the CA1 region of the hippocampus and evolution of status epilepticus has been studied. The evolution of seizures is closely correlated to the loss of paired-pulse inhibition. All 3 cholinergic-based models of status epilepticus have been studied using the paired-pulse inhibition technique. Pilocarpine reduces $GABA_A$ receptor-mediated paired-pulse inhibition in the CA1 region of the hippocampus in a dose-dependent fashion (31). Amygdala kindling results in reduction of GABA-mediated inhibition in CA1 hippocampus, which is further reduced by pilocarpine. Kainic acid, an analogue of the excitatory neurotransmitter glutamic acid, induces status epilepticus in experimental animals. Convulsant concentrations of kainic acid cause fading of IPSP in the CA1 region of the hippocampus (32).

Although studies using the paired-pulse inhibition method have shown the critical role of reduction of GABA-mediated inhibition in the pathogenesis of status epilepticus, they have not revealed the mechanisms underlying the disinhibition. Paired-pulse inhibition in the CA1 region of the hippocampus could be reduced by diminished release of GABA or by diminished postsynaptic $GABA_A$ receptor responsiveness. These possibilities are discussed in subsequent sections of this chapter.

## GABA LEVELS IN HIPPOCAMPUS RISE DURING STATUS EPILEPTICUS

Although the release of GABA from neurons during status epilepticus has not been studied, amino-acid neurotransmitter levels during status epilepticus have been measured. In status epilepticus induced by kainic acid, there are decreases in glutamate, aspartate, and glutamine concentrations and increases in GABA concentration in the hippocampus (33). Walton and colleagues have studied amino-acid neurotransmitter levels in status epilepticus induced by lithium and pilocarpine during various electrographic stages (34). Both aspartate and glutamate levels decline in the hippocampus, pyriform cortex, motor cortex, and entorhinal cortex during the early phase of status epilepticus and continue to do so in the late phase. GABA levels, on the other hand, rise in early status epilepticus and continue to do so in the late stages. It is difficult to interpret these observations because increased GABA levels could represent increased synthesis, diminished release, or diminished breakdown of this neurotransmitter. Similar considerations pertain to glutamate and aspartate. More recent electrophysiologic studies have further suggested that extracellular GABA levels may be increased (35).

## $GABA_A$ RECEPTOR FUNCTION IN THE HIPPOCAMPUS DIMINISHES DURING STATUS EPILEPTICUS

Recently, the possibility that the reduction of GABA-mediated inhibition seen in status epilepticus is a consequence of changes in CA1 pyramidal neurons has been investigated. Several possible changes in CA1 pyramidal neurons could reduce the efficacy of GABA in producing chloride currents. The number of $GABA_A$ receptors could be reduced; the efficacy of GABA in opening the ion channel after binding could be reduced, or the chloride reversal potential or the driving force for chloride current could be reduced. In one study, status epilepticus was induced in 18- to 28-day-old rats with an injection of 3 meq/kg lithium chloride, followed 20 hours later with an injection of 25 mg/kg pilocarpine. Age-matched naïve littermates were used as controls. The animals were allowed to have seizures for 45 minutes and then were anesthetized. CA1 pyramidal neurons were acutely isolated by a method modified from that described originally (36). Whole-cell, perforated patch recordings of $GABA_A$ currents were made from acutely isolated CA1 pyramidal neurons from rats having status epilepticus or from naïve control rats. The "perforated patch" method was employed, and the electrode solution (except for the tip) contained the pore-forming antibiotic, amphotericin. Recordings of $GABA_A$ receptor currents were conducted in whole-cell voltage-clamp mode. These experiments showed that marked reductions of $GABA_A$ receptor currents in CA1 pyramidal neuron occurred during status epilepticus that produced loss of GABA-mediated inhibition. A third of all CA1 pyramidal neurons isolated from animals undergoing status epilepticus showed no response to GABA, in contrast to 7% of neurons isolated from naïve animals. These experiments also indicated that, during status epilepticus, $GABA_A$ receptor currents were reduced by reduction of both conductance and the chloride reversal potential.

These findings suggest that the $GABA_A$ receptor is modified during an episode of status epilepticus. $GABA_A$ receptors are regulated by numerous positive (barbiturates, benzodiazepines, and neurosteroids) and negative (picrotoxin, bicuculline, and Zn++) allosteric modulators. The sensitivity of $GABA_A$ receptors to GABA and to allosteric modulators changes gradually during normal development, during development of chronic epilepsy, and following prolonged exposure to $GABA_A$ receptor agonists. Here we report the development of rapid functional plasticity of $GABA_A$ receptors occurring over 45 minutes of continuous seizures (status epilepticus) in rats. Seizures induced in rats by administration of lithium followed by pilocarpine were readily terminated by diazepam when administered early during the seizures. During status epilepticus, however, there was a substantial reduction of diazepam potency for termination of the seizures. To determine if the loss of sensitivity to diazepam was due to an alteration of $GABA_A$ receptor functional properties, whole-cell $GABA_A$ receptor currents were recorded from hippocampal dentate granule cells isolated acutely from control rats and from rats undergoing status epilepticus. $GABA_A$ receptor properties were characterized by determining GABA sensitivity and the sensitivity of $GABA_A$ receptors to regulation by benzodiazepines, barbiturates, and Zn++. When compared with those from naïve littermates, $GABA_A$ receptor currents from rats undergoing status epilepticus were less sensitive to diazepam and Zn++ but retained their sensitivity to GABA and pentobarbital. These studies suggest that the prolonged seizures of status epilepticus rapidly alter the functional properties of hippocampal dentate granule cell $GABA_A$ receptors (37).

The mechanism of reduction of $GABA_A$ receptor-mediated inhibition is being explored. $GABA_A$ receptors undergo a cycle of internalization and insertion into the cell membrane via a clathrin-dependent endocytic process (38). Internalization of the surface $GABA_A$ receptor correlates with a reduced response to GABA, whereas inhibition of internalization results in an increase in the amplitude of synaptic $GABA_A$ receptor currents (39). An activity-induced acceleration of the internalization of $GABA_A$ receptors from the cell surface could partially explain the reduction in GABA-mediated inhibition observed during the prolonged seizures of status epilepticus. The number of receptors at a synapse is an important determinant of synaptic strength (40), so a reduction in the total number of postsynaptic $GABA_A$ receptor could result in a decline in GABAergic inhibition.

This rapid loss of $GABA_A$-receptor benzodiazepine sensitivity during seizures has been difficult to explain. Recent studies have suggested that benzodiazepine-insensitive receptors are expressed in hippocampal neurons on extrasynaptic membranes. Furthermore, these receptors appear to mediate a novel form of inhibition called tonic inhibition. We tested whether, during status epilepticus, there is increased internalization of synaptic, diazepam-sensitive $GABA_A$ receptors, which leaves extrasynaptic diazepam-insensitive receptors on the neuronal surface. A combination of immunocytochemical and electrophysiologic studies has suggested that cultured hippocampal neurons express 2 types of $GABA_A$ receptors. One type containing $\alpha_1$, $\alpha_2$, $\beta_{2/3}$, and $\gamma_2$ receptor subunits form clusters present at GABAergic synapses and in extrasynaptic membrane. The second type of receptor, containing the $\alpha_4$, $\beta_1$, and $\delta$ subunits, is diffusely distributed in the extrasynaptic membrane (41,42). Using an in vitro model of status epilepticus combined with electrophysiologic and cellular imaging techniques, we found that prolonged epileptiform bursting results in a reduction in GABA-mediated synaptic inhibition. Furthermore, we found that the constitutive internalization of $GABA_A$ receptors is rapid and is accelerated by increased activity associated with seizures. Reduction of activity reduced the rate of internalization. These findings suggest that the rate of $GABA_A$-receptor internalization is regulated by neuronal activity, and its acceleration contributes to the reduction in inhibitory transmission observed during status epilepticus (43).

## NMDA RECEPTOR FUNCTION IS ENHANCED DURING LIMBIC STATUS EPILEPTICUS

Although abnormal GABAergic mechanisms are involved in the pathogenesis of status epilepticus, excitatory transmission mediated by glutamate is essential for spread of epileptiform activity. Glutamate activates multiple subtypes of postsynaptic excitatory amino-acid receptors during status epilepticus, but studies have focused on the N-methyl D-aspartate (NMDA) receptor. The role of non-NMDA receptors in status epilepticus is uncertain. Current evidence suggests NMDA activation sustains status epilepticus and may, in part, cause the characteristic neuropathologic changes in status epilepticus.

The NMDA-receptor channel is a nonselective cation channel, which is permeable to monovalent cations $Na^+$ and $K^+$ and the divalent cation $Ca^{++}$, and is blocked by physiologic concentrations of the divalent cation $Mg^{++}$(44). At negative membrane potentials, NMDA current is reduced due to a voltage-dependent open channel block produced by $Mg^{++}$ (44). The block is relieved by membrane depolarization, and, thus, NMDA-receptor current only flows through depolarized channels. Also unique to NMDA-receptor channels, a coagonist, glycine, must be bound to the receptor channel for activation. NMDA-receptor channels are also regulated by both oxidation and reduction and by pH, being active only at higher pH. The divalent cation $Zn^{++}$ also produces a fast open channel block that is similar to that produced by $Mg^{++}$, but that also produces a voltage-independent change in gating properties of NMDA-receptor channels, reducing the open duration and frequency of channel opening. Dissociative anesthetics, such as dizocilpine (MK-801), ketamine, and phencyclidine, also reduce NMDA-receptor currents by an open channel block mechanism, but the block is long lasting due to high affinity of the dissociative anesthetics for the NMDA-receptor channel (44).

NMDA-receptor antagonists fail to block initiation of status epilepticus. The NMDA-receptor antagonist MK-801 administered prior to or shortly after the onset of kainate-induced status epilepticus or lithium pilocarpine-induced status epilepticus do not control seizures (45-49). Although some authors have reported that seizures are less intense after NMDA-receptor antagonist administration (50), others have reported worsening of electrographic seizures by NMDA-receptor antagonists (45).

In an insightful study, Williamson and Lothman demonstrated that NMDA-receptor antagonists have a "use-dependent" action, ie, repeated seizures must occur before NMDA-receptor antagonists can act as anticonvulsants. Fully kindled rats with stable grade 5 behavioral seizures and a 50- to 60-second afterdischarge duration were given 5 kindling stimuli, 30 minutes apart, after MK-801 administration. The behavioral and electrographic seizures resulting from the first 2 stimuli did not change from baseline. In contrast, electrographic and behavioral seizures declined in a dose-dependent fashion in response to the third and fourth stimuli. The authors suggested that NMDA-receptor antagonists are effective anticonvulsants in a use-dependent fashion. They predicted that NMDA-receptor antagonists would be useful in prolonged, persistent, or recurrent seizures. The use-dependent action of MK-801 as an anticonvulsant is in keeping with the known properties of NMDA. During normal, low-frequency, excitatory neurotransmission, NMDA receptors are not activated, but the prolonged high-frequency neuronal activity of sustained status epilepticus is likely to create a suitable environment for greater NMDA activation and, thus, seizure perpetuation (51).

More recent studies have demonstrated that prolonged status epilepticus can be treated with ketamine, a clinically available NMDA-receptor antagonist, and ketamine is more effective in the treatment of prolonged status epilepticus, compared with early status epilepticus (52). NMDA-receptor function can be inhibited by multiple mechanisms, including competitive block by drugs such as 3-((R,S)-2-carboxypiperazin-4-yl)-propyl-1-phosphonic acid (CPP); by open channel block at the phencyclidine site by MK-801 or ketamine (53); and by action at the pH-sensitive site by ifenprodil (54). NMDA-receptor antagonists CPP, MK-801, and ifenprodil have been compared for their ability to terminate prolonged status epilepticus. These studies have suggested that noncompetitive NMDA-receptor antagonists are superior to competitive and allosteric inhibitors of NMDA-receptors in terminating prolonged status epilepticus induced by electrical stimulation (55).

The ability of NMDA-receptor antagonists to suppress status epilepticus varies from model to model. For example, the NMDA-receptor antagonist ketamine terminates diazepam-refractory status epilepticus generated by electrical stimulation (see previous information in this chapter), but it is ineffective when used alone in status epilepticus induced by cholinergic stimulation. Multiple doses of ketamine, ranging from ineffective to toxic, have been examined for their efficacy in terminating diazepam-refractory status epilepticus. The same range of ketamine doses has also been used in combination with 2 doses of diazepam. The principal finding of one study was that a combination of diazepam and ketamine rapidly terminates prolonged cholinergic stimulation-induced status epilepticus in a synergistic fashion. Diazepam shifts the ketamine dose-response (status epilepticus termination) relationship to the left and increases the maximal effect of ketamine. In summary, a combination of ketamine and diazepam might be a clinically useful treatment for NCSE (56).

## LONG-TERM CONSEQUENCES OF NONCONVULSIVE STATUS EPILEPTICUS

Current experimental studies on the consequences of prolonged NCSE focus on its potential to cause neuronal loss and on the late development of epilepsy.

### NEURONAL LOSS

Activation of NMDA-receptors and excitotoxic mechanisms are believed to be involved in the production of the neuropathologic changes of status epilepticus. Neuropathologic studies performed on patients dying during or shortly after an episode of status epilepticus show loss of CA1 pyramidal neurons, Purkinje cells in the cerebellum, and cortical neurons (57). There is growing evidence from serial magnetic resonance imaging studies in patients demonstrating that the hippocampus is injured during prolonged status epilepticus (58-60). A prospective study seeking to evaluate the effect of prolonged febrile seizures in children on hippocampal volume and other imaging characteristics is in progress.

Neuropathologic changes similar to those observed in humans can be replicated in experimental animals, including mammals, by prolonged seizures. Key areas of neuropathologic changes in experimental animals are the hippocampus, middle layers of the cerebral cortex, and the cerebellum. Cerebellar damage relates to hyperthermia, but neuronal loss in the hippocampus and the cortex is caused by the seizures themselves and is not related to hypoxia, ischemia, hyperthermia, or metabolic injuries during status epilepticus (61-63).

In rodents, neuronal loss occurs in experimental status epilepticus, whether the status epilepticus is induced by electrical stimulation, lithium-pilocarpine, or kainate (10). The noncompetitive NMDA-receptor antagonists ketamine, phencyclidine, and MK-801 protect against neuronal damage associated with electrical stimulation-induced, kainic acid-induced, and lithium/pilocarpine-induced status epilepticus (64). The competitive NMDA-receptor antagonist, CGP-40116 protects against neuronal damage produced during status epilepticus induced by lithium-pilocarpine (48). This neuroprotection cannot be completely attributed to anticonvulsant effects of these compounds because electrographic seizures often continue after their administration.

### PROLONGED SEIZURES AND EPILEPTOGENESIS: IS CELL LOSS NECESSARY?

A key consequence of status epilepticus in experimental animals is development of recurrent spontaneous seizures and epilepsy (65). Recurrent spontaneous seizures develop following status epilepticus induced by electrical stimulation, lithium-pilocarpine, and kainate (66-68). Neuronal loss and recurrent spontaneous seizures occur concurrently in many models of epilepsy, and this association has led to the hypothesis that neuronal loss is necessary for recurrent spontaneous seizures. This association, however, is weak. In several animal models, recurrent spontaneous limbic seizures have developed without characteristic neuropathologic findings of mesial temporal sclerosis. In 1 model, 20-day-old rat pups were subjected to prolonged seizures induced by lithium and pilocarpine, and the animals were examined as adults (69). Two thirds of the animals that were subjected to early-life status epilepticus developed recurrent spontaneous limbic seizures, which in some cases progressed to stage V

(Racine scale) seizures (70). The authors found no evidence of mesial temporal sclerosis or mossy fiber sprouting in two thirds of the animals with recurrent spontaneous seizures. In the remaining animals, CA1 and CA3 cell loss or mossy fiber sprouting or both were found. In another study, 10-day-old pups were subjected to prolonged febrile seizures and allowed to grow to adulthood, at which point video-EEG recordings were taken using a pair of hippocampal and cortical electrodes, and behavior was monitored for 5 hours each night (71). Recurrent spontaneous hippocampal seizures associated with behavioral manifestations of freezing and automatisms were recorded from one third of all animals studied. There was no evidence of neuronal loss or sprouting in any epileptic animal. Additionally, previous studies have raised questions about the relationship of cell loss and mossy fiber sprouting to the pathogenesis of recurrent spontaneous seizures (71). In kainate and electrical stimulation models of epilepsy, the extent of cell loss varies significantly from animal to animal, including examples of temporal lobe epilepsy without cell loss. Dissociation between epileptogenesis and mossy fiber sprouting has been described in these models.

The emerging evidence, therefore, suggests that cell loss and mossy fiber sprouting are not absolutely necessary for the generation of recurrent spontaneous limbic seizures, but these neuropathologic findings may indicate a more refractory or progressive form of temporal lobe epilepsy. Cell loss and sprouting are commonly seen in surgical specimens because patients refractory to medical therapies are selected for surgery.

## LONG-TERM CONSEQUENCES OF NONCONVULSIVE STATUS EPILEPTICUS AND ITS TREATMENT: A ROLE FOR HOMEOSTATIC PLASTICITY?

Emerging literature in cortical plasticity suggests that clinicians need to pay attention to another consequence of prolonged changes in neuronal activity that results in a set of neuronal changes collectively referred to as homeostatic plasticity (72). The homeostatic plasticity hypothesis proposes that neurons and neuronal circuits maintain a stable function in the face of perturbations such as changing neuronal activity, synaptic inputs, synapse formation, and proliferation. In order to maintain a stable function, neurons in the circuit adapt by changing synaptic strength and altering intrinsic conductances. The hypothesis has been tested in vitro and in vivo, in which global changes in neuronal activity induce changes in the strength of excitatory and inhibitory synapses and in intrinsic conductances.

The concept of homeostatic plasticity might have implications for NCSE and its treatment. A prolonged increase in neuronal activity occurring during NCSE may reset intrinsic conductances and synaptic transmission in homeostatic response to increased activity. Conversely, profound suppression of neuronal activity induced by anesthetics could activate compensatory mechanisms that would contribute to the refractoriness of seizures.

## ABSENCE STATUS EPILEPTICUS

Absence status epilepticus occurs in patients with generalized epilepsies. Absence status epilepticus in patients with primary generalized epilepsy is usually easy to control with benzodiazepines. Major advances have been made in understanding the pathophysiology of absence seizures, which might have some bearing upon the mechanisms of absence status epilepticus.

Seminal studies of Penfield and Jasper suggested that the neurobiologic mechanisms underlying generalized spike-wave and focal spikes were distinct. Although the neurobiology of focal spikes has been studied intensively for the past 30 years, major advances in understanding generalized spikes and waves are more recent (73,74). Current thinking about the pathogenesis of absence seizures dates to the landmark experiments of Jasper and Droogleever-Fortuyn, who demonstrated that electrical stimulation of the midline and intralaminar nuclei of the thalamus in cats at a stimulus frequency of 3 cycles per second could produce bilateral, synchronous, spike-wave discharges on the cortical EEG. The relevance of this finding to human epilepsy was demonstrated by Williams, who, utilizing depth electrode recordings from the thalamus of a child with absence seizures, observed that bilaterally synchronous 3-cycle-per-second, spike-wave discharges were present in that structure (75). More recent functional magnetic resonance imaging studies of typical absence seizures confirm the role of the thalamus in generating absence seizures (76).

Both human and animal data strongly suggest that generalized absence seizures arise from aberrant thalamocortical rhythms. To understand the proposed hypotheses of the pathogenesis of this disorder, it is necessary to review first the synaptic circuitry of the thalamus and cortex, the unique oscillatory thalamocortical rhythms generated by that circuitry, the cellular mechanisms underlying these neuronal oscillations, and the neurotransmitters involved in intrinsic thalamic, thalamocortical, and corticothalamic pathways.

The thalamocortical circuit is also the substrate of the neurobiology of sleep and was reviewed by Steriade (77). There are several reasons to believe that the neurobiologic mechanisms underlying sleep spindles and generalized spike-and-wave discharge are related (see later in this section). Thalamocortical oscillations are generated in the thalamus as the result of synaptic interactions in a network in which the main players are the inhibitory GABA-containing neurons of the reticular thalamic nucleus, thalamocortical cells, and cortical pyramidal neurons. Different areas of the cerebral cortex receive inputs from various dorsal thalamic nuclei. In turn, cortical neurons of layer 6 innervate topographically appropriate regions of both the dorsal thalamus and the reticular thalamic nucleus. The reticular cells receive excitatory inputs from axon collaterals of thalamic neurons that project to the cortex and of cortical neurons that project to the thalamus; they project back to the thalamus (but not to the cerebral cortex) and also innervate other cells of the reticular thalamic nucleus. In this manner, the reticular nucleus is uniquely positioned to influence the flow of information between the thalamus and the cerebral cortex.

Intracellular recordings of reticular and thalamocortical cells in vivo and in vitro, as well as computational modeling of thalamic cells, have shown a mirror (inverse) image in these 2 neuronal classes during oscillations. In reticular cells, rhythmic (7- to 14-Hz) bursts are generated by low-threshold Ca++ spikes and are superimposed on a slowly rising and decaying depolarizing envelope. The bursts of reticular cells inhibit large numbers of thalamocortical cells through their divergent GABA-containing axons, which leads to the appearance of rhythmic IPSP in thalamocortical neurons. Some of these IPSP result in enough removal of inactivation of the low-threshold $Ca^{++}$ current to be followed by a rebound low-threshold $Ca^{++}$ spike and an associated burst of action potentials. These periodic bursts in thalamocortical cells converge onto reticular neurons and facilitate their rhythmic oscillation. The bursts are also transferred to the cortex, where they induce excitatory postsynaptic potentials in cortical pyramidal cells, thereby generating the EEG spindle waves.

Isolation of the reticular nucleus from the rest of the thalamus and the cerebral cortex abolishes oscillations in the dorsal thalamus and the cortex, but it is important to note that the deafferented reticular thalamic nucleus can itself generate oscillations. Indeed, the reticular thalamic cells possess a unique assortment of ionic currents that allows them to oscillate individually. Axonal, and in some species dendrodendritic, interconnections between reticular cells may allow the coupling and interaction of these endogenous oscillators, thereby generating spindle oscillations in an isolated nucleus. This hypothesis is strengthened by simplified models of reticular thalamic neurons with mutual inhibition that exhibit synchronous oscillatory activity.

The spindle oscillations of natural sleep are related to the development of a pattern of oscillatory activity, the spike-and-wave EEG complexes, which are associated with absence seizures. Because the reticular thalamic nucleus is central to the genesis of spindle oscillations, decreasing or abolishing the inhibitory efficacy of reticular neurons upon thalamocortical cells would also decrease the incidence of epileptic spike-and-wave discharges. This hypothesis is supported by recent experiments showing that, in animal models of genetic absence epilepsy, thalamic injections of a selective agonist of $GABA_B$ receptors increase the incidence of spike-and-wave discharges, whereas injections of a $GABA_B$ antagonist decrease these seizures in a dose-dependent manner. The activation of $GABA_B$ receptors in thalamocortical cells enhances the removal of inactivation of the low-threshold $Ca^{++}$ spike and subsequently results in larger-than-usual rebound burst discharges in a greater-than-usual proportion of thalamocortical cells. These facilitated rebound bursts further excite reticular cells, which quickly results in the generalization of paroxysmal activity.

The other direct evidence linking generalized spike-and-wave discharges and thalamocortical oscillations comes from the studies on the mechanism of action of ethosuximide. Ethosuximide reduces low-threshold $Ca^{++}$ current in thalamic neurons in a dose-dependent fashion at clinically relevant concentrations (78). Another specific anti-absence drug, methadione, shares this property. The drugs known to suppress 3-Hz, generalized, spike-and-wave discharge also suppress low-threshold $Ca^{++}$ spikes in thalamic neurons. Thus, the low-threshold $Ca^{++}$ spike is critical for the generation of thalamocortical oscillations, so these oscillations are likely mechanisms for the generation of 3-Hz spikes and waves. What aberration of normal thalamocortical oscillations occurs to produce pathologic 3-Hz spike-and-wave discharges is not yet known.

## ATYPICAL ABSENCE SEIZURES

An interesting animal model of atypical absence seizures has been developed and is likely to be useful in understanding the mechanisms of atypical absence status epilepticus. A cholesterol biosynthesis inhibitor, AY-9944, when administered repeatedly to rat pups between ages P6 and P33, results in recurrent spontaneous absence seizures (79). These seizures are considered atypical because they exhibit slow spike-wave discharges on EEG, and ictal behavior manifests and ends slowly. Furthermore, the functional anatomy of atypical absence seizures appears to be distinct. Spike discharges in atypical absence seizures in experimental animals invade limbic structures such as the hippocampus, whereas typical absence seizures do not involve the hippocampus (80). It is unclear whether atypical absence status epilepticus develops in these animals, but this model might be adapted to study atypical absence status epilepticus.

## NONCONVULSIVE STATUS EPILEPTICUS IN CRITICALLY ILL PATIENTS

There are several studies of critically ill comatose patients found to be in NCSE. The pathophysiology of these seizures is uncertain. Currently, there are no well-validated animal models that can be used to study the pathophysiologic mechanisms underlying these phenomena.

## CONCLUSION

This chapter focuses on pathophysiologic mechanisms underlying NCSE and the consequent effects on neurons and neuronal circuits. It is important to recognize that the pathophysiology of NCSE is poorly understood due to several factors but, primarily, because a large number of seizure types, diseases, epilepsies, acute neurologic insults, and even medical illnesses can result in NCSE. These different types of NCSE result from seizures that involve different parts of the brain, activating different circuits and cell types. It is possible that all of these causes of NCSE converge upon a "final common pathway" of cellular and molecular changes resulting in neuronal plasticity or injury. Alternatively, it is possible that each seizure type elicits a unique cellular and molecular response in the circuit it activates. There is currently insufficient evidence to support or dismiss either possibility.

## REFERENCES


1. Volkmann J, Seitz RJ, Muller-Gartner HW, Witte OW. Extrarolandic origin of spike and myoclonus activity in epilepsia partialis continua: a magnetoencephalographic and positron emission tomography study. J Neuroimaging 1998;8:103-106.
2. Noachtar S, Ebner A, Witte OW, Seitz RJ. Palatal tremor of cortical origin presenting as epilepsia partialis continua. Epilepsia 1995;36:207-209.
3. Maeda Y, Oguni H, Saitou Y, Mutoh A, Imai K, Osawa M, Fukuyama Y, Hori T, Yamane F, Kubo O, Ishii K, Ishiwata K. Rasmussen syndrome: multifocal spread of inflammation suggested from MRI and PET findings. Epilepsia 2003;44:1118-1121.
4. Louis ED, Williamson PD, Darcey TM. Chronic focal epilepsy induced by microinjection of tetanus toxin into the cat motor cortex. Electroencephalogr Clin Neurophysiol 1990;75:548-557.
5. Brooks VB, Asanuma H. Action of tetanus toxin in the cerebral cortex. Science 1962;137:674-676.
6. Nilsen KE, Walker MC, Cock HR. Characterization of the tetanus toxin model of refractory focal neocortical epilepsy in the rat. Epilepsia 2005;46:179-187.
7. Collins RC. Use of cortical circuits during focal penicillin seizures: an autoradiographic study with [14C]deoxyglucose. Brain Res 197821;150:487-501.
8. Bergey GK, Bigalke H, Nelson PG. Differential effects of tetanus toxin on inhibitory and excitatory synaptic transmission in mammalian spinal cord neurons in culture: a presynaptic locus of action for tetanus toxin. J Neurophysiol 1987;57:121-131.
9. Lothman EW, Bertram EH, Bekenstein JW, Perlin JB. Self-sustaining limbic status epilepticus induced by 'continuous' hippocampal stimulation: electrographic and behavioral characteristics. Epilepsy Res 1989;3:107-119.
10. Lothman E. The biochemical basis and pathophysiology of status epilepticus. Neurology 1990;40:13-23.
11. Treiman DM, Walton NY, Kendrick C. A progressive sequence of electroencephalographic changes during generalized convulsive status epilepticus. Epilepsy Res 1990;5:49-60.
12. Fountain NB, Lothman EW. Pathophysiology of status epilepticus. J Clin Neurophysiol 1995;12:326-342.
13. Hosford DA. Animal models of nonconvulsive status epilepticus. J Clin Neurophysiol 1999;16:306-313.
14. Chapman AG, Meldrum BS, Siesjo BK. Cerebral metabolic changes during prolonged epileptic seizures in rats. J Neurochem 1977;28:1025-1035.
15. Lothman EW, Collins RC. Kainic acid induced limbic seizures: metabolic, behavioral, electroencephalographic and neuropathological correlates. Brain Res 1981;218:299-318.
16. Honchar MP, Olney JW, Sherman WR. Systemic cholinergic agents induce seizures and brain damage in lithium-treated rats. Science 1983;220:323-325.
17. Walton NY, Treiman DM. Experimental secondarily generalized convulsive status epilepticus induced by D,L-homocysteine thiolactone. Epilepsy Res 1988;2:79-86.
18. Mazarati AM, Wasterlain CG, Sankar R, Shin D. Self-sustaining status epilepticus after brief stimulation of the perforant path. Brain Res 1998;801:251-253.
19. Rafiq A, Zhang YF, DeLorenzo RJ, Coulter DA. Long-duration self-sustained epileptiform activity in the hippocampal- parahippocampal slice: a model of status epilepticus. J Neurophysiol 1995;74:2028-2042.
20. Mody I, Lambert JD, Heinemann U. Low extracellular magnesium induces epileptiform activity and spreading depression in rat hippocampal slices. J Neurophysiol 1987;57:869-888.
21. Lothman EW, Hatlelid JM, Zorumski CF. Functional mapping of limbic seizures originating in the hippocampus: a combined 2-deoxyglucose and electrophysiologic study. Brain Res 1985;360:92-100.
22. Handforth A, Ackermann RF. Functional [14C]2-deoxyglucose mapping of progressive states of status epilepticus induced by amygdala stimulation in rat. Brain Res 1988;460:94-102.
23. Handforth A, Treiman DM. Functional mapping of the early stages of status epilepticus: A 14C-2-deoxyglucose study in the lit hium-pilocarpine model in rat. Neuroscience 1995;64:1057-1073.

24. Handforth A, Treiman DM. Functional mapping of the late stages of status epilepticus in the lithium-pilocarpine model in rat: A 14C-2-deoxyglucose study. Neuroscience 1995;64:1075-1089.
25. VanLandingham KE, Lothman EW. Self-sustaining limbic status epilepticus. I. Acute and chronic cerebral metabolic studies: limbic hypermetabolism and neocortical hypometabolism. Neurology 1991;41:1942-1949.
26. Lothman EW, Bertram EH3, Stringer JL. Functional anatomy of hippocampal seizures. Prog Neurobiol 1991;37:1-82.
27. Rafiq A, DeLorenzo RJ, Coulter DA. Generation and propagation of epileptiform discharges in a combined entorhinal cortex/hippocampal slice. J Neurophysiol 1993;70:1962-1974.
28. Kapur J, Stringer JL, Lothman EW. Evidence that repetitive seizures in the hippocampus cause a lasting reduction of GABAergic inhibition. J Neurophysiol 1989;61:417-426.
29. Kapur J, Lothman EW. Loss of inhibition precedes delayed spontaneous seizures in the hippocampus after tetanic electrical stimulation. J Neurophysiol 1989;61:427-434.
30. Freund TF, Buzsáki G. Interneurons of the hippocampus. Hippocampus 1996;6:347-470.
31. Michelson HB, Kapur J, Lothman EW. Reduction of paired pulse inhibition in the CA1 region of the hippocampus by pilocarpine in naive and in amygdala-kindled rats. Exp Neurol 1989;104:264-271.
32. Westbrook GL, Lothman EW. Cellular and synaptic basis of kainic acid-induced hippocampal epileptiform activity. Brain Res 1983;273:97-109.
33. Chapman AG, Westerberg E, Premachandra M, Meldrum BS. Changes in regional neurotransmitter amino acid levels in rat brain during seizures induced by L-allylglycine, bicuculline, and kainic acid. J Neurochem 1984;43:62-70.
34. Treiman DM, Walton NY, Gunawan S. Brain amino acid concentrations during specific electroencephalographic stages of status epilepticus in the rat. Epilepsy Res Suppl 1992;8:283-294.
35. Naylor DE, Liu H, Wasterlain CG. Trafficking of GABA(A) receptors, loss of inhibition, and a mechanism for pharmacoresistance in status epilepticus. J Neurosci 2005;25:7724-7733.
36. Kay AR, Wong RK. Isolation of neurons suitable for patch-clamping from adult mammalian central nervous systems. J Neurosci Methods 1986;16:227-238.
37. Kapur J, Macdonald RL. Rapid seizure-induced reduction of benzodiazepine and Zn++ sensitivity of hippocampal dentate granule cell $GABA_A$ receptors. J Neurosci 1997;17:7532-7540.
38. Barnes EM, Jr. Assembly and intracellular trafficking of $GABA_A$ receptors. Int Rev Neurobiol 2001;48:1-29.
39. Kittler JT, Delmas P, Jovanovic JN, Brown DA, Smart TG, Moss SJ. Constitutive endocytosis of $GABA_A$ receptors by an association with the adaptin AP2 complex modulates inhibitory synaptic currents in hippocampal neurons. J Neurosci 2000;20:7972-7977.
40. Edwards FA, Konnerth A, Sakmann B. Quantal analysis of inhibitory synaptic transmission in the dentate gyrus of rat hippocampal slices: a patch-clamp study. J Physiol (Lond) 1990;430:213-249.
41. Mangan PS, Kapur J. Factors underlying bursting behavior in a network of cultured hippocampal neurons exposed to zero magnesium. J Neurophysiol 2004;91:946-957.
42. Sun C, Sieghart W, Kapur J. Distribution of alpha1, alpha4, gamma2, and delta subunits of $GABA_A$ receptors in hippocampal granule cells. Brain Res 2004;1029:207-216.
43. Goodkin HP, Yeh JL, Kapur J. Status epilepticus increases the intracellular accumulation of $GABA_A$ receptors. J Neurosci 2005;25:5511-5520.
44. McBain CJ, Mayer ML. N-methyl-D-aspartic acid receptor structure and function. Physiol Rev 1994;74:723-760.
45. Fariello RG, Golden GT, Smith GG, Reyes PF. Potentiation of kainic acid epileptogenicity and sparing from neuronal damage by an NMDA receptor antagonist. Epilepsy Res 1989;3:206-213.
46. Clifford DB, Olney JW, Benz AM, Fuller TA, Zorumski CF. Ketamine, phencyclidine, and MK-801 protect against kainic acid-induced seizure-related brain damage. Epilepsia 1990;31:382-390.
47. Clifford DB, Olney JW, Maniotis A, Collins RC, Zorumski CF. The functional anatomy and pathology of lithium-pilocarpine and high- dose pilocarpine seizures. Neuroscience 1987;23:953-968.
48. Fujikawa DG, Daniels AH, Kim JS. The competitive NMDA receptor antagonist CGP 40116 protects against status epilepticus-induced neuronal damage. Epilepsy Res 1994;17:207-219.
49. Rice AC, DeLorenzo RJ. N-methyl-D-aspartate receptor activation regulates refractoriness of

status epilepticus to diazepam. Neuroscience 1999;93:117-123.
50. Rice AC, DeLorenzo RJ. NMDA receptor activation during status epilepticus is required for the development of epilepsy. Brain Res 1998;782:240-247.
51. Williamson JM, Lothman EW. The effect of MK-801 on kindled seizures: implications for use and limitations as an antiepileptic drug. Ann Neurol 1989;26:85-90.
52. Borris DJ, Bertram EH, Kapur J. Ketamine controls prolonged status epilepticus. Epilepsy Res 2000;42:117-122.
53. Collingridge GL, Lester RA. Excitatory amino acid receptors in the vertebrate central nervous system. Pharmacol Rev 1989;41:143-210.
54. Mott DD, Doherty JJ, Zhang S, Washburn MS, Fendley MJ, Lyuboslavsky P, Traynelis SF, Dingledine R. Phenylethanolamines inhibit NMDA receptors by enhancing proton inhibition. Nature Neuroscience 1998;1:659-667.
55. Yen W, Williamson J, Bertram EH, Kapur J. A comparison of three NMDA receptor antagonists in the treatment of prolonged status epilepticus. Epilepsy Res 2004;59:43-50.
56. Martin BS, Kapur J. A combination of ketamine and diazepam synergistically controls refractory status epilepticus induced by cholinergic stimulation. Epilepsia 2008;49:248-255.
57. DeGiorgio CM, Tomiyasu U, Gott PS, Treiman DM. Hippocampal pyramidal cell loss in human status epilepticus. Epilepsia 1992;33:23-27.
58. VanLandingham KE, Heinz ER, Cavazos JE, Lewis DV. Magnetic resonance imaging evidence of hippocampal injury after prolonged focal febrile convulsions. Ann Neurol 1998;43:413-426.
59. Korngut L, Young GB, Lee DH, Hayman-Abello BA, Mirsattari SM. Irreversible brain injury following status epilepticus. Epilepsy Behav 2007;11:235-240.
60. Heinrich A, Runge U, Kirsch M, Khaw AV. A case of hippocampal laminar necrosis following complex partial status epilepticus. Acta Neurol Scand 2007;115:425-428.
61. Brierley JB, Horton RW, Meldrum BS. Physiological observations during prolonged epileptic seizures in primates and their relation to subsequent brain damage. J Physiol (Lond) 1972;222:69P-70P.
62. Meldrum BS, Vigouroux RA, Brierley JB. Systemic factors and epileptic brain damage. Prolonged seizures in paralyzed, artificially ventilated baboons. Arch Neurol 1973;29:82-87.
63. Meldrum BS, Brierley JB. Prolonged epileptic seizures in primates. Ischemic cell change and its relation to ictal physiological events. Arch Neurol 1973;28:10-17.
64. Prasad A, Williamson JM, Bertram EH. Phenobarbital and MK-801, but not phenytoin, improve the long-term outcome of status epilepticus. Ann Neurol 2002;51:175-181.
65. Buckmaster PS. Laboratory animal models of temporal lobe epilepsy. Comp Med 2004;54: 473-485.
66. Lothman EW, Bertram EH, Kapur J, Stringer JL. Recurrent spontaneous hippocampal seizures in the rat as a chronic sequela to limbic status epilepticus. Epilepsy Res 1990;6:110-118.
67. Coulter DA. Chronic epileptogenic cellular alterations in the limbic system after status epilepticus. Epilepsia 1999;40(suppl 1):S23-33; discussion S40-1; S23-33.
68. Wuarin JP, Dudek FE. Electrographic seizures and new recurrent excitatory circuits in the dentate gyrus of hippocampal slices from kainate-treated epileptic rats. J Neurosci 1996;16: 4438-4448.
69. Raol YS, Budreck EC, Brooks-Kayal AR. Epilepsy after early-life seizures can be independent of hippocampal injury. Ann Neurol 2003;53:503-511.
70. Racine RJ. Modification of seizure activity by electrical stimulation. II. Motor seizure. Electroencephalogr Clin Neurophysiol 1972;32: 281-294.
71. Dube C, Richichi C, Bender RA, Chung G, Litt B, Baram TZ. Temporal lobe epilepsy after experimental prolonged febrile seizures: prospective analysis. Brain 2006;129:911-922.
72. Turrigiano GG, Nelson SB. Hebb and homeostasis in neuronal plasticity. Curr Opin Neurobiol 2000;10:358-364.
73. Snead OC, III. Basic mechanisms of generalized absence seizures. Ann Neurol 1995;37:146-157.
74. Huguenard JR, McCormick DA. Thalamic synchrony and dynamic regulation of global forebrain oscillations. Trends Neurosci 2007;30: 350-356.
75. Williams D. The thalamus and epilepsy. Brain 1965;88:539-556.
76. Labate A, Briellmann RS, Abbott DF, Waites AB, Jackson GD. Typical childhood absence seizures are associated with thalamic activation. Epileptic Disord 2005;7:373-377.

77. Steriade M, McCormick DA, Sejnowski TJ. Thalamocortical oscillations in the sleeping and aroused brain. Science 1993;262:679-685.
78. Coulter DA, Huguenard JR, Prince DA. Specific petit mal anticonvulsants reduce calcium currents in thalamic neurons. Neurosci Lett 1989;98:74-78.
79. Cortez MA, McKerlie C, Snead OC, III. A model of atypical absence seizures: EEG, pharmacology, and developmental characterization. Neurology 2001;56:341-349.
80. Velazquez JL, Huo JZ, Dominguez LG, Leshchenko Y, Snead OC, III. Typical versus atypical absence seizures: network mechanisms of the spread of paroxysms. Epilepsia 2007;48:1585-1593.

PART II

# FOCAL NONCONVULSIVE STATUS EPILEPTICUS

CHAPTER 8

# FRONTAL LOBE NONCONVULSIVE STATUS EPILEPTICUS

PIERRE THOMAS AND BENJAMIN ZIFKIN

In patients with nonconvulsive status epilepticus (NCSE), electroencephalography (EEG) enables diagnosis of an ictal state, as well as differentiation into the 2 main electroclinical varieties of NCSE: absence status (AS) and complex partial status epilepticus (CPSE).

AS (which will be addressed in Chapter 12) consists of a confusional state of variable intensity, ranging from simple cognitive slowing to catatonic stupor, that lasts for hours to days and is associated in half of cases with eyelid myoclonus (1-4). The literature, however, describes a type of AS "with focal characteristics" seen in patients with symptomatic or cryptogenic partial epilepsy. Patients may exhibit EEG findings showing asymmetric bilateral complexes (5-7). As will be discussed later in this chapter, such cases may represent a type of frontal lobe nonconvulsive status epilepticus (FLNCSE).

CPSE consists of a "prolonged epileptic episode in which fluctuating or frequently recurring focal electrographic epileptic discharges, arising in temporal or extratemporal regions, result in a confusional state with variable clinical symptoms" (8). Although temporal and extratemporal CPSE have classically been considered separately, such a rigid topographic distinction is difficult and even inappropriate, considering the diversity of the epileptogenic networks involved. Even so, one of the most characteristic presentations of temporal CPSE has been linked to disorganization of activity in the amygdala and hippocampus (9). It is characterized by a cycle of repeated complex partial seizures with altered awareness and stereotyped automatisms, interrupted by a more subtle disorder of awareness and reactive automatisms. This is, however, rare. More frequently, there is a continuous confusional state without any marked cycling, which has been attributed to disorganization of extratemporal function, especially of the frontal lobe (10).

In 1985, Williamson and colleagues reported depth-electrode studies in 8 patients with CPSE and found a frontal-lobe origin in 5 (11). These could be unilateral or bilateral and involve lateral, medial, or orbital frontal areas. In 1988, Rohr-Le Floch and colleagues found that 18 of 60 patients with NCSE had frontal NCSE, described as "frontal status"(12). In these patients, cognitive disturbances occurred at the same time as the continuous or recurrent ictal EEG activity over 1 or both frontopolar areas. Diagnostic criteria were also the presence of prolonged cognitive disturbance, at times with focal ictal signs. The EEG had to include adequate coverage of the frontal regions. Apart from the distribution of the EEG abnormalities, these patients also had some important, but subtle, clinical features: there was little change in level of awareness, but there could be mood changes with some disinhibition. Brain lesions were found in 11 of 18 patients (61%).

We prospectively studied all cases of CPSE presenting at our institution from 1991 to 1996 and meeting the following criteria for inclusion as FLNCSE: (1) alteration of cognitive function with or without confusion, lasting at least 1 hour; (2) motor seizure manifestations limited to slight and unforced head and eye deviation or focal low-amplitude myoclonus or both; (3) video-EEG confirmation of NCSE with a brief standardized neuropsychological evaluation performed during the episode of NCSE; (4) ictal EEG discharges beginning strictly over frontopolar, lateral, or medial frontal electrodes (Fp1, Fp2, F3, F4, Fz); and (5), if the ictal discharges were more widespread, involving anterior temporal or inferior frontal electrodes F7 or F8, the ictal single-photon computed tomographic scan (SPECT) showed clear hyperperfusion of 1 frontal region when compared to a postictal scan (13).

Of 44 patients with NCSE seen over 5 years, 10 (23%) fulfilled these criteria. Their mean age was 56.4 years (range 32-74 years). Seven were men, and 6 had no history of epilepsy. Two major types of FLNCSE, based on electroclinical presentation, emerged from this study.

Type 1 FLNCSE occurred in 7 patients. It was characterized by mild disturbance of cognitive function and by mood disturbances with a normal level of alertness and with no postictal amnesia. Four of these patients were emotionally disinhibited, moderately hypomanic, abnormally talkative, and inappropriately familiar. The other 3 showed indifference, lack of facial expression, and reduced speech, motivation, and spontaneous activity. Neurologic examination showed perseveration, confabulation, and impaired programming of complex activities such as bimanual tasks, serial subtraction, and drawing of alternate patterns (Figure 8-1). At the onset of the ictal EEG discharge, 4 subjects had additional findings: forced thinking, ipsilateral or contralateral head turning, slight myoclonia of the corners of the mouth, or negative motor events with loss of postural tone. The EEG showed unilateral frontopolar or frontocentral ictal activity starting with rapid, low-amplitude, recruiting rhythm, lasting from 45 to 230 seconds (average 159 seconds) (Figure 8.2A). These events were restricted to 1 frontal or frontotemporal area, with no contralateral epileptiform activity (Figure 8.2B). Normal background rhythm was recorded in 5 of 7 cases. Because of the relatively subtle clinical findings, we thought that this type 1, also reported by others (14-16), was better described as a simple partial status epilepticus with affective or cognitive features than as a CPSE. Table 8.1 shows the diagnoses initially made in the emergency department prior to the EEG.

FLNCSE type 2 occurred in 3 patients with cyclic spatiotemporal disorientation, behavior disturbance, and motor and verbal perseverations. This led to marked alteration of aware-

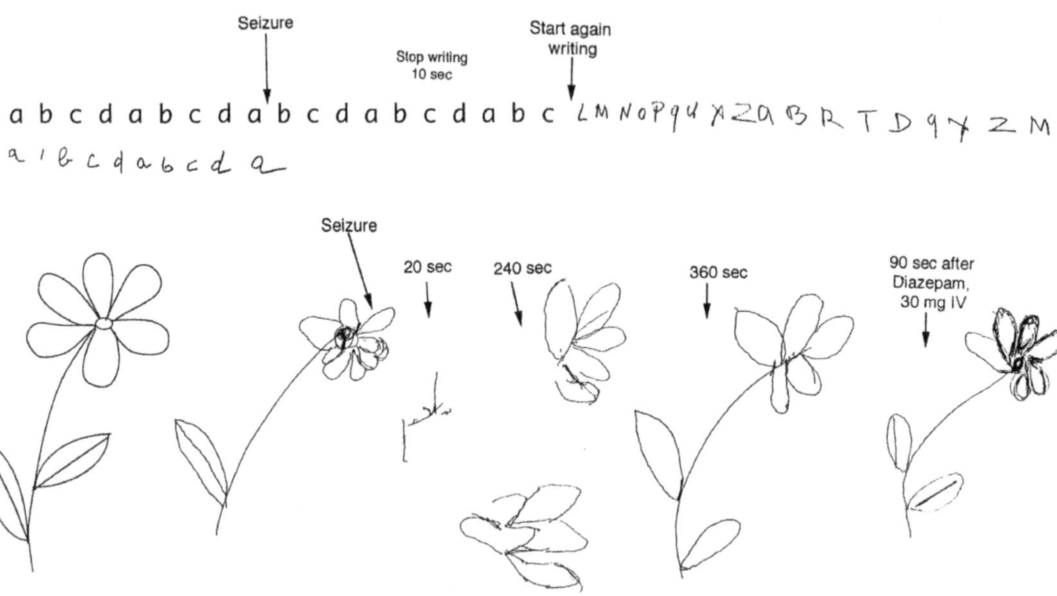


**Figure 8.1** Neuropsychologic testing during an episode of type 1 frontal nonconvulsive status epilepticus. Note the suspension of activity at seizure onset, then the motor perseverations. Performance improves after intravenous administration of diazepam.

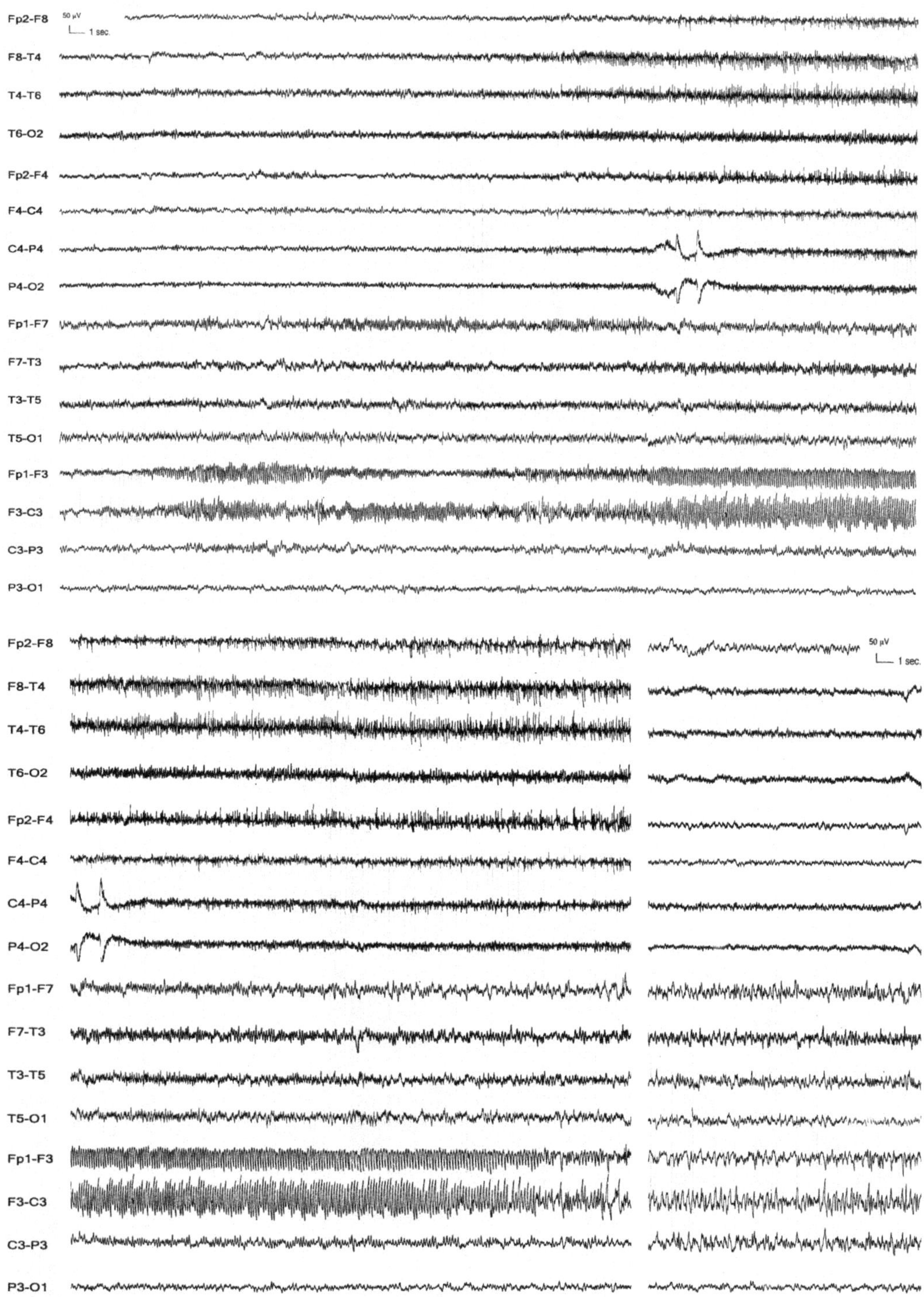


**Figure 8.2** Type 1 frontal nonconvulsive status epilepticus in a 36-year-old patient with a left frontal low-grade astrocytoma. At onset of seizure (A), note the prolonged, left frontal, 12-Hz, rhythmic spike activity. At the end of seizure, there is strict ipsilateral unihemispheric spread of ictal activity (B). The patient showed affective disinhibition without change in awareness.

TABLE 8.1 DIFFERENTIAL DIAGNOSES OF TYPE 1 FRONTAL LOBE NONCONVULSIVE STATUS EPILEPTICUS

- Transient global amnesia
- Prolonged postictal state
- Interictal psychosis
- Malingering
- Psychogenic nonepileptic seizure
- Depression
- Hysteria
- Antiepileptic drug overdose
- Psychotropic drug overdose
- Psychotropic drug withdrawal
- The amnesia-and-automatism syndrome after use of a short half-life benzodiazepine
- Akinetic mutism after a frontal-lobe stroke

ness with postictal catatonic stupor and amnesia. The EEG showed abnormal background activity and prolonged ictal activity averaging 255 seconds. This involved both frontotemporal or frontocentral regions simultaneously (Figure 8.3). Some patients showed progression over several minutes from an initial unilateral frontopolar focus to bilateral asymmetric discharges or even to bilateral synchronous spike-and-wave or polyspike-and-wave discharges similar to those seen in AS with focal characteristics.

In 6 of the 10 patients, ictal SPECT showed unilateral frontopolar hyperperfusion (2 cases) associated with medial or lateral frontal hyperperfusion (3 cases). One patient with an apparent bilateral anterior medial frontal hyperperfusion had only unilateral hyperperfusion over the right anteromedial and orbital frontal regions after subtraction of ictal and interictal SPECT and 3-dimensional modeling using his magnetic resonance imaging results (Figure 8.4).

In this series, 6 of the 10 patients had frontal lobe lesions. Three had tumors: 2 oligodendrogliomas and 1 ethmoidal lymphoma. The other 3 had previous frontal lobe surgery, 2 for meningiomas and 1 for a brain abscess. Contributing factors in the other patients included neurosyphilis, nonketotic hyperglycemia, high doses of psychotropic drugs, and hyponatremia in an alcoholic patient.

Benzodiazepines were ineffective as sole treatment in 8 of 10 patients. Six were controlled by intravenous administration of phenytoin, and 1 received 600 mg of carbamazepine orally as further treatment. One patient was not controlled by valproate and then intravenously administered phenobarbital and required barbiturate general anesthesia. All patients received maintenance antiepileptic drug treatment. There were no recurrences, and no short-, medium-, or long-term cognitive sequelae could be found. Two patients died within a

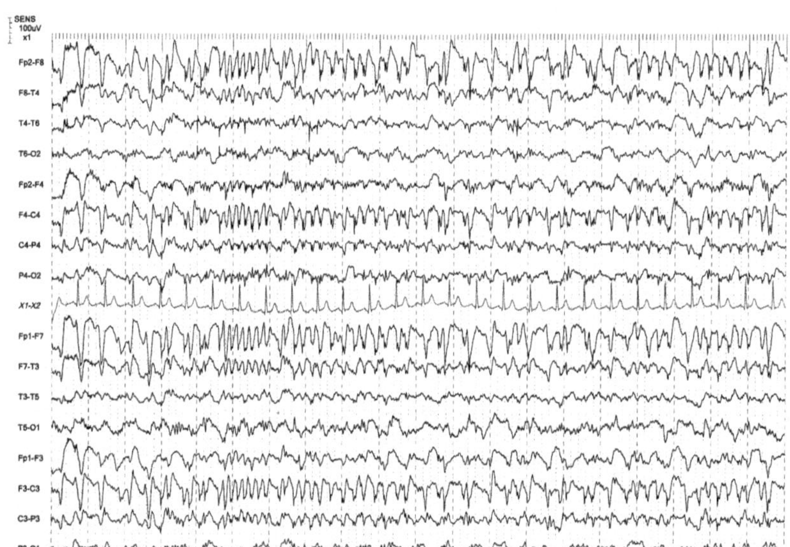


**Figure 8.3** Type 2 frontal nonconvulsive status epilepticus in a 56-year-old patient with cryptogenic partial epilepsy and severe confusion. Recurring bifrontal seizures start with a 5-Hz spike-wave pattern, a rapid decrease in frequency, and then merging of discharges.

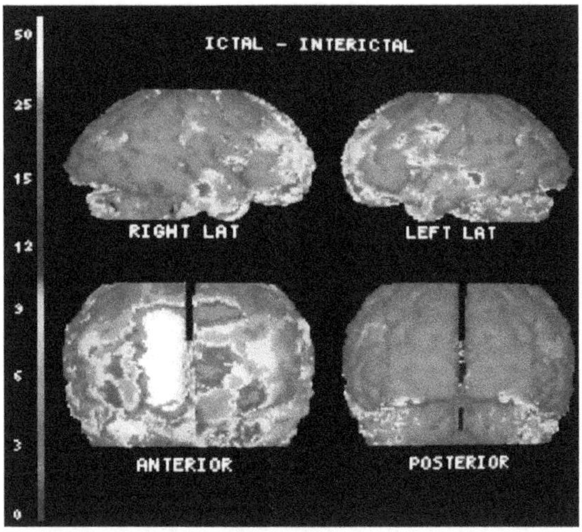


**Figure 8.4** Three-dimensional analysis of ictal and postictal single-photon emission computed tomography subtraction in a patient with type 2 nonconvulsive status epilepticus of frontal origin, showing a 50% increase in perfusion with prominent involvement of the right antero-mesial and orbito-frontal structures. Reprinted with permission (13).

year, 1 from the cause of the NCSE, an ethmoidal lymphoma. Six had karyotypes that ruled out ring chromosome 20.

## LITERATURE REVIEW

Apart from the studies cited in the previous section of the chapter (11-13), others have described similar events, with bilateral but clearly asymmetric ictal activity over anterior head regions or with ictal discharges localized over the frontal lobe. Because these cases of AS with focal features were so similar to extratemporal CPSE, it was suggested that the degree of ictal disorganization of frontal lobe functions could explain both, the first one representing simply a more developed form of the second.

The similarities between AS and frontal CPSE led to what Shorvon described as a "nosographic labyrinth" (8), and very similar or even identical entities have been reported using several different terms: borderline cases of petit mal status (5), transitional petit mal status (2), absence status with focal characteristics (7), acute prolonged confusion as a frontal-onset ictal state (17), nonconvulsive confusional frontal status (18), CPSE of frontal origin (19), and acute confusional state with frontal origin (20). We have chosen to call this frontal NCSE, using a term that describes localization only and that intentionally avoids implying any marked alteration of consciousness.

We reviewed 70 reported cases in 25 studies in which the inclusion criteria were approximately those that we used (Table 8.2) (5-7,11-15,17-33). The average age of patients was 36 years, ranging from 13 to 84 years. About 60% were women. In more than one third of cases, NCSE occurred with no history of epilepsy. A focal frontal lesion was present in approximately 35%. More recent work reports a distinct subgroup of patients with a mosaic state of ring chromosome 20 (30,31,34). Only 2 additional patients had ictal SPECT, showing similar unilateral frontal hyperperfusion (26,30).

The change in awareness in FLNCSE is variable. In type 1, isolated cognitive and behavior changes without marked changes in alertness are frequent, found in more than half of cases in the largest series (12). Many authors have reported changes in mood with unconcerned and disinhibited behavior or with indifference and perplexity at the same time as the unilateral frontal EEG discharges (6,7,11,17,21). Other patients have had more marked changes in consciousness associated with asymmetric bifrontal activity (17,24,29,30). In most cases, these observations of AS with focal characteristics are no different from those of type 2 FLNCSE except that there has been no confirmation of focal frontal origin with metabolic imaging (18,26,29). Table 8.3 provides an attempt to compare the main characteristics of FLNCE with AS and temporal lobe CPSE.

## EPILEPTOGENIC NETWORKS AND FRONT LOBE NONCONVULSIVE STATUS EPILEPTICUS

The most singular EEG finding in type 1 FLNCSE is low-amplitude rapid activity at the

**TABLE 8.2** NONCONVULSIVE STATUS EPILEPTICUS OF FRONTAL ORIGIN IN 70 PATIENTS

| Author, year, reference no. | Number of pts [Age] | Preexisting epilepsy | Ictal EEG | Impairment of consciousness | Etiologic factors |
|---|---|---|---|---|---|
| Hess et al, 1971 (5) | 2 (pts 1, 2) [15,16] | Yes | Recurrent bifrontal discharges followed by slow waves | Slight (pt1)<br>Severe (pt 2) | Unknown |
| Kugoh & Hosokawa, 1977 (14) | 1 [33] | Yes | Recurrent L frontal discharges | Slight | L Fr posttraumatic cyst |
| Gall et al, 1978 (6) | 1 (pt 4) [44] | Yes | Continuous R Fr PSW | Slight | Unknown |
| Geier, 1978 (21) | 2 (pts 2, 3) [22, 18] | Yes | Continuous bifrontal SW | Slight | Unknown |
| Picornell-Darder et al, 1978 (15) | 1 [18] | No | R fronto-central recurrent discharges | Slight | R subdural hematoma |
| Niedermeyer et al, 1979 (7) | 2 [23, 74] | Yes | L Fr (pt 1) and R Fr (pt 2) continuous discharges | Slight | Unknown |
| Melamed et al, 1979 (22) | 1 [37] | No | NA | Severe | L orbito-Fr meningioma |
| Aguglia et al, 1983 (17) | 1 [63] | No | L Fr discharges, then diffuse continuous PSW | Slight | Unknown |
| Berkovic et al, 1985 (18) | 1 (pt 2) [NA] | No | L Fr discharges, then continuous PSW | NA | Left Fr mass lesion |
| Williamson et al, 1985 (11) | 5 (pts 1, 2, 3, 4, 6) [19-47, mean 27.3] | Yes | Onset of seizures (depth electrodes): L Fr (pt 1), L medial Fr (pt 2), bilateral Fr (pts 3,4), L orbito-Fr (pt 6). | Slight (pt1)<br>Moderate (pts 2,3)<br>Severe (pts 4,6) | Unknown |
| Lim et al, 1986 (23) | 1 (pt 2)[67] | No | Continuous R fronto-central discharges | Severe | Unknown |
| Tomson et al, 1986 (24) | 2 (pts 4, 5) [66,52] | Yes | Continuous L (pt 4) and R (pt 5) fronto-central discharges | Severe (pt 4)<br>Severe (pt 5) | Unknown |
| Rey & Papy, 1987 (20) | 3 (pts 2, 3, 4) [84, 75, 79] | No (pt 3,4)<br>Yes (pt 2) | Continuous bifrontal delta activity (pt 2)<br>Bifrontal SW (pt 3)<br>Recurrent L Fr discharges (pt 4) | Moderate (pt 2,3)<br>Severe (pt 4) | Unknown |
| Rohr-Le Floch et al, 1988(12) | 18 [20-78, mean 36.5] | No (13 pts)<br>Yes (5 pts) | Recurrent L Fr discharges: 3 pts<br>Recurrent discharges with a L Fr (2 pts), R Fr (2 pts) or bifrontal (2 pts) predominance<br>Continuous rhythmic theta activity with a R Fr (2 pts), L Fr (2 pts), or bifrontal (3 pts) predominance.<br>R Fr continuous SW: 2 pts | Slight (8 pts)<br>Moderate to Severe (10 pts) | Fr astrocytoma: 2 pts<br>Fr meningioma: 2 pts<br>Fr hematoma: 2 pts<br>Depressed Fr skull fracture: 2 pts<br>Fr arachnoid cyst: 1 pt<br>Fr depth electrode procedure: 1 pt<br>8 pts: unknown |

| | | | | | |
|---|---|---|---|---|---|
| Takeda, 1988 (19) | 1 [47] | Yes | Recurrent R Fr discharges | Slight | R Fr contusion |
| Striano et al, 1990 (25) | 1 [26] | Yes | Recurrent R Fr discharges | Severe | R Fr astrocytoma |
| Fujiwara et al, 1991 (26) | 1 [27] | Yes | R Fr discharges, then continuous bifrontal PSW | Slight | Alcohol |
| Masnou et al, 1994 (27) | 1 [41] | Yes | Continuous bifrontal rhythmic theta activity | Slight | Unknown |
| Thomas & Andermann, 1994 (28) | 1 [81] | No | R Fr discharges followed by PSW | Severe | Unknown |
| Kudo et al, 1995 (29) | 4 (pts 1, 2, 3 , 4) [43, 33, 43, 27] | Yes | R Fr discharges followed by continuous, diffuse PSW | Slight (pts 1,3)<br>Moderate (pts 2,4) | Unknown |
| Inoue et al, 1997 (30) | 5 (pts 1, 2, 3, 5, 6 ) [14, 13, 21, 31, 25] | Yes | R Fr discharges followed by diffuse SW (pts 1, 6)<br>Bilateral Fr discharges (pts 2, 5)<br>Continuous rhythmic delta activity with a R Fr predominance (pt 3) | Slight (pts 5)<br>Moderate (pt 3, 6)<br>Severe (pt 1,2) | Ring chromosome 20 (all pts)<br>R Fr dysplasia (pt 2)<br>Unknown (pt 3) |
| Thomas et al, 1999 (13) | 10 [65, 32, 48, 74, 51, 53, 47, 61, 73, 60] | No (6 pts)<br>Yes (4 pts) | Unilateral discharges beginning with low voltage fast activity (pts 1-7)<br>Bilateral, assymetrical or symmetrical recurrent Fr discharges (pts 8 -10) | Slight (pt 1-7)<br>Severe (pt 8-10) | Cerebral tumor (pts 3,6, 9)<br>Hyperosmolarity (pt 1)<br>Fr lobe surgery (pt 2,4,5)<br>Psychotropic drugs (pt 8)<br>Neurosyphilis (pt 7)<br>Alcohol (pt 10) |
| Petit et al, 1999 (31) | 3 [9, 14, 43 ] | Yes | Bifrontal continuous sharp theta activity and SW (pt 1)<br>Diffuse flattening, then Fr slow waves (pt 2)<br>Rhythmic bifrontal slow waves (pt 3) | Slight to Moderate | Ring chromosome 20 (all pts) |
| Fernandez-Torre et al, 2000 (32) | 1 [53] | Yes | Recurrent, L Fr polar discharges with secondary bilateralization | Moderate | L Fr hematoma |
| Morioka et al, 2002 (33) | 1 [35] | No | Recurrent R seizures | Moderate | R Fr hematoma |

***Abbreviations:*** *EEG refers to electroencephalography; Fr, frontal lobe; L, left; R, right; SW, spike-waves; PSW, polyspike-waves; pt(s), patient(s); NA, not available.*

**TABLE 8.3** COMPARISON OF THE MAIN CLINICAL CHARACTERISTICS OF VARIOUS TYPES OF NONCONVULSIVE STATUS EPILEPTICUS

| | FLNCSE Type 1 | FLNCSE Type 2 | ASE | TL CPSE mesial | TL CPSE lateral |
|---|---|---|---|---|---|
| Impairment of consciousness | Mild | Usually severe | Mild, moderate or severe | Moderate or severe | Moderate or severe |
| Fluctuations of consciousness | Yes | No | Yes | Yes (waxing and waning) | Sometimes |
| Temporo-spatial disorientation | Rare | Yes | Yes | Yes | Yes |
| Bilateral eyelid myoclonias | No | No | Yes, ~ 50% | No | No |
| Verbal fluency | Usually normal | Reduced | Reduced | Reduced | Dysphasia |
| Oro-alimentary automatisms | No | No | No | Yes (lip-smacking, swallowing) | Rare |
| Simple gesture automatisms | No | Yes | Yes | Yes | Yes |
| Complex gesture automatisms | No | Sometimes | Rare | Sometimes | Yes |
| Fugue state (poriomania) | No | Not documented | Yes (Rare) | Yes (Rare) | Yes (Rare) |
| Perseverations | Yes | Yes | Yes | Rare | Rare |
| Confabulations | Yes | No | Rare | No | Rare |
| Echolalia/palilalia | Yes | No | Rare | No | Rare |
| Indifferent/perplex attitude | Yes ~ 50 % | Yes | Yes | No | No |
| Ironic/hilarious attitude | Yes ~ 50% | No | No | No | No |
| Anxious/aggressive behavior | No | No | No | Frequent (agitated, fearful) | Frequent |
| Psychotic behavior | No | No | No | Frequent (fluctuates) | Frequent |
| Hallucinations types | No | No | No | Frequent (delusions) | Frequent, various |
| Lateralized motor manifestations | No | Sometimes (version) | No | Frequent | Frequent, various types |
| Amnesia of the episode | No | Yes | Often partial | Yes | Often partial |

*Adapted from Ref 12: Rohr-Le-Floch et al., 1988.*

***Abbreviations:*** *FLNCSE, frontal lobe nonconvulsive status epilepticus; ASE, absence status epilepticus; TL CPSE, temporal lobe complex partial status epilepticus; ~ 50%, occurs in approximately half the cases.*

onset of the ictal periods (Figure 8.5). This is usually localized to a frontopolar electrode (Fp1 or Fp2) or a lateral frontal one (F3 or F4). We have never documented onset in type 1 FLNCSE with spike-and-wave or polyspike-and-wave activity in these regions. It is possible that, given the frequency of frontal lesions in these patients, the phenomena of secondary bilateral synchrony often found in frontal-lobe epilepsies are blocked by a structural lesion. In both scalp- and depth-electrode recording, the low-amplitude fast activity is very suggestive of an underlying disorganization of cortical function, whereas spike-and-wave activity indicates some degree of organization of cortical activity (35).

In our experience, the unilateral fast activity of type 1 FLNCSE is usually asymptomatic, perhaps because the epileptogenic zone is in a clinically silent area. Electroclinical correlation then becomes useful only after the discharges have spread within the frontal lobe. The clinical pattern then becomes apparent with dysfunction of a striatofrontal network, combining signs of a relatively mild frontal disturbance and memory disorder. Cortical functions such as language and praxic and gnostic functions are usually preserved. This pattern of cognitive disturbance resembles that described by the neuropsychologists of the Salpêtrière group as "loss of psychic self-activation" found in patients with extrapyramidal vascular lesions (36). Thus, this clinical pattern, functionally comparable to that of bipallidal lesions, could be produced by the recruitment of networks linking the prefrontal association cortex and the striatum by the unilateral frontopolar discharge, involving disorganization of a prefrontal-pallidal-thalamo-cortical loop.

A further argument in favor of basal ganglia involvement in frontal NCSE is provided by an [18F] fluoro-l-DOPA positron emission tomography study of 14 patients with mosaic ring chromosome 20 and 10 control subjects (37). There was a significant bilateral symmetric reduction in ligand binding in the putamen and caudate regions of the affected group, suggesting that dysfunction of dopaminergic neurotransmission in those regions could result in the inability of striatal structures to interrupt the epileptic discharges.

Recent neurophysiologic studies suggest other hypotheses (38). Niedermeyer and Lopes da Silva studied the dynamics of intracranial fast activity of the transition to the ictal state in frontal and frontotemporal areas (35). There was a marked reduction in correlation among the network structures at the seizure onset, associated with the appearance of 24- to 80-Hz gamma activity, typical of ictal activity in these regions. There was a rapid return of spatial coherence of these signals to preictal values in the postictal period. These data suggest that the epileptic discharge can transiently block the interstructural relations of the network in which it occurs and, thus, disrupt normal network function. These findings, as the authors note (38), update the 19th century ideas of Hughlings Jackson, for whom the loss of function of highest cortical centers permitted the "release" of centers phylogenetically lower in the central nervous system (39). In the case of frontal seizures and NCSE, the emergence of stereotyped and rather simple behaviors would not be due to the disorganization of one or another network but, instead, to the activation of subcortical

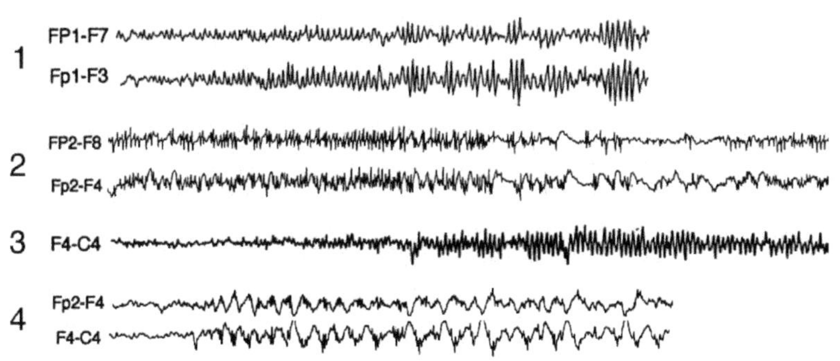


**Figure 8.5** Low-amplitude fast activity recorded at seizure onset in 4 patients with type 1 frontal nonconvulsive status epilepticus.

networks freed from the inhibitory influence of higher centers.

## CONCLUSIONS

FLNCSE is a diagnostic challenge. Prompt EEG and neuropsychologic testing will confirm the diagnosis. This may be especially difficult in type 1 frontal NCSE, in which consciousness is only mildly disturbed, if at all. Type 2 frontal NCSE can present more dramatically and in the same manner as an extratemporal CPSE or may be mistaken for AS with asymmetric anterior EEG discharges. Although type 1 may develop into type 2, this is rare in our experience. FLNCSE most often occurs in patients with no history of epilepsy and indicates a frontal lesion in more than one third of cases. If imaging is noncontributory, it may be important to exclude a ring chromosome 20 syndrome, especially in patients with mild mental retardation. Treatment with benzodiazepines alone is often ineffective, and intravenous administration of fosphenytoin is often needed. Some patients may require general anesthesia, with (13) or without barbiturates (32). The role of other antiepileptic drugs remains unclear. Further comment on treatment may be found in Chapter 20.

Many questions remain unanswered: What is the true incidence of this syndrome? Which epileptogenic networks are involved? Are there idiopathic forms in childhood? Does frontal NCSE without etiologic explanation presage cognitive decline in the elderly? Only further prospective studies can resolve these questions, but such investigations are difficult to organize and perform because of the difficulties in making an early positive diagnosis and the heterogeneity of the clinical and EEG presentation.

## REFERENCES

1. Andermann F, Robb JP. Absence status. A reappraisal following review of thirty-eight patients. Epilepsia 1972;13:177-187.
2. Guberman A, Cantu-Reyna G, Stuss D, Broughton R. Nonconvulsive generalized status epilepticus: clinical features, neuropsychological testing and long-term follow-up. Neurology 1986;36:1284-1291.
3. Thomas P, Zifkin B, Andermann F. Absence status. In: Wasterlain CG, Treiman DM, eds. Status Epilepticus: Mechanisms and Management. Cambridge, MA: MIT Press; 2006:91-108.
4. Thomas P, Snead OC III. Absence status epilepticus. In: Engel J Jr, Pedley T, eds. Epilepsy: a Comprehensive Textbook, Vol. 1, 2nd ed. Philadelphia, PA: Lippincott Williams and Wilkins; 2008:693-703.
5. Hess R, Scollo-Lavizzari G, Wyss FE. Borderline cases of petit mal status. Eur Neurol 1971;5:137-154.
6. Gall MV, Scollo-Lavizzari G, Becker H. Absence status in the adult. New results including computerized transverse axial tomography. Eur Neurol 1978;17:121-128.
7. Niedermeyer E, Fineyre F, Riley T, Uematsu S. Absence status (petit mal status) with focal characteristics. Arch Neurol 1979;36:417-421.
8. Shorvon S. Status Epilepticus: its Clinical Features and Treatment in Children and Adults. Cambridge, England: Cambridge University Press; 1994.
9. Treiman DM, Delgado-Escueta AV. Complex partial status epilepticus. In: Delgado-Escueta AV, Wasterlain CG, Treiman DM, Porter RJ, eds. Status Epilepticus. Adv Neurol. Vol 34. New York, NY: Raven Press; 1983:69-81.
10. Delgado-Escueta AV, Treiman DM. Focal status epilepticus: modern concepts. In: Lüders H, Lesser RP, eds. Epilepsy: Electroclinical Syndromes. London, England: Springer-Verlag; 1987:347-391.
11. Williamson PD, Spencer DD, Spencer SS, Novelly RA, Mattson RH. Complex partial status epilepticus: a depth electrode study. Ann Neurol 1985;18:647-654.
12. Rohr-Le Floch J, Gauthier G, Beaumanoir A. États confusionnels d'origine épileptique: intérêt de l'EEG fait en urgence. Rev Neurol 1988;144:425-436.
13. Thomas P, Zifkin B, Migneco O, Lebrun C, Darcourt J, Andermann F. Nonconvulsive status epilepticus of frontal origin. Neurology 1999;52:1174-1183.
14. Kugoh T, Hosokawa K. Mental dullness associated with left frontal continuous focal discharges. Folia Psych Neurol Japon 1977;31:473-480.
15. Picornell-Darder I, Conde M, Carbonell J. État de mal post-traumatique à symptomatologie uniquement psychique. Rev EEG Neurophysiol 1978;8:341-344.

16. Thomas P, Mottin Y. État de mal frontal non convulsif. Rev Neurol 1997;153:421-426.
17. Aguglia U, Tinuper P, Farnarier G. État confusionnel critique à point de départ frontal chez le sujet âgé. Rev EEG Neurophysiol 1983; 13:174-179.
18. Berkovic SF, Andermann F, Aubé M, Rémillard G-M, Gloor P. Nonconvulsive confusional frontal status. Epilepsia 1985;26:529.
19. Takeda A. Complex partial status epilepticus of frontal lobe origin. Jap J Psychiatry 1988;42:525-530.
20. Rey M, Papy JJ. États d'obnubilation critique d'origine frontale: un diagnostic clinique difficile. Rev Electroencephalogr Neurophysiol 1987;17:377-385.
21. Geier S. Prolonged psychic epileptic seizures: a study of the absence status. Epilepsia 1978;19:431-445.
22. Melamed E, Lavy S, Argov Z, Feinsod M. Absence and automatisms associated with an orbitofrontal meningioma. J Clin Psychiatry 1979;40:44-45.
23. Lim L, Yagnik P, Schraeder P, Wheeler S. Ictal catatonia as a manifestation of non convulsive status epilepticus. J Neurol Neurosurg Psych 1986;49:833-836.
24. Tomson T, Svanborg E, Wedlund JE. Nonconvulsive status epilepticus: high incidence of complex partial status. Epilepsia 1986;27:276-285.
25. Striano S, Barbieri F, Bilo L, Ruosi P, Soricellis M. Recurrent frontal status epilepticus with polymorphic clinical features. A case report. Acta Neurol (Napoli) 1990;12:193-199.
26. Fujiwara T, Watanabe M, Matsuda K, Senbongi M, Yagi K, Seino M. Complex partial status epilepticus provoked by the ingestion of alcohol: a case report. Epilepsia 1991;32:650-656.
27. Masnou P, Salefranque F, Megas H, Vidart JN. Activité critique subintrante et épilepsie frontale : rôle dans la genèse de troubles du comportement. Epilepsies 1995;6:235-239.
28. Thomas P, Andermann F. Absence status in elderly patients is most often situation-related. In: Malafosse A, Genton P, Hirsch E, Marescaux C, Broglin D, Bernasconi R, eds. Idiopathic Generalized Epilepsies: Clinical, Experimental and Genetic Aspects. London, England: John Libbey; 1994:95-109.
29. Kudo T, Sato K, Yagi K, Seino M. Can absence status epilepticus be of frontal lobe origin? Acta Neurol Scand 1995;92:472-477.
30. Inoue Y, Fujiwara T, Matsuda K, Kubota H, Tanaka M, Yagi K, Yamamori K, Takahashi Y. Ring chromosome 20 and nonconvulsive status epilepticus. A new epileptic syndrome. Brain 1997;120:939-953.
31. Petit J, Roubertie A, Inoue Y, Genton P. Nonconvulsive status in the ring chromosome 20 syndrome: a video illustration of 3 cases. Epileptic Disord 1999;1:237-241.
32. Fernandez-Torre JL, Gonzalez C, Sanchez JM. Nonconvulsive status epilepticus of frontal origin. A case report. Rev Neurol 2000;30:1040-1043.
33. Morioka T, Nishio S, Ikezaki K, Inamura T, Kawamura T, Fukui K. Unilateral striatal damage following status epilepticus of ipsilateral frontal lobe origin. Seizure 2002;11:261-265.
34. Locharernkul C, Ebner A, Promchainant C. Ring chromosome 20 with nonconvulsive status epilepticus: electroclinical correlation of a rare epileptic syndrome. Clin Electroencephalogr Neurosci 2005;36:151-160.
35. Niedermeyer E, Lopes da Silva F. Electroencephalography: Basic Principles, Clinical Applications, and Related Fields, 4th ed. Baltimore, MD: Williams & Wilkins; 1999.
36. Laplane D, Levasseur M, Pillon B, Dubois B, Baulac M, Mazoyer B, Tran Dinh S, Sette G, Danze F, Baron JC. Obsessive-compulsive and other behavioural changes with bilateral basal ganglia lesions. A neuropsychological, magnetic resonance imaging and positron tomography study. Brain 1989;112:699-725.
37. Biraben A, Semah F, Ribeiro MJ, Douaud G, Remy P, Depaulis A. PET evidence for a role of the basal ganglia in patients with ring chromosome 20 and epilepsy. Neurology 2004;63:73-77.
38. Wendling F, Bartolomei F, Bellanger JJ, Bourien J, Chauvel P. Epileptic fast intracerebral EEG activity: evidence for spatial decorrelation at seizure onset. Brain 2003;126:1449-1459.
39. Jackson JH. Evolution and dissolution of the nervous system. In: Taylor J, ed. Selected Writings of John Hughlings Jackson. Vol 2. London, England: Hodder & Stoughton; 1932:45-75.

CHAPTER 9

# PARIETAL LOBE NONCONVULSIVE STATUS EPILEPTICUS

JENNIFER HOPP AND ALLAN KRUMHOLZ

Prompt diagnosis and aggressive control are critical for promoting survival and improving outcomes for patients with convulsive status epilepticus (1), but, until very recently, a similar emphasis has not been valid for patients with nonconvulsive status epilepticus (NCSE) (2). This, however, appears to be changing. Increasingly, greater attention is being directed to the rapid diagnosis and vigorous management of patients with NCSE as this disorder is better understood, identified more frequently, and recognized to pose some risks for morbidity and mortality similar to those of convulsive status epilepticus (2,3). Neither our understanding of the broad clinical spectrum of NCSE nor our approaches to its treatment, however, are as well defined and established as they are for convulsive status epilepticus (3,4).

Although partial NCSE was initially considered to arise solely from the temporal lobes, it soon became apparent that many patients had seizures arising from the frontal lobes (2-7). In this chapter, we consider an unusual variant of localized or partial NCSE that originates from parietal regions of cortex and may therefore be termed parietal lobe NCSE, focusing on in its clinical presentations, diagnosis, and management.

## PARIETAL LOBE FUNCTION

To appreciate how parietal seizures or parietal NCSE may present clinically, an understanding of the normal anatomy and function of the parietal lobe is helpful. Essentially, the parietal lobe is important for functions, including sensation, such as of touch and pain; information processing; spatial orientation; and language comprehension. The cortical regions designated as the parietal lobe appear to integrate information from different sensory modalities, as in the determination of spatial location of objects. This particular function enables regions of the parietal cortex to map or incorporate objects perceived visually into body-coordinate positions (8-10).

Anatomically, the parietal lobe is located anterior to the occipital lobe and posterior to the frontal lobe. The central sulcus separates the parietal lobe from the frontal lobe, and the parieto-occipital sulcus separates the parietal and occipital lobes. The parietal lobe can be subdivided into the superior parietal lobule and the inferior parietal lobule, separated by the intraparietal sulcus. The parietal lobe includes Brodmann areas 3, 5, 7, 39, and 40 (Figure 9.1) (10).

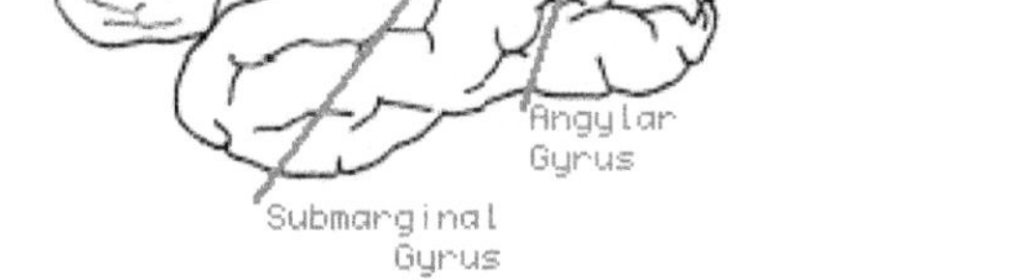


**Figure 9.1** Normal anatomy and structure of the parietal lobe showing its relation to other brain regions and organization, including Brodmann areas.

These areas of the parietal lobe appear to serve special functions. The postcentral gyrus is the primary sensory area involved in body sensation, which is somatotopically organized in the sensory homunculus. Stimulation of this area typically results in sensations of tingling and numbness, whereas lesions of this area cause loss of contralateral sensation. The superior parietal lobule is involved with the interaction and perception of the individual in surrounding space, and a lesion in this area may result in contralateral neglect. The supramarginal and angular gyri of the inferior parietal lobule are involved with the integration of information for speech and perception. Lesions in these areas can result in difficulty with object recognition and language comprehension (8-10).

What we understand about the parietal lobe and its functions derives, in large measure, from meticulous clinical observations. Many functions that we now reliably attribute to the parietal lobes were first suspected based on physicians' observations of individual patients with lesions in this region. For example, in 1924, Josef Gerstmann described an unusual pattern of clinical dysfunction that initiated a new understanding and appreciation of parietal function and impairment (Figure 9.2). In particular, what is now termed Gerstmann syndrome is characterized by (1) finger agnosia, (2) right-left disorientation, (3) agraphia or dysgraphia, and (4) dyscalculia (8).

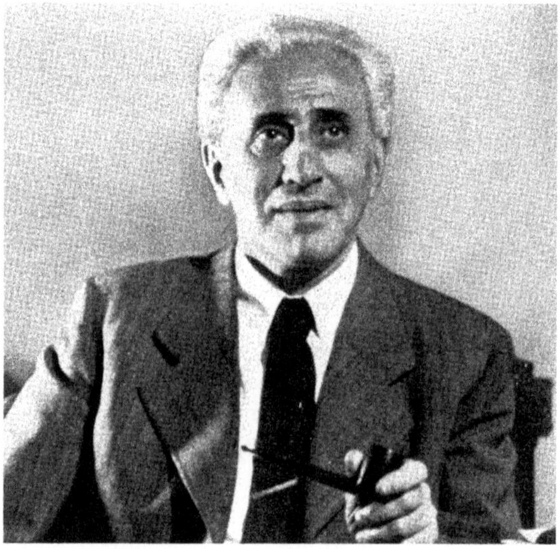

**Figure 9.2** Josef Gerstmann

Gerstmann syndrome is characterized by various global disturbances in function caused by a focal or lateralized parietal lesion. In other instances of parietal lobe dysfunction, the deficit may lateralize to the contralateral side of the body, as in a hemisensory deficit, or to contralateral space, as with hemi-inattention or neglect.

Some examples of the specific manifestations of perceptual and visual-spatial dysfunction that can be observed with parietal lobe dysfunction are depicted in Figures 9.3 and 9.4. These are dysfunctions that lateralize to the contralateral parietal lobe, as opposed to those that cause more global or bilateral difficulties, as in Gerstmann syndrome (8).

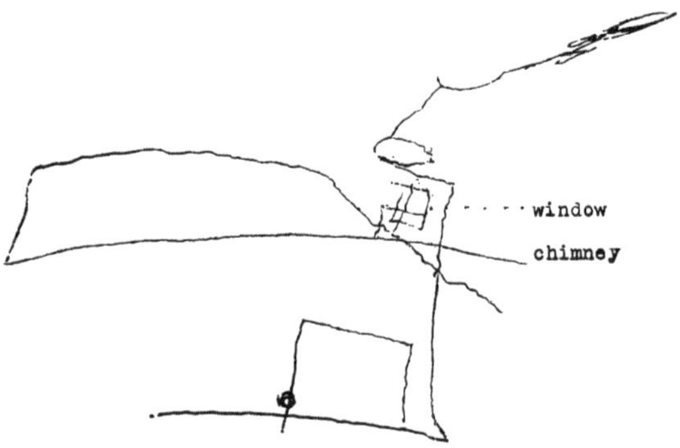


**Figure 9.3** This drawing of a house shows neglect of the left side of the image and disorientation in a patient with a right parietal disorder.

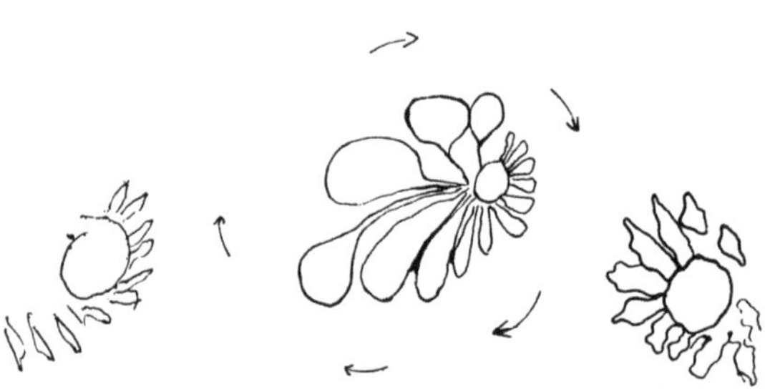

**Figure 9.4** Drawings by patients. The figure on the far left demonstrates incompleteness of the left side of a daisy head—drawn by a patient with a right parietal lesion. The drawing in the middle shows distortion of the left-sided petals of a daisy head; this patient had a right parietal lesion. The right-most drawing of a daisy head shows inadequacies on the right side of the image. This patient had a left parietal deficit.

## PARIETAL LOBE SEIZURES

Clinical manifestations of seizures arising from parietal lobe vary and may be difficult to recognize. The seizures are characteristically identified and categorized by the presenting aura or early symptom because the subsequent spread of seizure activity may not accurately localize the site of initial seizure onset (11-15). A further confusing factor is that the seizure may actually start in a clinically subtle or "silent" area of cortex, with the initial clinical symptoms due to the spread of seizure activity to other areas of cortex that are more likely to produce observable signs or symptoms, such as motor convulsions. The incidence of seizures arising from the parietal lobe is not well established, but these seizures are thought to be relatively rare, with some series providing estimates of 1.4% of seizures in patients with epilepsy (11,12).

Seizures arising in the postcentral gyrus of the parietal lobe are most common and are typically described by patients as manifested by either positive or negative sensations. Descriptions have included sensations of "pins and needles, tickling, pricking, sensation of crawling under the skin"(13). These sensations are usually contralateral to the ictal onset but may be ipsilateral or bilateral. More general feelings of a widespread body "aura" have been attributed to activation of the supplementary sensorimotor area (13). In patients with parietal lobe epilepsy, it is common for sensory auras to precede other seizure manifestations, as might be expected from reports of typical patterns of spread for seizures. Motor phenomena typically follow sensory auras in parietal lobe seizures. In these cases, the descriptions of sensory involvement often correspond to the known sensory homunculus, with a kind of sensory "jacksonian march," often followed by motor activity. Duration of these seizures is typically brief, and patients must not be amnestic of the aura in order to report these parietal localizing sensations.

Paresthesias have been described as the most common manifestation of seizures of parietal onset. For example, somatosensory auras were the most common parietal seizure manifestation in one series of 72 patients undergoing presurgical evaluation for intractable epilepsy (14). Specifically, "tingling" was the most common symptom reported by 76% of patients in that retrospective study, and the upper extremity was the most common site of involvement in 37 of 72 patients (14).

Reports of pain and perceptions of heat or cold during a seizure are less common and may be difficult to distinguish from each other. A perception of heat has been reported more commonly than that of cold (15), and studies by Penfield and Jasper using electrical stimulation suggest the onset in the perisylvian region (9).

Another rare presentation of parietal lobe epilepsy involves seizures with sexual phenomena. They have been reported as originating primarily in the paracentral lobule near the primary somatosensory area, but the frontal lobe and the mesial temporal lobe have also been linked to these seizures (11). Interestingly, parietal seizures with sexual phenomena appear to differ from those of temporal origin by semiology. Seizures involving sexual phenomena from the temporal lobe typically consist of sexual automatisms and are often described by patients as pleasurable (11), whereas seizures of parietal onset that include sexual symptoms are often described as unpleasant or frightening (11). These seizures often begin with unilateral paresthesias or numbness in the genitals or breasts and may be followed by clonic activity, presumably with spread of the seizure (11).

Psychiatric phenomena have been associated with temporal and frontal seizures and also with seizures of parietal lobe onset, including anxiety and panic. Alemayehu and colleagues have described 2 patients with right parietal tumors whose seizures consisted of symptoms of fear; intracranial electroencephalography (EEG) confirmed seizure onset with parietal cortical discharges (16). Both patients had been given a diagnosis of panic attacks before the electrophysiologic or EEG confirmation of the site of seizure origin.

> *One patient had stereotyped seizures described as the sudden onset "of*

> *dizziness, palpitations, and irrational fear which lasted several minutes. At times, she felt 'far away,' but there was no accompanying alteration of awareness." The authors note that "on one occasion, she ran out of her home in her nightgown."*

Other descriptions of auras involving the parietal lobe include disturbances of body image, such as a feeling of floating or of movement, "butterflies," and "a thought in the stomach"(17). In addition, the feeling of inability to move has been associated with involvement of the secondary sensory areas on the suprasylvian border of the parietal lobe. Occasionally, the seizure semiology may suggest parietal involvement, but it may also represent spread from the frontal or temporal lobes, as has been described by Feinberg and colleagues (18), whose patient reported symptoms consistent with an alien hand syndrome but who had EEG abnormalities in the right frontotemporal region.

> *I can't control this arm [her left]...it just does what it wants to do ... [the left hand] belonged to someone else ... [left arm is] a buddy ... a nickname I gave to the figure that was attached to me.*

The most commonly reported sites of sensory auras include the whole body, upper limb, and upper limb and face (15). Many other clinical manifestations are attributed to parietal lobe onset (11,13). Data from intraoperative mapping and cortical mapping also further the understanding of anatomic localization of seizures of parietal lobe onset. Jackson, Penfield, and Jasper delineated sensory seizures according to localization, describing rolandic, sensory cortex, and supplementary sensory area seizures (9).

With regard to the pathology associated with parietal lobe seizures, there are both lesion and nonlesion causes, as defined by imaging. In particular, in a large series of patients from the Montreal Neurological Institute with parietal lobe epilepsy, 29% had tumors as the cause of seizures (9). Gliosis, vascular malformations, hamartomas and cortical dysplasias, and prior cerebral infarcts were other common causes of parietal-onset seizures. Magnetic resonance imaging may show these focal lesions (16), and ictal single-photon emission computed tomography (SPECT) and interictal positron emission tomography may provide corroborative evidence of the localization of seizure onset. Interictal EEG may show just hemispheric lateralizing findings, rather than more localizing parietal lobe abnormalities (15,20).

Because of the often subtle clinical findings and seizure manifestations of parietal seizures, the lack of consistent imaging correlates, and the often unconvincing or poorly localizing EEG abnormalities in many patients with parietal lobe seizures, the differential diagnosis of sensory auras and seizures suggesting parietal lobe epilepsy must remain broad. That differential may include nonepileptic psychogenic seizures and transient manifestations from cerebral ischemia or vascular disease. More lasting or permanent parietal lobe dysfunction suggests structural lesions such as strokes or tumors, whereas transient or fluctuating deficits are more typical of symptomatic localization-related epilepsy.

## PARIETAL LOBE NONCONVULSIVE STATUS EPILEPTICUS

Prolonged ictal sensory changes are rare and uncommonly reported, so it is not surprising that there have been few well-documented case reports of patients in what might reasonably be regarded as parietal NCSE. Penfield and Jasper (9) described sensory auras that persisted, similar to those of epilepsia partialis continua, without spread to motor regions and suggested that this presentation of symptoms could occur within the context of focal status epilepticus. Focal parietal status epilepticus has been reported as occurring with persistence of sensory auras, similar to those described earlier in this chapter with parietal seizures. Even prolonged auras are often followed by spread to contiguous and distant regions, leading to impairment or loss of consciousness, motor activity, and other clinical phenomena. Moreover, recognition of somatosensory seizures requires that patients are able to report symptoms suspicious for parietal lobe involvement, and such reporting also requires that patients are not amnestic for the auras and sensory symptoms associated with the seizure.

## CASE REPORTS

There are several reports of known or suspected cases of patients with reasonably confirmed parietal NCSE (20-27) (Table 9.1). These reports illustrate typical symptoms, as well as EEG and imaging correlates.

Thomas and colleagues reported ictal asomatognosia associated with hemiparesis in a patient with concurrent right, parieto-temporal, 4-Hz, continuous spike-wave discharges (24). She had a history of recurrent "prolonged confusional states" but, on a routine office visit at 2:10 in the afternoon, was noted to have new clinical symptoms: "at the reception desk, she complained of having lost her handbag, which she was still holding with her left upper limb." A video-EEG study was begun at 2:45 pm and "showed continuous, high-amplitude, rhythmic spike-waves localized over the right temporo-parieto-occipital areas. Her clinical state was described by the authors (24).

> *Vigilance was normal, and the patient was oriented to time and space. She had no aphasia, subtracted sevens without a single error, and knew her name, address, telephone number, and the names and ages of her grandchildren. Slight head and eye deviation toward her left was associated with a left upper limb underutilization without left segmental loss of muscle strength. She had indifference and a left spatial neglect when she was asked to cross circles on paper.*

Although most cases of prolonged parietal seizure activity include descriptions of concomitant clinical symptoms, Wright and colleagues have reported a case of postictal prosopagnosia that followed a prolonged period of NCSE. This presentation was thought to represent postictal manifestations of parietal involvement during the seizure activity that was associated with a left fusiform gyrus malformation seen on imaging (27).

In some cases, clinical symptoms appear to involve more than 1 region. A 52-year-old man in complex partial status epilepticus involving the parietal lobe was described by Lukovits and colleagues (21) as presenting with variable semiology.

> *[The patient] presented with headache, personality changes, a right homonymous hemianopia, and mild receptive aphasia ... [and] ... motor neglect ... When asked to write, he put the pen in his mouth like a cigarette.*

His EEG, performed 3 hours after "onset of his change in behavior showed continuous high-voltage, semirhythmic, sharp-and-slow waves in the left posterior temporal and parietal regions" (21).

## DIAGNOSIS

The diagnosis of parietal lobe NCSE depends on identification of symptoms or signs of long-lasting (typically 30 minutes or more) parietal lobe impairment or dysfunction, which may be either stable or fluctuating, due to epileptic seizures. The diagnosis is based on reports or observations of prolonged, persistent somatosensory phenomena or cognitive impairments clinically consistent with parietal lobe dysfunction due to epilepsy. Parietal lobe functions that may be impaired due to NCSE are varied, as was described earlier in this chapter. Of particular importance in parietal NCSE, one should anticipate that the deficits will vary and fluctuate more over short periods rather than remain fixed or stable, as they might after a static lesion such as tumor or stroke.

The EEG is very important for confirming the epileptic nature of a functional disturbance

**TABLE 9.1** SELECTED CASES OF REPORTED PARIETAL NONCONVULSIVE STATUS EPILEPTICUS

| Sex and age, y | Symptoms and Findings | Imaging results | EEG results | Treatment | Outcome | Etiology | Ref |
|---|---|---|---|---|---|---|---|
| M 62 | Alteration of consciousness with rightward eye and head deviation; right facial twitching | MRI: normal SPECT: left posterior parietal hyperperfusion | Left posterior sharp waves | Glucose control | Repeat studies normal at 20 days; recurrence in 2 years | Nonketotic hyperglycemia | Huang et al, 2005 (22) |
| F 69 | Asomatognosia, "she complained of having lost her handbag, which she was still holding with her left upper limb." | MRI: "enlargement of the right ventricular system without any focal lesion" | "High-amplitude, 4-Hz, rhythmic spike-waves, with ... amplitude gradient from right temporo-parieto-occipital to central regions" | PHT | Improved – seizure free | "Anton-Babinski syndrome of non-vascular origin"; history of epilepsy | Thomas et al, 1998 (24) |
| F 77 | Confusion, agitation, visual and auditory hallucinations; saccadic eye movements and hyperreflexia. Formal neuro-psychological testing: language dysfunction with perseveration, comprehension difficulty and Balint syndrome | MRI: hyperintense signal changes bilaterally | Rhythmic sharp-waves right parieto-occipital lobe | IV fluids, furosemide, IV PHT, CBZ | Improved | Hypercalcemia | Kumpfel T et al., 2000[26] |
| F 61 | Asomatognosia and alien hand | MRI: right GBM | Continuous right frontotemporal spikes | IV diazepam | Improved | GBM | Feinberg TE et al., 1998[18] |
| M 75 | Confusion | n/a | "frequent and recurrent seizure activity arising from the right | IV PHT, IV PB, IV propofol, IV thiopental | Cardiac arrest following prior improvement | No prior history of seizures; hypoxia; unclear | Fernandez-Torre et al., 2006[26] |

| | | | | | | | |
|---|---|---|---|---|---|---|---|
| | | | temporo-occipital junction and spreading rapidly to the temporal areas" | | | | |
| M 52 | Homonymous hemianopia, motor neglect, hyperreflexia, visual agnosia | CT: ring enhancing hypo-dense mass | "continuous, high-voltage, semirhythmic, sharp-and-slow waves over the left posterior temporal parietal" region | IV lorazepam, IV PHT | Improved; EEG normal at 2 months | IV contrast | Lukovitz et al., 1996[21] |
| F 67 | "almost continuous" déjà vu with "peculiar bodily feelings, e.g. tingling in the left side of her face, a feeling of floating in the air looking down on her body and a feeling of a compulsion to do things;" prosopagnosia | MRI: lesion, fusiform gyrus | "focal right temporal abnormality and generalized spike and wave discharges" on initial EEG | Not listed | Not listed | "benign vascular lesion such as venous angioma" | Wright et al., 2006[27] |
| F 25 | Memory difficulties, aphasia, apraxia of right hand; paresthesias of right arm and face; confusion | PET hyper-metabolism in left parietal lobe, hypometabolism in frontal lobes, left more than right; 1.5-T MRI: normal; 3-T MRI: small focal cortical dysplasia | Slowing "over anterior derivations … more pronounced on the left, but no epileptic activity" | LTG, PHT, clobazam; LTG increased | Seizure-free 10 days after hospital admission | Possible cortical dysplasia | Paesschen et al., 2007[36] |

***Abbreviations:*** *M, male; MRI, magnetic resonance imaging; CT, computerized axial tomography scan; SPECT, single-photon emission computed tomography; F, female; PHT, phenytoin; IV, intravenous CBZ, carbamazepine; PB, phenobarbital; status epilepticus, status epilepticus; GBM, glioblastoma multiforme; EEG, electroencephalogram.*

as due to NCSE, particularly in parietal lobe NCSE (3,28). The diagnosis is most secure when an EEG obtained during the period of functional impairment or concern shows some form of continuous or waxing-and-waning pattern of epileptiform activity. Moreover, this epileptiform activity characteristically coincides with the parietal neurologic dysfunction attributed to NCSE and typically subsides with cessation of the clinical symptoms, as for example after medication treatment (2,3,28).

The EEG should not be considered the sole basis for diagnosing parietal lobe NCSE and must be considered within the presenting clinical context. There are epileptiform disturbances or encephalopathies of other types associated with spikes or sharp-waves on the EEG that should be distinguished from typical NCSE. Patients with structural lesions such as strokes or tumors may have associated epileptiform activity, such as periodic lateralized epileptiform discharges, that may be surrogates of the severity of brain injury, with the epileptiform discharges themselves not clearly the cause of the impaired function (3). A diagnosis of NCSE is most secure when there is good evidence that the epileptiform activity on the EEG is judged to be the cause of the impaired function (3). This is not always easy to determine but should be a central consideration in establishing a diagnosis of parietal lobe NCSE. Brain imaging, such as SPECT scanning, may also provide confirming or corroborative data to help make the diagnosis of parietal NCSE when the symptoms do not provide adequate localization or convincing evidence (29-31).

In some patients, treatment with antiepileptic drugs, such as benzodiazepines, in conjunction with EEG monitoring and clinical assessment can help demonstrate that epileptiform activity is actually causing functional impairment, thereby confirming a clinical diagnosis of NCSE. Indeed, if the epileptic activity is abolished with antiepileptic therapy and the patient simultaneously improves clinically and symptoms resolve, that is compelling evidence that the process in question is indeed NCSE (3). For some subtle manifestations of parietal lobe dysfunction, such as visual-spatial disorientation, however, determining the resolution of clinical symptoms may be difficult, particularly in situations in which there is substantial postictal confusion or lethargy.

Ictal SPECT may help to identify an area of seizure activity in 70% to 90% of patients with epilepsy (29-31). This is a relatively new technology for which there is not as much experience as with EEG, but it can identify active seizure regions in focal or localized status epilepticus. In general, there is an area of increased metabolic activity during the seizure or status epilepticus and decreased metabolic activity postictally (29-31).

## MANAGEMENT OF PARIETAL NCSE

The medical treatment of patients with parietal lobe NCSE is similar to that for other localization-related or partial NCSE. Imaging studies, including ictal SPECT and positron emission tomography, however, may not provide definitely epileptic or seizure-localizing findings, and EEG often shows lateralizing, but not necessarily localizing, abnormalities. Therefore, identification of the area of seizure onset often depends on the patient's report of auras and other clinical symptoms. In addition, because parietal NCSE may consist of a prolonged aura without spread to adjacent regions, there may be no other associated symptoms and limited imaging or EEG changes, as has been reported in other cases of simple partial seizures (28).

Therapy should be prompt and appropriate but need not be overly aggressive because the morbidity and mortality in most patients with NCSE is not as severe as for convulsive status epilepticus (1,3). Antiepileptic drug therapy should be initiated with continuous video-EEG monitoring to determine the effects of therapy in patients who may have subtle or difficult-to-assess symptoms, such as those of parietal lobe dysfunction. Outcomes in patients with convulsive status epilepticus and NCSE are largely dependent on the etiology of the status (2,3,32,33). Still, there is evidence that some patients with complex partial status epilepticus (and at least 1 patient with parietal lobe NCSE

[26]) had status epilepticus associated with long-lasting or permanent neurologic deficits (2,3).

Surgical resection of the involved area of cortex has been reported, but it is not first-line therapy because of the difficulty in the localization of the ictal onset and because of surgical risks (34,35). Focal cortical resection of the right mesial parietal region has been performed on a 4-year-old girl who presented with an aura of left hand pain followed by tonic activity, who had failed both medical management and multiple subpial transection (35). This resulted in seizure freedom without significant neurologic deficit 2 years postoperatively (35). Other series have suggested that 20% of nontumor and 75% of tumor cases of parietal lobe epilepsy may be rendered seizure-free by resective surgery (33,34). Because parietal lobe surgery carries a risk of a fixed sensory deficit, the risk-benefit ratio must be considered, and medical treatment options should be exhausted before proceeding to surgery.

## CONCLUSIONS

Parietal NCSE is not a well-recognized or common entity. It fits in the general category of partial NCSE and may present as compex partial status epilepticus. Described above are the clinical features expected in such cases, with documentation of a number of examples that may fall under the general rubric of parietal lobe NCSE. Clinical features that suggest parietal NCSE include parietal lobe dysfunction, such as focal hemisensory symptoms, left-right disorientation, dysmorphopsias, and confusion persisting for longer than 30 minutes. Once suspected clinically, parietal lobe NCSE is best confirmed by EEG localization of epileptiform changes consistent with a focal status epilepticus. Alternatively, SPECT scanning or other imaging may support a diagnosis of focal parietal status epilepticus. Treatment follows the principles of management of other forms of partial NCSE but not necessarily the more intensive treatment often proposed for convulsive status epilepticus (1,2).

## REFERENCES


1. Dodson WE, DeLorenzo RJ, Pedley TA, Shinnar S, Treiman DM, Wannamaker BB. Treatment of convulsive status epilepticus: recommendations of the epilepsy foundation of America working group on status epilepticus. JAMA 1993;270:854-9.
2. Krumholz A, Sung GY, Fisher RH, Barry E, Bergey GK, Grattan LM. Complex partial status epilepticus accompanied by serious morbidity and mortality. Neurology 1995;45:1499-504.
3. Krumholz A. Epidemiology and evidence for mortality and morbidity in nonconvulsive status epilepticus. J Clin Neurophysiol 1999;16:314-322.
4. Shorvon S. Status epilepticus: its clinical features and treatment in children and adults. Cambridge, England: Cambridge University Press; 1994.
5. Kaplan PW. History of status epilepticus. In: Drislane FW, ed. Status Epilepticus: a Clinical Perspective. Totowa, NJ: Humana Press; 2005:3-10.
6. Drislane FW. Types of status epilepticus: definitions and classification. In: Drislane FW, ed. Status Epilepticus: a Clinical Perspective. Totowa, NJ: Humana Press; 2005:11-31.
7. Gastaut H. Classification of status epilepticus. In: Delgado-Escueta AV, Wasterlain CG, Treiman DM, Porter RJ, eds. Status Epilepticus. Adv Neurol. Vol. 34. New York, NY: Raven Press; 1983:15-35.
8. Critchley M. The Parietal Lobes, 3rd ed. New York, NY: Hafner Publishing Company, Inc.; 1969.
9. Penfield W, Jasper HH. Epilepsy and the Functional Anatomy of the Human Brain, 2nd ed. Boston, MA: Little, Brown; 1954.
10. Kolb B, Whishaw I. Fundamentals of Human Neuropsychology, 3rd ed. New York, NY: WH Freeman & Co.;1990:354-364.
11. Sveinbjornsdottir S, Duncan JS. Parietal and occipital epilepsy: a review. Epilepsia 1993;34:493-521.
12. Siegel AM, Williamson PD. Parietal lobe epilepsy. Adv Neurol 2000;84:189-199.
13. Tuxhorn I, Kerdar MS. Somatosensory Auras. In: Lüders HO, Noachtar S, eds. Epileptic Seizures: Pathophysiology and Clinical Semiology. Philadephia, PA: Churchill Livingstone; 2000:286-297.

14. Tuxhorn I. Clinical characteristics of somatosensory auras. Epilepsia 1997;38(suppl 3): 221.
15. Mauguiére F, Courjon J. Somatosensory epilepsy: A review of 127 cases. Brain 1978;101:307-332.
16. Alemayehu S, Bergey GK, Barry E, Krumholz A, Wolf A, Fleming CP, Frear EJ. Panic attacks as ictal manifestations of parietal lobe seizures. Epilepsia 1995;36:824-830.
17. Manford M, Shorvon SD. Prolonged sensory or visceral symptoms: an under-diagnosed form of non-convulsive focal (simple partial) status epilepticus. J Neurol Neurosurg Psychiatry 1992;55:714-716.
18. Feinberg TE, Roane DM, Cohen J. Partial status epilepticus associated with asomatognosia and alien hand-like behaviors. Arch Neurol 1998;55:1574-1576.
19. Salanova V, Andermann F, Rasmussen T, Olivier A, Quesney LF. Parietal lobe epilepsy: Clinical manifestations and outcome in 82 patients treated surgically between 1929 and 1988. Brain 1995;118:607-627.
20. Cascino GD, Hulihan JF, Sharbrough FW, Kelly PJ. Parietal lobe lesional epilepsy: electroclinical correlation and operative outcome. Epilepsia 1993;34:522-527.
21. Lukovits T, Fadul CE, Pipas JM, Williamson PD. Nonconvulsive status epilepticus after intravenous contrast medium administration. Epilepsia 1996;37:1117-1120.
22. Huang CW, Hsieh YJ, Pai MC, Tsai JJ, Huang CC. Nonketotic hyperglycemia-related epilepsia partialis continua with ictal unilateral parietal hyperperfusion. Epilepsia 2005;46:1843-1844.
23. Fazekas F, Kapeller P, Schmidt R, Stollberger R, Varosanec S, Offenbacher H, Fazekas G, Lechner H. Magnetic resonance imaging and spectroscopy findings after focal status epilepticus. Epilepsia 1995;16:946-949.
24. Thomas P, Giraud K, Alchaar H, Chatel M. Ictal asomatognosia with hemiparesis. Neurology 1998;51:280-282.
25. Kumpfel T, Lechner C, Auer K, Kraft E, Lydtin H, Trenkwalder C. Nonconvulsive status epilepticus with marked neuropsychiatric manifestations and MRI changes after the treatment of hypercalcemia. Acta Neurol Scand 2000; 102:337-339.
26. Fernandez-Torre JL, Figols J, Martinez-Martinez M, Gonzalez-Rato J, Calleja J. Localisation-related nonconvulsive status epilepticus: Further evidence of permanent cerebral damage. J Neurol 2006;253:392-395.
27. Wright H, Wardlaw J, Young AW, Zeman A. Prosopagnosia following nonconvulsive status epilepticus associated with a left fusiform gyrus malformation. Epilepsy Behav 2006;9:197-203.
28. Williamson PD, Spencer S. Clinical and EEG features of complex partial seizures of extratemporal origin. Epilepsia 1986;27(Suppl 2):546-563.
29. Ho SS, Berkovic SF, Newton MR, Austin MC, McKay WJ, Bladin PF. Parietal lobe epilepsy: clinical features and seizure localization by ictal SPECT. Neurology 1994;44:2277-2284.
30. Newton MR, Austin MC, Chan JG, McKay WJ, Rowe CC, Berkovic SF. Ictal SPECT using technetium-9m- HMPAO: methods for rapid preparation and optimal deployment of tracer during spontaneous seizures. J Nucl Med 1993;34:666-670.
31. Hwang DI, Kim JH, Park SW, Han MH, Yu IK, Lee SH, Lee DS, Lee SK, Chung CK, Chang KH. Comparative analysis of MR imaging, positron emission tomography, and ictal single-photon emission CT in patients with neocortical epilepsy. Am J Neuroradiol 2001;22:937-946.
32. Barry E, Hauser WA. Status epilepticus: the interaction of epilepsy and acute brain disease. Neurology 1993;43:1473-1478.
33. Salanova V, Andermann F, Rasmussen T, Olivier A, Quesney LF. Tumoural parietal lobe epilepsy. Brain 1995;118:1289-1304.
34. Olivier A, Boling W. Surgery of parietal and occipital epilepsy. Adv Neurol 2000;84:533-575.
35. Ng Y, Kim HL, Wheless JW. Successful neurosurgical treatment of childhood complex partial status epilepticus with focal resection. Epilepsia 2003;44:468-471.
36. Van Paesschen W, Porke K, Fannes K, Vandenberghe R, Palmini A, Van Laere KV, Dupont P. Cognitive deficits during status epilepticus and time course of recovery: A case report. Epilepsia 2007;48:1979-1983.

# CHAPTER 10

# TEMPORAL LOBE NONCONVULSIVE STATUS EPILEPTICUS

HEINZ GREGOR WIESER AND MICHAEL FISCHER

The term aura usually refers to that portion of a seizure that is subjectively experienced before loss of consciousness and for which memory is retained. In older terminology, a simple partial seizure without motor phenomena is identical to an aura, but, when consciousness is lost, the aura is, in fact, the first symptom of a psychomotor or complex partial seizure (1). The term *isolated aura* (or *aura in isolation*) is often found in outcome classifications and in driver's license regulations. Although an epileptic aura is always based on an epileptic seizure discharge, not all electrographic epileptic seizure discharges are accompanied by an aura, eg, circumscribed hippocampal discharges (or afterdischarges induced by electrical stimulation) might completely escape subjective and objective clinical detection. To the best of our knowledge, Scott and Masland first described somatosensory hallucinations as a continuous symptom, ie, as an aura continua (2). The term *aura continua* can be found in Karbowski as a synonym for continuous psychomotor status (3,18). Wolf used it as synonym for status epilepticus of focal sensory seizures or for hallucinosis (4-6).

The question of whether temporal lobe psychomotor seizures could also occur in a prolonged condition, as in status epilepticus, and whether such activity could be the underlying cause for prolonged twilight states was, for a long time, controversial. As late as 1963, Landolt noted "... finally there remain those cases that we personally know from the literature only, for example, the case of Gastaut and that of Schorsch, in whom obviously the 'generalized state of twilight attacks' continued for days resulting in a twilight state. We have to ask us [sic], however, if these cases have not been petit mal status." From Landolt's statement (7), it becomes very clear that petit mal status (ie, absence status) was sharply delineated from psychomotor status epilepticus, which is a distinction that was no longer respected with the widely used term *nonconvulsive status epilepticus* (NCSE). Trousseau, Prichard, Bright, Hughlings Jackson, and Charcot all provided descriptions of NCSE (8-16). A fuller historic account of NCSE can be found in Chapter 1.

The most important early literature dealing with psychomotor status epilepticus focused on the phenomenologic description of this condition, as evidenced by the review of Wolf, who discussed 7 cases and added 2 of his own (4). In his description, Wolf followed Janz, who distinguished the discontinuous form, characterized by the occurrence of psychomotor attacks that follow each other at 2- to 10-minute intervals, from the continuous form (17). Under the continuous form, Janz described 2 variants: (1) long-lasting sensory, somatosensory, or "psychic" seizures and (2) epileptic twilight states with productive-psychotic signs and symptoms.

In his 1979 symposium on status psychomotoricus, Karbowski referred to 36 published cases of psychomotor status in which the electroencephalogram (EEG) was sufficiently described and illustrated, and added 8 of his own cases (18). Seven additional publications appeared in 1978 (19-25).

## CLASSIFICATION

The most recent proposal of the International League Against Epilepsy Classification Core Group (26), an attempt to complete the earlier work of the Task Force on Classification and Terminology, differentiates "self-limited epileptic seizure types" from "status epilepticus." Under "status epilepticus," this report lists 9 headings: (1) epilepsia partialis continua of Kojevnikov; (2) supplementary motor area status epilepticus; (3) aura continua; (4) dyscognitive focal (psychomotor, complex partial) status epilepticus; divided into (A) mesial temporal and (B) neocortical; (5) tonic-clonic status epilepticus; (6) absence status epilepticus; (7) myoclonic status epilepticus; (8) tonic status epilepticus and (9) subtle status epilepticus.

The explanatory text says that category 3, aura continua, is a rare but well-described manifestation of focal epilepsy. The symptoms depend on the localization. The attacks are usually without impairment of consciousness. The symptoms wax and wane, often for hours, and may be associated with a motor component, depending on the spread. Dysesthesia, painful sensations, and visual changes are examples. Limbic aura continua is the most common clinical pattern. Fear, an epigastric rising sensation, or other features may recur every few minutes for many hours, or for more than a day, without going on to seizures with impairment of awareness. Electrographic correlation is variable. The diagnosis must be entertained, particularly in patients with well-established epilepsy.

The explanatory text for the mesial temporal subtype of the dyscognitive focal (psychomotor, complex partial) status epilepticus is as follows: "Focal status epilepticus, predominantly involving mesial limbic structures, consists of serial dyscognitive focal ictal events without return of clear consciousness in between. Onset can be limited to one side or can alternate between hemispheres."

Dyscognitive focal status epilepticus often evolves from, or alternates with, aura continua, so that much overlap between aura continua and psychomotor status exists in the literature, and cases are finally categorized according to their full semiology (ie, as psychomotor status, although, for a certain period of time, they would fulfill the criteria of an aura continua [27,28]).

Therefore, with regard to the new proposed International League Against Epilepsy classification, temporal NCSE comprises and overlaps with aura continua, dyscognitive focal (psychomotor, complex partial) status epilepticus, and subtle status epilepticus. See also Chapter 2 on the classification of NCSE.

## PATHOPHYSIOLOGY

In humans, the underlying pathophysiology of the various subtypes of NCSE has not been investigated in detail, so most remain speculation.

An aura continua reflects the intrinsic epileptogenic properties of a discharging epileptogenic neuronal network that remains "well controlled" with regard to spread. Obviously, in such a condition, there is no further propagation of the epileptic discharge and no further neuronal recruitment (ie, no relevant increase of the number of epileptically involved neurons). A hippocampal epileptic focus causing electrographic focal status epilepticus may be limited to a volume of less than 1 cm in diameter (29). Metaphorically, the "critical mass" necessary for the spread of the discharge is not reached. To a certain degree, however, waxing and waning occurs. The aura content is the product of the "interpretive cortex" (30), which deals with this discharging "epileptic focus." Mechanistically, status epilepticus represents the failure of the natural seizure-suppressing mechanisms responsible for seizure termination (31). Proposed operational definitions of status epilepticus do not adequately reflect the underlying mechanisms involved in status epilepticus. As Engel rightly pointed out, mechanisms that prevent active inhibition—desynchronization of hypersynchronous discharges and depolarization block—have to be considered. In addition, progressive features that contribute to subsequent functional and structural brain disturbances and maturational factors may be important (26).

Several of our patients who have undergone selective amygdalohippocampectomy (32) because of drug-resistant mesial temporal lobe epilepsy, and in whom this operation was successful without further explicit seizures, experienced persisting auras in the first postoperative months. Moreover, a few patients claimed that the feeling of an impending seizure would, with some fluctuation of intensity, persist for hours or even days and, thus, mimic an aura continua. In such cases, one might assume that the removal of amygdala and hippocampal formation suppressed manifest psychomotor seizures, but the temporal and insular neocortex were still "epileptically disturbed" and able to produce prolonged aura phenomena. The so-called "running down" phenomenon of such postoperatively persisting auras lends further support to the idea that, for the full expression of psychomotor seizures, both the mesial limbic and neocortical cortexes are necessary. Such a view differentiates between the epileptogenic zone and the seizure-onset zone with a further conceptual differentiation of the seizure-onset zone into an "actual" and "potential" seizure-onset zone (33).

The clinical pathophysiology of aura continua remains unclear. A modification of the electrographic characteristics of focal status epilepticus by adequately addressed sensory stimuli has been documented in a long-lasting musical aura continua with circumscribed discharges in the right Heschl gyrus (27). Antiepileptic drugs may play a role by changing seizure threshold and preventing spread. A de novo right temporal NCSE was reported during tiagabine adjunctive therapy in a 30-year-old woman with infantile-onset epilepsy due to a left temporal gliotic area (34). Similar observations have been described with the use of levetiracetam (35) and other antiepileptic drugs.

There are a number of animal models of temporal lobe complex partial status epilepticus, including kainic acid in the mouse, lithium and pilocarpine, and electrical stimulation of the hippocampus or amygdala in the rat (36-41), that provide insight into the mechanisms underlying temporal lobe complex partial status epilepticus. A fuller treatment of these issues is given in Chapter 7. These models, centered in the limbic system, provide a good experimental basis for suggesting that psychomotor status epilepticus may induce long-term sequelae (40) and provide possible mechanisms for neuronal damage and long-term epileptogenesis (41-52). There is experimental evidence for cerebral reorganization and possible opportunities for the use of protective agents (53-58).

Thus, from experimental evidence, it might be concluded that long-term consequences of status epilepticus in the limbic system include alterations in patterns of expression of neurotransmitter receptors and in the function of excitatory and inhibitory synapses, cell loss, and circuit rearrangements within the limbic system. This brain damage can contribute to the development of epilepsy, ie, a condition of recurrent spontaneous seizures. Conversely, development of an epileptic condition enhances the susceptibility of the limbic system to trigger status epilepticus discharges.

## LOCALIZATION

Theoretically, each part of the cortex, and probably deep nuclei as well, can give rise to long-lasting localized epileptiform discharges. According to their functional specialization, the epileptic dysfunction of a localized ganglionic structure of the brain may give rise to "positive" or "negative" symptoms of a particular quality. The symptoms and signs are often the result of the interpretation of the not-discharging "healthy" brain, which is confronted with a pathologic "bombardment" or an epileptic dysfunctional network. This implies that the localization of the cortex in which symptoms are produced (the "symptomatogenic zone") and the localization in which the epileptiform discharges are generated (the "primary epileptogenic zone" or, better, the "seizure-onset zone") are not necessarily concordant.

An intriguing question is whether certain brain regions are more predisposed than others to such a circumscribed and long-lasting epileptiform discharge behavior. By analogy with epilepsia partialis continua and dyscognitive focal (psychomotor) or limbic status, it is reasonable to assume that certain brain regions are, in fact, predisposed to this discharge behavior. From posttraumatic epilepsy, it is well known that the central and mesiotemporal lobe cortexes are more seizure prone than are other cortexes, but it is less clear whether region-specific differences exist to limit seizure discharges in time.

It is obvious that limbic aura continua and mesial temporal dyscognitive focal status epilepticus involve the limbic system, with the hippocampal formations and nuclei amygdalae as their core structures.

The hippocampal formation has been shown to be able to discharge in a status-like manner during depth recordings. Discharge associated signs and symptoms might be subtle (electrical status epilepticus with minor symptoms) but consistent with hemisphere-specific deficits in tachistoscopic lexical recognition tasks and face-matching tasks, respectively (29). (See Case 1 and Figure 10.1). This is in line with more recent $H_2{}^{15}O$ positron emission tomography data attributing associative functions (ie, associative binding) to the hippocampal formation (59-62).

The nuclei amygdalae are candidates for explaining the rich and multifaceted signs and symptoms observed in limbic seizures and limbic status epilepticus. This is because nearly all cortical areas of the temporal lobe, major parts of the frontal lobe, and the insular cortex project to the amygdala (63). Some amygdaloid nuclei receive several cortical sensory projections with substantial convergence of cortical input. It is well documented that visual, auditory, olfactory, and, to some extent, taste information reaches the amygdala. Somatosensory input is less clear, but there is reason to believe that all 5 modalities have some convergence in the dorsomedial part of the lateral nucleus of the amygdala. For example, the dorsomedial part of the lateral nucleus receives projections from the orbitofrontal area, which responds to olfactory stimulation; this part is also the major amygdaloid projection zone of the cortical taste area. In addition, there are posterior insular cortex projections to this area carrying visceral, and probably other somatic information. Moreover, auditory input from the temporal polar cortex projects powerfully to this region. Visual projections are directed primarily to the dorsolateral part of the lateral nucleus (64).

Efferent fibers from the amygdala are the stria terminalis and, to a lesser degree, the ventro-fugal bundle, with overlapping targeting areas in the medial and rostral hypothalamus and regio septalis, as well as the posterior part of the magnocellular Ncl dorso-medialis thalami. The latter connects the amygdala with the orbitofrontal cortex and constitutes a part of the second circuit (besides the Papez circuit), ie, the basolateral limbic circuit, formulated by Yakovlev and reemphasized by Livingston and Escobar (65,66).

Except for a few illustrations with prolonged discharges in the anterior cingulate

## CASE 1

This case is discussed in detail in reference 29. In short, this woman was admitted at age 26 because of medically refractory psychomotor seizures during the previous 3 years, with frequent secondary generalization. She had experienced isolated epigastric auras since 3 years of age and several episodes of long-lasting (up to 10 days) isolated gustatory aura continua. Ictal semiology was fairly constant and typically consisted of an unpleasant gustatory or epigastric aura or both, followed by arrest, progressive clouding of consciousness, salivation, and oroalimentary automatisms with marked flushing and then cyanosis. Following a left selective amygdalohippocampectomy at age 27, the patient was seizure free, and antiepileptic medication could be withdrawn. Because she had a secondary generalized seizure 3 days after childbirth at age 35 and some isolated gustatory auras, carbamazepine was reintroduced. With this antiepileptic treatment, she is again aura

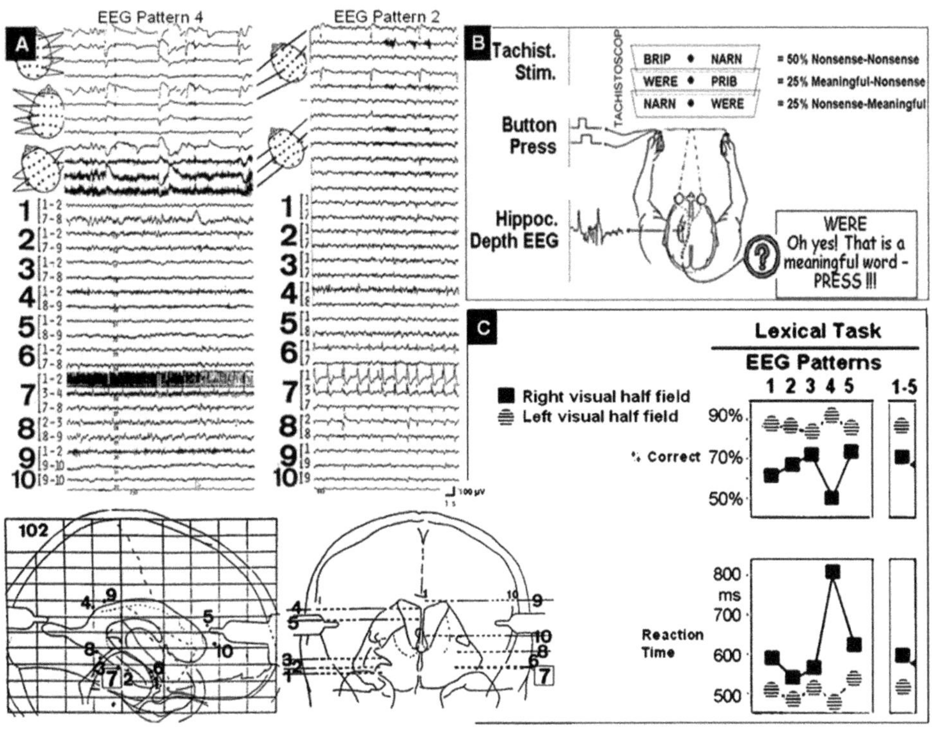


**Figure 10.1** Illustration of left hippocampal electrical status activity during the lexical decision task. A Combined scalp- and depth-electrode electroencephalogram (EEG) showing the high-frequency spike ("tonic" = EEG pattern 4) and slow "clonic" (EEG pattern 2) discharge of the left hippocampus (inner contacts of electrode 7). Note that the left EEG section is a bipolar recording and the right EEG section is a common average reference recording. The scalp EEG does not pick up the hippocampal activity. There is moderate propagation to the homolateral amygdala (6/1-2), and this synchronized epileptiform activity also affects the common intracerebral average reference, giving rise to some "erroneous" activity with opposite polarity in the scalp EEG.

The test situation during the tachistoscopically presented lexical decision task is shown in panel (B): 50% of the stimuli consists of 2 matched nonsense words (example: BRIP–NARN); 50% of the stimuli pairs consist of a nonsense word and a matched meaningful high-frequency filler word (example: WERE), either in the left (25%) or in the right (25%) visual hemifield. (C) Results of lexical decision task during left hippocampal status activity. Overall result (right, 1-5) and breakdown according to the left hippocampal EEG pattern. 1: Normal and flat. 2: Slow "clonic" sharp-waves < 1/second. 3: Fast "clonic" sharp-waves > 1/second; 4: High-frequency "tonic" spike discharge. 5: Tonic-clonic. Note that the number of correct button presses during tonic discharges drops to chance level (50% correct responses) when stimuli addressed the left hemisphere with its hippocampus epileptically discharging (ie, right visual hemifield stimuli), whereas the percentage of correct responses to stimuli addressing the right hemisphere (ie, left visual hemifield) in general was high (87%), indicating a reversed hemispheric language dominance during this left hippocampal status, and even showed a kind of additional compensatory improvement during left hippocampal tonic discharges (EEG pattern 4). Measurement of reaction time (mean of both hands) likewise resulted in a marked increase but only for stimuli addressing the epileptically disturbed left hemisphere during tonic hippocampal discharges. Reprinted with permission from Lippincott Williams & Wilkins (Modified from [29] and [159]).

gyrus associated with confusion and emotional and autonomic signs and symptoms, and a few cases with kakosmia from frontal orbital cortexes, there is little evidence for the existence of isolated limbic status epilepticus in areas other than the temporal lobe (32,67,68).

## CLINICAL MANIFESTATION OF THE LIMBIC AURA CONTINUA

Typically, an aura lasts seconds to minutes, is stereotypic, and evolves to other ictal clinical features, including loss of awareness. If an aura occurs in isolation, ie, is self-limited in time and without further progression, it is more appropriately called a focal-onset seizure without spread (simple partial seizure in the older terminology). Rarely, such symptoms last hours to days (and according to a recent report, exceptionally even years) and are then called aura continua, ie, represent a form of focal status.

Psychic seizures were referred to by Jackson as so-called dreamy states, including déjà-vu experiences and ictal reminiscences (69-72). Jackson subsequently referred to such events as "psychical." Gowers reported on 25 patients with "psychical auras," with 10 having an "emotional aura;" all of these patients had fear (73). Penfield introduced the term "experiential" to describe such mental phenomena and divided the patients' experiences into illusions and hallucinations, which could be predominantly visual, auditory, or both, or an "unclassified" experience such as a dream, a flashback, or a memory without further description. Lennox referred to 3 categories of "psychic seizures," which are (1) dream states, feeling of unreality, or illusions; (2) hallucinations; and (3) mild confusion or disorientation, a feeling of strangeness without loss of memory or consciousness. Experiential means that the mental phenomena have a relevance to the patient's past; Gloor specified that they typically combine elements of perception, memory, and affect (74). Mesial temporal lobe seizures may present as anxiety disorders (75). The principal ictal "psychic phenomena" may be listed as follows: perceptual hallucinations (visual, auditory, olfactory, gustatory, rarely vertiginous), mnemonic (déjà/jamais vu/entendu/vécu, memory recall, memory gaps/amnesia), emotional (fear, sadness, pleasure, sexual emotion, emotional distress, anger), and other (change in reality, depersonalization, feeling of other presence, doppelgänger—heautoscopy (out-of-body experience), forced thinking, and distortion of body image (32,76-78) (Case 2 and Figure 10.2). The epileptogenic (or symptomatogenic?) zone of these experiential phenomena can be localized to the amygdala, hippocampus, parahippocampal gyrus, and temporal neocortex (79).

Ictal depression and anxiety in temporal lobe epilepsy is common (80). Henriksen, as well as McLachlan and Blume, described status epilepticus with fear as the outstanding clinical expression (81,82). A large body of literature exists on this topic (83-84). Ictal laughter (85) is usually associated with hypothalamic pathology, mainly hamartoma, in which gelastic seizures are the hallmark.

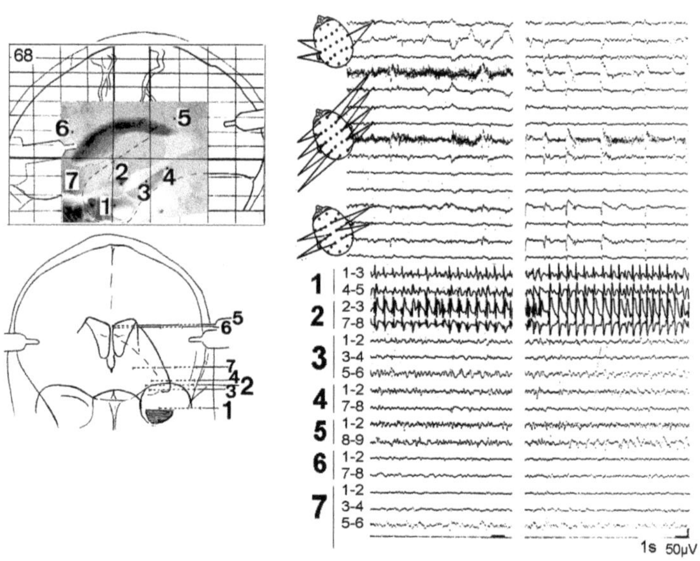


**Figure 10.2** Simultaneous scalp- and depth-electrode electroencephalogram (EEG) during a rage attack of 6 minutes' duration. The second and fourth minute are shown. The ictal, rhythmic, and clonic 1/second discharge is restricted to the depth electrodes 1 and 2 (electrode 2 targeting the left amygdala) and is not seen in the scalp EEG. Note the contrast medium–filled cyst after ventriculography Reprinted with permission from Georg Thieme Verlag (Modified from Wieser 1979 [76] and 1983 [67]).

**CASE 2**

Since age 9, this 45-year-old man has experienced 2 types of psychomotor seizures: (1) paroxysmal speech disturbances and (2) fits of rage leading to brawls and consequently to internments. For years he was thought to be an aggressive "psychopath," although the episodes were suggestive of epileptic seizures: he abruptly raised his hands and raved, or suddenly became speechless, or indiscriminately attacked and hit anyone around. Except for head trauma at age 4, his medical history was unremarkable. Radiographic studies under stereotactic conditions (répèrage as a precondition for stereo-electroencephalography) showed a left temporal-basal cyst extending to the temporal horn. Histologic examination of the removed brain tissue (parts of the left anterior basal temporal lobe together with the lesion) revealed a small capillary hemangioblastoma. Following surgical treatment, the patient had no further aggressive outbursts and was seizure free for a period of 4.5 years. Then, after head trauma, seizures recurred, and he again underwent surgery at age 35 with removal of the left hippocampus, with moderate seizure outcome.

For many authors, the so-called interictal personality and behavior syndrome of temporal lobe epilepsy, as well as other described personality peculiarities, are also intimately linked with an active temporal lobe epilepsy (86,87).

The causal relationship, however, usually remains a guess because very localized ongoing epileptic discharges in deep brain regions cannot be picked up on the routine scalp EEG. Pontius has reported on motiveless firesetting and has implicated partial limbic seizure kindling by revived memories of fires in what she called "limbic psychotic trigger reaction" (88,89).

Olfactory symptoms can be localized to anterior perforate, prepiriform cortex, lateral olfactory gyrus, periamygdalar cortex, entorhinal cortex, amygdala, septal nuclei, and hypothalamus (70,72,90). Mesial temporal limbic status with olfactory symptoms has been documented (91).

Gustatory symptoms can be localized to the parietal operculum near insula, anterior insula, and probably to the anterior mesial structures (14,92). A "gustatory aura continua" was the leading symptom of case 4 in our 1985 paper (29), with left hippocampal status activity in the depth EEG (see Case 2 and Figure 10.2). It was also associated with subtle higher cognitive deficits detected with a tachistoscopically presented lexical decision task. Seshia and McLachlan reported on 1 patient with a long-lasting metallic taste for 2 years (a 46-year-old with left temporal seizure origin, symptoms abolished after surgery, and oligodendroglioma) and another with foul taste for 5 years (a 34-year-old with right temporal seizure origin, symptoms abolished after surgery, and mesial temporal sclerosis) (93).

Auditory symptoms can be localized to auditory cortex and Heschl gyrus with a tonotopical organization. Schiffter and Straschill, as well as Wieser, described aura continua musicalis (27,94). A report on Wieser's patient was published under the heading "psychomotor status epilepticus" because of the aura continua with musical hallucinations (the patient experienced a song that was well known and familiar to her) in "endless repetition" and with stereo-EEG–documented restricted epileptiform discharges near Heschl's gyrus, with spread to the ipsilateral mesiobasal limbic structures, accompanied by alteration of consciousness. The beginning of this electrical epileptic status activity was accompanied by only musical hallucinations. Most cases with simple auditory hallucinations described in the literature do not fulfill the criteria of an aura continua (18,95). Blanke and colleagues described a patient with epilepsy (due to left parieto-temporal brain damage) suffering from the paroxysmal unilateral experience of hearing a person in her near extrapersonal space, associated with a deficit in spatial auditory perception and other paroxysmal disorders of somatognosia (96).

Vertigo can be localized to the vestibular cortex in the superior temporal gyrus rostral to the auditory cortex (14,76). Penfield and Jasper (14) described vertiginous aura continua (Case M. Bu.).

Manford and Shorvon reported on 4 patients with epigastric sensations (described as "butterflies," or "a thought in the stomach"), lasting up to several days, without associated behavior impairment (97).

Painful epileptic seizures are likewise uncommon but have been described (98-100). Direct evidence that long-lasting pain occurs as aura continua (ie, as a special form of focal status) is scanty, but this possibility should not be discarded. Indeed, Seshia and McLachlan report on 2 patients with long-lasting aura continua and "pain" (93). The first was a 21-year-old with nose pain for 2 years and a left temporal seizure origin. The symptom was abolished after surgery, without pathology in the resected tissue. The second patient was a 43-year-old with epigastric pain and a right temporal seizure origin; the symptom was abolished after resection of a glioma. Certain forms of pain per se might be closely linked to basic epileptic phenomena (101). The positive therapeutic effect of antiepileptic drugs in such circumstances is well known.

A special subtype in children, the so-called abdominal aura continua (abdominal epilepsy, recurring abdominal pain) has been described (102-104). Umbilical sensations in children and long-lasting borborygmi, widened pupils, pilomotor phenomena, goose-flesh or periodic shivering, and so on, also have been described (67,76,105-110). Finally, French authors have used a category of "erratic" for other rare manifestations and boundary conditions (28).

The main clinical features of autonomic seizures are abdominal sensations, apnea, hyperventilation, palpitations, arrhythmias and bradyarrhythmias, tachycardia, chest pain, cyanosis, erythema, flushing, genital sensations and orgasm, miosis/mydriasis/hippus, lacrimation, perspiration, pilomotor excitation ("gooseflesh"), urinary urgency and incontinence, and vomiting. Psychomotor seizures with autonomic symptoms as the leading feature are well known (111). Under the category of NCSE, Rabending and Fischer describe ictal bradycardia and asystole (112). Zijlmans and colleagues determined the prevalence of heart-rate changes and electrocardiographic abnormalities during epileptic seizures in 281 seizures in 81 patients (113). Electrocardiographic abnormalities were found in 26% of seizures (44% of patients), and long seizure duration increased the occurrence of electrocardiographic abnormalities. Nishiguchi and colleagues described a boy with occipital lobe epilepsy, showing a prolonged QTc in the ictal ECG (114).

In the Panayiotopoulus syndrome, Panayiotopoulus and Koutroumanidis documented recurrent autonomic status epilepticus with emesis (115-118). Autonomic status epilepticus is often accompanied by certain peculiarities of personality and behavior, and, therefore, we have described autonomic phenomena in the context of limbic dyscontrol syndrome (86,119). Common overt or subtle behavior changes include irritability, fear, panic, and sometimes existential emptiness or some other form of pathologic self-perception.

One of Seshia and McLachlan's patients suffered for 8 years from epigastric fear that started after surgery (with a left temporal seizure origin, and mesial temporal sclerosis). A particularly rare ictal or status symptom is aggression (120). We have described and illustrated a depth-EEG–recorded rage attack of 6 minutes' duration accompanied by restricted left amygdalar, rhythmic, 1-per-second, epileptiform discharges (Figure 99 in (67); see Case 2 and Figure 10.1). Limbic encephalitis might be associated with autonomic aura continua, and pilomotor status epilepticus has been recently reported in a case with voltage-gated potassium channel, antibody-positive, nonparaneoplastic limbic encephalitis (121).

## CLINICAL MANIFESTATIONS OF THE "MESIAL TEMPORAL DYSCOGNITIVE FOCAL STATUS EPILEPTICUS"

Dyscognitive focal status epilepticus often begins with a history of recurrent or prolonged simple partial seizures, or it may follow or precede a generalized convulsive seizure. Patients with mesial temporal lobe status epilepticus often are confused and exhibit variable responsiveness. Memory of the event is usually impaired. Behavior may fluctuate or be quite bizarre (see Case 3 and Figures 10.3 to 10.5). Often, patients exhibit clinical automatisms, as with typical psychomotor seizures, including repetitive lip-smacking, fumbling, or swallowing movements. Subtle nystagmus may be observed. The range of confusion can be great. Some patients present with mildly diminished responsiveness, and others with frank stupor or in a catatonic state. Aphasia and other localizing signs and symptoms (eg, dystonic hand posturing) may accompany mesial temporal dyscognitive focal status.

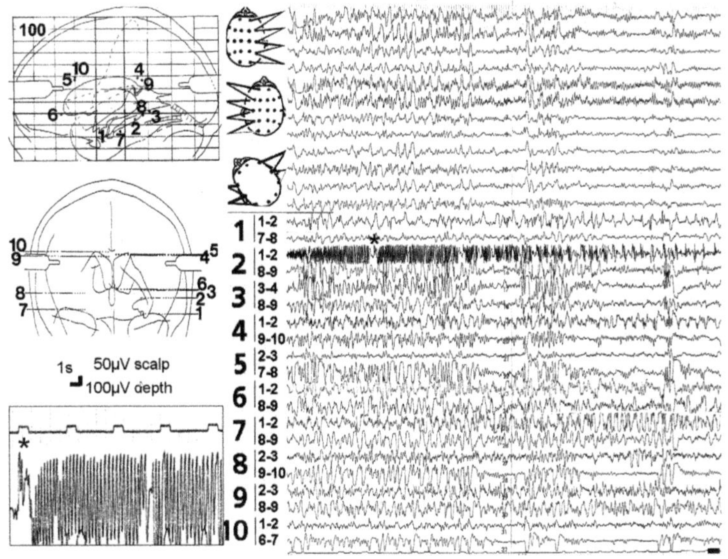


**Figure 10.3** Simultaneous scalp- and depth-electroencephalograms during an intermittent left hippocampal status epilepticus. Note the 14/second spike discharge seen in 2/1-2 (left hippocampus).

Onset can be sudden or insidious. In the best documented cases, the psychomotor status condition evolved gradually with minor symptoms (aura continua) in the beginning. The type of aura continua depended on the initially circumscribed discharge localization, reflecting the functional anatomy of the brain. In those circumstances in which the seizure-onset zone was in the neocortex, the hallucinations were often unimodal at the beginning (ie, visual if the EEG discharge was in the visual, and acoustic if the discharge was in the acoustic, cortex). With progressive spread of the ongoing epileptic discharges into mesial temporolimbic core structures, the quality of the hallucinations became more complex, and polymodal complex hallucinations, autonomous-vegetative signs, and signs and symptoms in the emotional and affective sphere prevailed. On the other hand, a recognizable seizure event might be at the beginning, and the psychomotor status manifests itself as a postictal twilight state, with ongoing discharges in some (usually temporolimbic) structures.

The typical overall gestalt of a dyscognitive focal mesial temporal lobe status is that of a fluctuating, waxing-waning condition with alterations of restless, sometimes fearful, and agitated behavior with memory flashbacks; experiential hallucinations; delusions; and hallucinations. Automatisms can be present. This contrasts with the more monotonous 3-per-second spike-slow-wave, petit mal status (spike-wave stupor), with clouded consciousness and slowed and impaired thinking. Nowack and Shaikh suggest that complex partial status epilepticus can progress through stages (defined by EEG) analogous to those described by Treiman in generalized convulsive status epilepticus (122,123).

Some authors have designated subtypes of partial NCSE according to the prevailing signs and symptoms (28,81,124). In dyscognitive focal status, the following categories of signs and symptoms can prevail: somatosensory signs and symptoms with dysesthesia as well as visual, acoustic, olfactory, gustatory, and autonomic phenomena. Abdominal status epilepticus is a special subtype that has been described

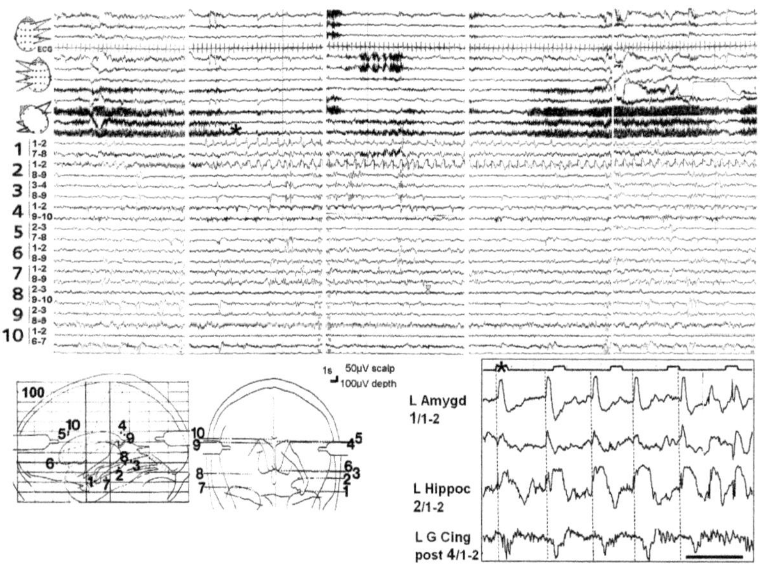


**Figure 10.4** Electroencephalography sections during a prolonged, mainly rhythmic, sharp-wave discharge of about 1.3/second in the left amygdala and left hippocampus, with spread to the posterior cingulate gyrus (4/1-2).

in children. Scott and Masland have described somatosensory hallucinations as a "continuous symptom" (2).

The predominance of dysphasic or aphasic signs and symptoms is far less frequent, but well-documented as the sole manifestation of focal status (125-138). Kirshner and colleagues described aphasia due to partial status epilepticus of the basal temporal language area (139), and Ozkaya and colleagues (140) aphasic status epilepticus with PLEDs in a bilingual patient with a clinical course that supports the belief that a second language area for a second language learned in later stages of life is located in an area different from that for the native language.

## DIFFERENTIAL DIAGNOSIS

An ongoing continuous or recurrent intermittent epileptic discharge might be suspected, and consequently proven with EEG and response to antiepileptic drug treatment in an epileptic person with known focal pathology. If the prolonged aura symptoms consist of phenomena that fit well with the localization of the epileptic discharge in terms

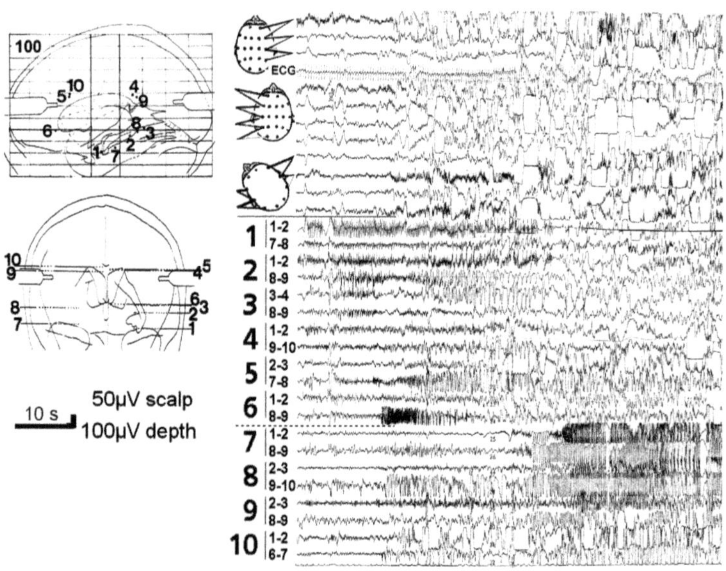


**Figure 10.5** During the intermittent left limbic electroencephalographic status activity (see Figures 10.3 and 10.4), some seizures evolved into full-blown psychomotor seizures, as illustrated here: The initial epileptic discharge predominates in the left amygdala (1/1-2) and left hippocampus (2/12). Then it spreads to the left posterior parahippocampal gyrus (3/3-4) before it affects the left frontal lobe (marked in 6/8-6). Later, with approximately 15 seconds delay, the right temporal structures are the main discharging structures (7/1-2 = right hippocampus).

**CASE 3**

Since age 9, this 41-year-old right-handed woman suffered initially from absence-like spells and later from frequent classic "psychomotor seizures" with an olfactory aura combined with a sense of diminished vision and hearing and with fear. The results of several neurologic examinations, including cranial computed tomographic (CT) scans, were all normal. A wide variety of antiepileptic drugs were tried without success. The years between age 11 and 16 were largely marked by a change in behavior and a social decline. Psychodynamic factors were thought to be responsible, and psychotherapy and family therapy were initiated, again without apparent success. This initially bright pupil declined in school very rapidly and was forced to leave school at age 15. She then spent more than a year in psychiatric hospitals. She developed aggressive behavior, rejected authority, and neglected hygiene. Shoplifting and episodes of sexual exhibition occurred. In repeatedly performed electroencephalograms (EEG) at this time (including mobile long-term EEG monitoring at age 15 years), several instances of a left temporal seizure focus were found interictally, and, on a single day, 29 psychomotor attacks were recorded, consisting of short arrest with motionless staring, occasionally followed by gestural automatisms and head deviation. She was amnestic for many of these attacks but always remembered initial fear and diminished vision and hearing. While hospitalized in an epilepsy clinic, she reportedly had "petit mal status" of 30 minutes duration, which was interrupted with clonazepam. At age 16 years, she was admitted for depth-EEG recording with a view toward epilepsy surgery. At that time, neurologic examination was normal except for an unusual amount of synkinetic movements. She was oriented in time and space but was slow and fearful, showed concentration difficulties, and had impaired verbal memory with word-finding difficulties on formal testing. The results of CT scans and the entire neuroradiologic examination under stereotactic conditions, including bilateral carotid angiography, were normal. During stereo-EEG with 18.6 hours of analysis time, 91 left mesiobasal limbic epileptic discharges were recorded. Taking into account the duration of the discharges, 11% of the analysis time was covered by high-frequency "tonic" or "tonic-clonic" discharges of the hippocampal formation alone or in combination with the ipsilateral amygdala. The average discharge interval was 12 minutes (range 8-16). Only 2 of these seizure discharges spread to the ipsilateral neocortical temporal and frontal areas (associated with an aura and head deviation) or later to the contralateral temporal lobe (associated with marked impairment of consciousness, prolonged automatisms, and amnesia). Following a selective amygdalohippocampectomy at age 16, the patient was seizure free, and a dramatic improvement in her behavior and personality was witnessed. She studied, married, and has 2 children.

of functional specialization of the brain, the diagnosis might be straightforward. In the absence of clear-cut EEG findings, however, an aura continua (in particular, if expressing itself with strange and unusual phenomena) might be difficult to diagnose. Not infrequently, convincing ictal discharges cannot be detected without intracranial recordings (see Figures10.1-10.4). Such invasive techniques, of course, are only justified in the context of surgical epilepsy therapy. Long-lasting autonomic, emotional, and psychic phenomena and personality changes, in which the mesial temporal lobe (in particular the amygdala) and the insular and frontal cortexes are candidate areas for suspected discharges, pose a problem. Circumscribed discharges at such localizations are difficult to detect in routine scalp EEG.

Limbic aura continua can mimic psychoses (postictal, recurrent intermittent psychoses, schizophrenia, schizophrenia-like illness), hallucinations or illusions due to a loss of primary sensation, drug-induced flashbacks, and sleep disorders (nightmares, night terrors, and REM sleep behavior disorder) (141,142). Prolonged autonomic ictal features can mimic psychiatric (panic attacks), paroxysmal autonomic dysfunction, endocrine (carcinoid, pheochromocytoma, hypoglycemia), cardiac, and gastrointestinal disorders (142,143). Of importance is the differential diagnosis of limbic encephalitis, both paraneoplastic and nonparaneoplastic. Nonparaneoplastic limbic encephalitis may have antibodies to voltage-gated potassium channels.

Acute intermittent porphyria should not be forgotten (144) and can be checked for with analysis of porphyrinogens in blood, urine, and stool.

Criteria for the diagnosis of dyscognitive focal (psychomotor, complex partial) status epilepticus are (1) recurrent psychomotor (complex partial) seizures without full recovery of consciousness between seizures, or a continuous "epileptic twilight state" with cycling between unresponsiveness and partially responsive phases (lasting longer than 30 minutes); (2) ictal EEG with recurrent epileptiform patterns like those seen in isolated complex partial seizures (see Figure 10.6); (3) with exceptions, an observable effect of an intravenously administered antiepileptic drug on both ictal EEG and clinical manifestations of the status; and (4) interictal EEG with a consistent epileptiform focus, usually in 1 or both temporal lobes (adapted with modifications from [145,146]).

Psychomotor or limbic status should certainly be distinguished from absence status. The primary criteria for classical absence status are (1) prolonged change of consciousness or behavior function (greater than 30 minutes), (2) generalized epileptic EEG abnormality (in classic cases, 3/second spike-slow waves) that is definitively changed from the preictal state, and (3) a prompt observable effect of an intravenously administered antiepileptic drug on both ictal EEG and clinical manifestations of the status (adapted from [146,147]). Nevertheless, many cases are borderline or atypical (148).

Epileptic behavior disturbances and psychoses might be due to prolonged nonconvulsive seizure activity. The idea that some abnormal mental states in epilepsy might be a form of focal status epilepticus is intriguing. Usually, epileptic psychosis is divided broadly into ictal, postictal, and interictal categories, each with distinctive features (83). Whereas postictal psychosis is usually associated with delirium, altered consciousness, and amnesia, interictal psychosis is characterized by clear consciousness, retained memory, and less severe behavior disturbances. Ictal psychosis in psychomotor status with fluctuating or frequently recurring focal electrographic epileptic discharges, arising in temporal or extratemporal regions, usually presents itself as a confusional state with a variable clinical state. It is said that extratemporal (in particular frontal) focal status has fewer cycling symptoms and that severe confusion is less pronounced in comparison with temporal lobe status. Fronto-orbital polar status epilepticus is said to be particularly subtle in clinical symptoms.

In an attempt to reexamine interictal psychoses based on the DSM IV Psychosis Classification and International Epilepsy Classification, Kanemoto and colleagues confirmed a close correlation between temporal lobe epilepsy and interictal psychoses. Within the temporal lobe epilepsy group, early epilepsy onset and a history of prolonged febrile convulsions were significantly associated with interictal psychosis. Within the symptomatic localization-related epilepsy group, complex partial seizures, autonomic aura, and temporal EEG foci were closely associated with psychoses. There was also a significantly higher incidence of ictal fear and secondary generalization in the group with localization-related epilepsies with (as opposed to without) interictal psychotic states (149). Temporal lobe epileptic activity may mimic dementia (150).

The differential diagnosis includes toxic or metabolic encephalopathy, delirium, psychiatric conditions, and transient global amnesia. Furthermore, limbic encephalitis—both paraneoplastic (151) and nonparaneoplastic—and herpes simplex encephalitis can be challenging differential diagnoses. Creutzfeldt-Jakob disease can present with focal or regional EEG abnormalities that might mimic NCSE (152-154). Also, psychogenic status epilepticus has to be considered (155,156), as well as metastatic central nervous system disease (157). In a recent review of NCSE in children, acute hypoxic-ischemic injury was the most frequent etiology (5 of 19; 26%), followed by exacerbation of underlying metabolic disease (21%), acute infection (16%), and change in antiepileptic drug regimen (16%) (158).

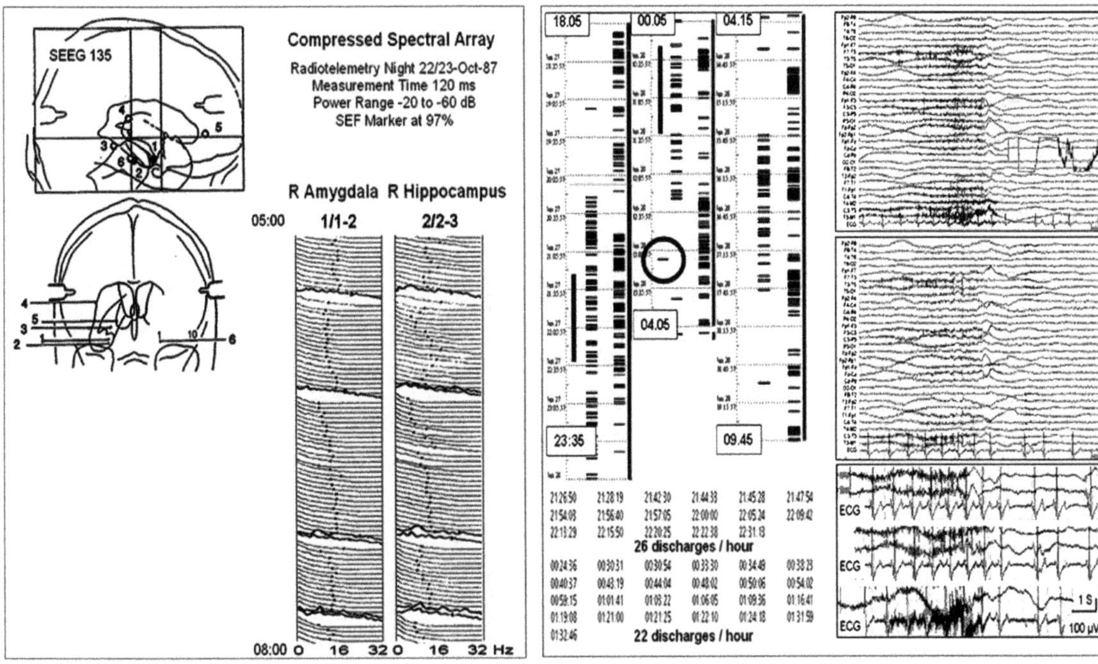


**Figure 10.6** Two examples depicting frequently recurring seizures. Left: Radiotelemetric seizure monitoring of stereo-electroencephalography (EEG) with 2 to 3 minutes of right mesiobasal seizure discharges nicely depicted by online compressed spectral array analyzing the depth-recorded activity in the right amygdala and hippocampus (inner contacts of depth electrodes 1 and 2; depth electrodes have 10 contacts numbered from inside out). The patient underwent right selective amygdalohippocampectomy at age 42 and is seizure and aura free since then (follow-up 9 years). Right: Intermittent left temporal status epilepticus with marked spread and a tendency for generalization in a 27-year-old woman monitored by scalp EEG telemetry with automatic seizure-detection algorithms. The times indicated by the vertical black bars were visually analyzed in detail and showed a discharge frequency of 26 and 22 epileptic discharges per hour, respectively. They were short lived (approximately 6 seconds' duration) and were not accompanied by any clear-cut clinical seizure symptoms. Only 1 discharge led to an awakening and button press (circled). Note the stereotyped electrocardiographic changes with acceleration of the heartbeat during the discharge and a bradycardia at the end of all seizure discharges (depicted for 3 discharges at the bottom).

## REFERENCES

1. Dreifuss F. Classification of epileptic seizures. In: Engel JJ, Pedley TA, eds. Epilepsy: A Comprehensive Textbook. Philadelphia, PA: Lippincott-Raven Publishers; 1997:517-524.
2. Scott JS, Masland RL. Occurrence of continuous symptoms in epilepsy patients. Neurology 1953;3:297-301.
3. Karbowski K. Epileptische Anfälle. Heidelberg, Germany: Springer; 1985.
4. Wolf P. [Clinical course and psychopathology of the status psychomotoricus]. Nervenarzt 1970;41:603-610.
5. Wolf P. Systematik von Status kleiner Anfälle in psychopathologischer Hinsicht. Mit Kasuistiken einiger seltener Zustandsbilder. In: Wolf P, Köhler GK, eds. Psychopathologische und pathogenetische Probleme psychotischer Syndrome bei Epilepsie. Bern, Switzerland: Hans Huber Verlag; 1980:32-52.
6. Wolf P. Halluzinationen im Rahmen epileptischer Psychosen. In: Karbowski K, ed. Halluzinationen bei Epilepsien und ihre Differential-

diagnose. Bern, Switzerland: Hans Huber Verlag; 1982:58-66.

7. Landolt H. Die Dämmer- und Verstimmungszustände bei Epilepsie und ihre Elektroenzephalographie. Z Gesamte Inn Med 1963;185:411-430.
8. Trousseau A. Clinique Médicale de l'Hôtel Dieu de Paris. Paris: Baillière et fils; 1868.
9. Prichard JC. A treatise on Diseases of the Nervous System. London, England: Underwood; 1822.
10. Bright R. Reports of Medical Cases, Selected with a View of Illustrating the Symptoms and Cure of Diseases by a Reference to Morbid Anatomy. London, England: Taylor; 1831.
11. Charcot JM. Clinical Lectures on the Diseases of the Nervous System. London, England: New Sydenham Society; 1889.
12. Taylor J. Selected Writings of John Hughlings Jackson. On Epilepsy and Epileptiform Convulsions. London, England: Hodder and Stoughton; 1931.
13. Clark LP, Prout TP. Status epilepticus: a clinical and pathological study in epilepsy. Am J Insanity 1903/04;60:291-306.
14. Penfield W, Jasper HH. Epilepsy and Functional Anatomy of the Human Brain. Boston, MA: Little Brown; 1954.
15. Lennox WG. The petit mal epilepsies—their treatment with tridione. JAMA 1945;129:1069-1074.
16. Lennox WG, Lennox MA. Epilepsy and Related Disorders. Boston, MA: Little, Brown Company; 1960.
17. Janz D. Die Epilepsien. Stuttgart, Germany: Thieme; 1969.
18. Karbowski K. Status psychomotoricus. Klinische und elektroenzephalographische Aspekte. In: Karbowski K, ed. Status Psychomotoricus und seine Differentialdiagnose. Bern, Switzerland: Hans Huber; 1980:39-71.
19. Ambrosetto G, Forti A, Spire JP, Tassinari CA. Studio elettroclinico di due casi di sato di male epilettico partiale. Bull Italian League against Epilepsy 1978;23:307-311.
20. Engel J, Jr., Ludwig BI, Fetell M. Prolonged partial complex status epilepticus: EEG and behavioral observations. Neurology 1978;28:863-869.
21. Mayeux R, Lueders H. Complex partial status epilepticus: case report and proposal for diagnostic criteria. Neurology 1978;28:957-961.
22. Oller Daurella L, Oller Ferrer-Vidal L, Russi A, Conill J. [Los estados de mal de crisis parciales complejas]. Bull Italian League against Epilepsy 1978;23:209-211.
23. Perri Di R, Messina C. Studio elettroclinico di due casi di "stato di male temporale." Bull Italian League against Epilepsy 1978;23:203-208.
24. Picornell Darder I, Conde M, Carbonell J. [Post-traumatic status epilepticus with only mental symptomatology]. Rev Electroencephalogr Neurophysiol Clin 1978;8:341-345.
25. Roger J, Dravet C, Bureau M. États de mal partiel chez l'enfant et l'adolescent. Bull Italian League against Epilepsy 1978;23:195-201.
26. Engel J, Jr. Report of the ILAE classification core group. Epilepsia 2006;47:1558-1568.
27. Wieser HG. Temporal lobe or psychomotor status epilepticus. A case report. Electroencephalogr Clin Neurophysiol 1980;48:558-572.
28. Wieser HG. Simple partial status epilepticus. In: Engel JJ, Pedley TA, eds. Epilepsy: A Comprehensive Textbook. Philadelphia, PA: Lippincott-Raven Publishers; 1997: 709-723.
29. Wieser HG, Hailemariam S, Regard M, Landis T. Unilateral limbic epileptic status activity: stereo EEG, behavioral, and cognitive data. Epilepsia 1985;26:19-29.
30. Penfield W. The interpretive cortex; the stream of consciousness in the human brain can be electrically reactivated. Science 1959;129: 1719-1725.
31. Wasterlain CG, Treiman DM. Status epilepticus: mechanisms and management. Boston, MA: MIT Press; 2006.
32. Wieser HG, Yasargil MG. Selective amygdalohippocampectomy as a surgical treatment of mesiobasal limbic epilepsy.Surg.Neurol.1982; 17:445-457.
33. Lüders HO, Kahane P. Definition and localization of the epileptic zone. Epileptic Disord 2006;8(Suppl 2):1-76.
34. Imperiale D, Pignatta P, Cerrato P, Montalenti E, Ravetti C, Benna P. Nonconvulsive status epilepticus due to a de novo contralateral focus during tiagabine adjunctive therapy. Seizure 2003;12:319-322.
35. Atefy R, Tettenborn B. Nonconvulsive status epilepticus on treatment with levetiracetam. Epilepsy Behav 2005;6:613-616.
36. Arabadzisz D, Antal K, Parpan F, Emri Z, Fritschy JM. Epileptogenesis and chronic seizures in a mouse model of temporal lobe epilepsy are associated with distinct EEG patterns and selective neurochemical alterations

in the contralateral hippocampus. Exp Neurol 2005;194:76-90.
37. Mazarati A, Lu X. Regulation of limbic status epilepticus by hippocampal galanin type 1 and type 2 receptors. Neuropeptides 2005;39:277-280.
38. Lothman EW, Bertram EH, Bekenstein JW, Perlin JB. Self-sustaining limbic status epilepticus induced by 'continuous' hippocampal stimulation: electrographic and behavioral characteristics. Epilepsy Res 1989;3:107-119.
39. Bertram EH, Lothman EW, Lenn NJ. The hippocampus in experimental chronic epilepsy: a morphometric analysis. Ann Neurol 1990;27:43-48.
40. Nairismagi J, Grohn OH, Kettunen MI, Nissinen J, Kauppinen RA, Pitkanen A. Progression of brain damage after status epilepticus and its association with epileptogenesis: a quantitative MRI study in a rat model of temporal lobe epilepsy. Epilepsia 2004;45:1024-1034.
41. Krsek P, Mikulecka A, Druga R, Hlinak Z, Kubova H, Mares P. An animal model of nonconvulsive status epilepticus: a contribution to clinical controversies. Epilepsia 2001;42:171-180.
42. Olney JW, deGubareff T, Sloviter RS. "Epileptic" brain damage in rats induced by sustained electrical stimulation of the perforant path. II. Ultrastructural analysis of acute hippocampal pathology. Brain Res Bull 1983;10:699-712.
43. Sloviter RS. "Epileptic" brain damage in rats induced by sustained electrical stimulation of the perforant path. I. Acute electrophysiological and light microscopic studies. Brain Res Bull 1983;10:675-697.
44. Shimosaka S, So YT, Simon RP. Distribution of HSP72 induction and neuronal death following limbic seizures. Neurosci Lett 1992;138:202-206.
45. Lowenstein DH, Shimosaka S, So YT, Simon RP. The relationship between electrographic seizure activity and neuronal injury. Epilepsy Res 1991;10:49-54.
46. Gorter JA, Goncalves Pereira PM, van Vliet EA, Aronica E, Lopes da Silva FH, Lucassen PJ. Neuronal cell death in a rat model for mesial temporal lobe epilepsy is induced by the initial status epilepticus and not by later repeated spontaneous seizures. Epilepsia 2003;44:647-658.
47. van Eijsden P, Notenboom RG, Wu O, de Graan PN, van Nieuwenhuizen O, Nicolay K, et al. In vivo 1H magnetic resonance spectroscopy, T2-weighted and diffusion-weighted MRI during lithium-pilocarpine-induced status epilepticus in the rat. Brain Res 2004;1030:11-18.
48. Wasterlain CG, Liu H, Mazarati AM, Baldwin RA, Shirasaka Y, Katsumori H, Thompspm KW, Sankar R, Pereira de Vasconselos A, Nehlig A. Self-sustaining status epilepticus: a condition maintained by potentiation of glutamate receptors and by plastic changes in substance P and other peptide neuromodulators. Epilepsia 2000;41(suppl 6):S134-143.
49. Coulter DA, DeLorenzo RJ. Basic mechanisms of status epilepticus. Adv Neurol 1999;79:725-733.
50. Seegers U, Potschka H, Löscher W. Transient increase of P-glycoprotein expression in endothelium and parenchyma of limbic brain regions in the kainate model of temporal lobe epilepsy. Epilepsy Res 2002;51:257-268.
51. Suopanki J, Lintunen M, Lahtinen H, Haltia M, Panula P, Baumann M, Tyynela J. Status epilepticus induces changes in the expression and localization of endogenous palmitoyl-protein thioesterase 1. Neurobiol Dis 2002;10:247-257.
52. Rogawski MA, Gryder D, Castaneda D, Yonekawa W, Banks MK, Lia H. GluR5 kainate receptors, seizures, and the amygdala. Ann N Y Acad Sci 2003;985:150-162.
53. Towne AR, Garnett LK, Waterhouse EJ, Morton LD, DeLorenzo RJ. The use of topiramate in refractory status epilepticus. Neurology 2003;60:332-334.
54. Blumkin L, Lerman-Sagie T, Houri T, Gilad E, Nissenkorn A, Ginsberg M, Watemberg N. Pediatric refractory partial status epilepticus responsive to topiramate. J Child Neurol 2005;20:239-241.
55. Foster JA, Puchowicz MJ, McIntyre DC, Herkenham M. Activin mRNA induced during amygdala kindling shows a spatiotemporal progression that tracks the spread of seizures. J Comp Neurol 2004;476:91-102.
56. Mohapel P, Ekdahl CT, Lindvall O. Status epilepticus severity influences the long-term outcome of neurogenesis in the adult dentate gyrus. Neurobiol Dis 2004;15:196-205.
57. Morimoto K, Fahnestock M, Racine RJ. Kindling and status epilepticus models of epilepsy: rewiring the brain. Prog Neurobiol 2004;73:1-60.
58. Zhang G, Raol YH, Hsu FC, Coulter DA, Brooks-Kayal AR. Effects of status epilepticus

on hippocampal $GABA_A$ receptors are age-dependent. Neuroscience 2004;125:299-303.
59. Henke K, Buck A, Weber B, Wieser HG. Human hippocampus establishes associations in memory. Hippocampus 1997;7:249-256.
60. Henke K, Weber B, Kneifel S, Wieser HG, Buck A. Human hippocampus associates information in memory. Proc Natl Acad Sci U S A 1999;96:5884-5889.
61. Henke K, Weber B, Schwedler K. PET studies of memory. Schweiz Arch Neurol Neurochir Psychiatr 1999;150:89-96.
62. Henke K, Treyer V, Weber B, Nitsch RM, Hock C, Wieser HG, Buck A. Functional neuroimaging predicts individual memory outcome after amygdalohippocampectomy. Neuroreport 2003;14:1197-1202.
63. Ben-Ari Y, ed. The Amygdaloid Complex. INSERM symposium 20; 1981; Amsterdam, Netherlands: Elsevier/North-Holland Biomedical Press; 1981:516.
64. Wieser HG. Temporal lobe epilepsies. In: Meinardi H, ed. The Epilepsies, part II. Handbook of Clinical Neurology. Amsterdam, Netherlands: Elsevier; 2000:53-96.
65. Yakovlev PI. Motility, behavior and the brain. Stereodynamic organization and neural coordinates of behavior. J Nerv Ment Dis 1948;107:313-335.
66. Livingston KE, Escobar A. Anatomical bias of the limbic system concept. A proposed reorientation. Arch Neurol 1971;24:17-21.
67. Wieser HG. Depth recorded limbic seizures and psychopathology. Neurosci Biobehav Rev 1983;7:427-440.
68. Williamson PD. Complex partial status epilepticus. In: Engel JJ, Pedley TA, eds. Epilepsy: a Comprehensive Textbook. Philadelphia, PA: Lippincott-Raven Publishers; 1997:681-699.
69. Jackson JH. On temporary mental disorders after epileptic paroxysms. In: Taylor J, ed. Selected Writings of John Hughlings Jackson. London, England: Staples Press; 1875:119-134.
70. Jackson JH, Beevor C. Case of tumor of the right temporo-sphenoidal lobe, bearing on the localization of the sense of smell and on the interpretation of a particular variety of epilepsy. Brain 1890:346-357.
71. Jackson JH, Colman WS. Case of epilepsy with tasting movements and "dreamy state": very small patch of softening in the left uncinate gyrus. Brain 1898:580-590.
72. Jackson JH, Stewart P. Epileptic attacks with a warning of crude sensation of smell and with intellectual aura (dreamy state) in a patient who had symptoms pointing to gross organic disease of the right temporo-sphenoidal lobe. Brain 1899:334-549.
73. Gowers WR. Epilepsy and Other Convulsive Diseases: Their Causes, Symptoms and Treatment. London, England: Chirchill J, Chirchill A; 1881.
74. Gloor P. Experiential phenomena of temporal lobe epilepsy. Facts and hypotheses. Brain 1990;113:1673-1694.
75. Young GB, Chandarana PC, Blume WT, McLachlan RS, Munoz DG, Girvin JP. Mesial temporal lobe seizures presenting as anxiety disorders. J Neuropsychiatry Clin Neurosci 1995;7:352-357.
76. Wieser HG. "Psychische Anfälle" und deren stereoelektroenzephalographisches Korrelat. Z Elektroenzephalogr Elektromyogr 1979; 10:197-206.
77. Fish DR. Psychic seizures. In: Engel JJ, Pedley TA, eds. Epilepsy: a Comprehensive Textbook. Philadelphia, PA: Lippincott-Raven Publishers; 1997:543-548.
78. Brugger P, Agosti R, Regard M, Wieser HG, Landis T. Heautoscopy, epilepsy, and suicide. J Neurol Neurosurg Psychiatry 1994;57:838-839.
79. Gloor P, Olivier A, Quesney LF, Andermann F, Horowitz S. The role of the limbic system in experiential phenomena of temporal lobe epilepsy. Ann Neurol 1982;12:129-144.
80. Weil AA. Ictal depression and anxiety in temporal lobe diaorders. Am J Psychiatry 1956;113:149-157.
81. Henriksen GF. Status epilepticus partialis with fear as clinical expression. Report of a case and ictal EEG findings. Epilepsia 1973;14:39-46.
82. McLachlan RS, Blume WT. Isolated fear in complex partial status epilepticus. Ann Neurol 1980;8:639-641.
83. Trimble MR, Bolwig TG. The Temporal Lobes and the Limbic System. Petersfield, England: Wrightson Biomed Publ; 1992.
84. Smith DB, Treiman D, Trimble MR. Neurobehavioral Problems in Epilepsy. Advances in Neurology. Vol 55. New York, NY: Raven Press; 1991.
85. Müller D, Müller J. Lachen als epileptische Manifestation. Jena, Germany: Gustav Fischer; 1980.

86. Waxman SG, Geschwind N. The interictal behavior syndrome of temporal lobe epilepsy. Arch Gen Psychiatry 1975;32:1580-1586.
87. Wieser HG, Landis T. Is the "interictal behaviour syndrome of temporal lobe epilepsy" really an "interictal" phenomenon? Neurol Psychiatr 1983:70-78.
88. Pontius AA. Motiveless firesetting: implicating partial limbic seizure kindling by revived memories of fires in "Limbic Psychotic Trigger Reaction." Percept Mot Skills 1999;88:970-982.
89. Pontius AA, Wieser HG. Can memories kindle nonconvulsive behavioral seizures in humans? Case report exemplifying the "limbic psychotic trigger reaction." Epilepsy Behav 2004;5:775-783.
90. Jackson JH. On a particular variety of epilepsy ("intellectual aura"), one case with symptoms of organic brain disease 1899. In: Taylor J, ed. Selected Writings of John Hughlings Jackson. New York, NY: Basic Book Inc; 1958:308-317; 385-405.
91. Wieser HG. Zur Frage der lokalisatorischen Bedeutung epileptischer Halluzinationen. In: Karbowski K, ed. Halluzinationen bei Epilepsien und Differentialdiagnose. Bern, Switzerland: Hans Huber Verlag; 1982:67-92.
92. Hausser-Hauw C, Bancaud J. Gustatory hallucinations in epileptic seizures. Electrophysiological, clinical and anatomical correlates. Brain 1987;110 :339-359.
93. Seshia SS, McLachlan RS. Aura continua. Epilepsia 2005;46:454-455.
94. Schiffter R, Straschill M. [Case report of a patient with sensory status epilepticus]. Nervenarzt 1977;48:321-325.
95. Penfield W, Perot P. The Brain's record of auditory and visual experience. A final summary and discussion. Brain 1963;86:595-696.
96. Blanke O, Ortigue S, Coeytaux A, Martory MD, Landis T. Hearing of a presence. Neurocase 2003;9:329-339.
97. Manford M, Shorvon SD. Prolonged sensory or visceral symptoms: an under-diagnosed form of non-convulsive focal (simple partial) status epilepticus. J Neurol Neurosurg Psychiatry 1992;55:714-716.
98. Wilkinson HA. Epileptic pain. An uncommon manifestation with localizing value. Neurology 1973;23:518-520.
99. Young GB, Blume WT. Painful epileptic seizures. Brain 1983;106:537-554.
100. Siegel AM, Williamson PD, Roberts DW, Thadani VM, Darcey TM. Localized pain associated with seizures originating in the parietal lobe. Epilepsia 1999;40:845-855.
101. Fromm GH, Faingold C, Browning RA, Burnham WM. Epilepsy and the Reticular Formation. Neurology and Neurobiology. New York, NY: Alan R. Liss Inc; 1987.
102. Schaeffler L, Karbowski K. Recurring paroxysmal abdominal pains of cerebral origin. Schweiz Med Wochenschr 1981;111:1352-1360.
103. Mitchell WG, Greenwood RS, Messenheimer JA. Abdominal epilepsy. Cyclic vomiting as the major symptom of simple partial seizures. Arch Neurol 1983;40:251-252.
104. Peppercorn MA, Herzog AG. The spectrum of abdominal epilepsy in adults. Am J Gastroenterol 1989;84:1294-1296.
105. Brody JA, Odom GL, Kunkle EC. Pilomotor seizures: report of a case associated with a central glioma. Neurology 1960;49:385-388.
106. Van Buren JM. The abdominal aura. A study of abdominal sensations occurring in epilepsy and produced by depth stimulation. Electroencephalogr Clin Neurophysiol 1963;15:1-19.
107. Wieser HG. [Stereo-electroencephalographic correlates of motor seizures]. Z Elektroenzephalogr Elektromyogr Verwandte Geb 1981;12:1-13.
108. Wieser HG. Ictal manifestations of temporal lobe seizures. Adv Neurol 1991;55:301-315.
109. Green JB. Pilomotor seizures. Neurology 1984;34:837-839.
110. Stodieck SR, Wieser HG. Autonomic phenomena in temporal lobe epilepsy. J Autonom Nerv Syst 1986;(Suppl):611-621.
111. Wieser HG, Williamson PD. Ictal semiology. In: Engel JJ, ed. Surgical Treatment of the Epilepsies. New York, NY: Raven Press; 1993:161-171.
112. Rabending G, Fischer W. [Epileptic psychosis and nonconvulsive status epilepticus with ictal bradycardia and asystole]. Psychiatr Neurol Med Psychol (Leipz) 1986;38:184-188.
113. Zijlmans M, Flanagan D, Gotman J. Heart rate changes and ECG abnormalities during epileptic seizures: prevalence and definition of an objective clinical sign. Epilepsia 2002;43:847-854.
114. Nishiguchi M, Shima M, Takahashi Y, Matsuoka H, Fujimoto S, Taira K, Yoshioka A. [A boy with occipital lobe epilepsy showing pro-

longed QTc in the ictal ECG]. No To Hattatsu 2002;34:523-527.
115. Panayiotopoulus CP. Panayiotopoulos Syndrome: a Common and Benign Childhood Epileptic Syndrome. London, England: John Libbey; 2002.
116. Panayiotopoulus CP. Autonomic seizures and autonomic status epilepticus peculiar to childhood: diagnosis and management. Epilepsy Behav 2004;5:286-295.
117. Koutroumanidis M, Rowlinson S, Sanders S. Recurrent autonomic status epilepticus in Panayiotopoulos syndrome: video/EEG studies. Epilepsy Behav 2005;7:543-547.
118. Tedrus GM, Fonseca LC. Autonomic seizures and autonomic status epilepticus in early onset benign childhood occipital epilepsy (Panayiotopoulos syndrome). Arq Neuropsiquiatr 2006;64:723-726.
119. Girgis M, Kiloh LG. Limbic Epilepsy and the Dyscontrol Syndrome. Developments in Psychiatry. Amsterdam, Netherlands: Elsevier/North-Holland Biomed Press; 1980.
120. Delgado-Escueta AV, Mattson RH, King L, Goldensohn ES, Spiegel H, Madsen J, Crandall P, Dreifuss F, Porter RJ. Special report. The nature of aggression during epileptic seizures. N Engl J Med 1981;305:711-716.
121. Wieser S, Kelemen A, Barsi P, Vincent A, Borbely C, Rasonyi G, Mueller S, Hess K, Wieser HG, Halasz P. Pilomotor seizures and status in non-paraneoplastic limbic encephalitis. Epileptic Disord 2005;7:205-211.
122. Treiman DM. Status epilepticus. Baillieres Clin Neurol 1996;5:821-839.
123. Nowack WJ, Shaikh IA. Progression of electroclinical changes in complex partial status epilepticus: filling in the blanks. Clin Electroencephalogr 1999;30:5-8.
124. Gastaut H. Classification of status epilepticus. In: Delgado-Escueta AV, Wasterlain C, Treiman D, Porter RJ, eds. Status Epilepticus. Adv Neurol. Vol 34. New York, NY: Raven Press; 1983:15-35.
125. Vernea JJ. Partial status epilepticus with speech arrest. Proc Aust Assoc Neurol 1974;11:223-228.
126. Gastaut H. Aphasia: the sole manifestation of focal status epilepticus. Neurology 1979;29:1638.
127. Hamilton NG, Matthews T. Aphasia: the sole manifestation of focal status epilepticus. Neurology 1979;29:745-748.
128. Dinner DS, Lueders H, Lederman R, Gretter TE. Aphasic status epilepticus: a case report. Neurology 1981;31:888-891.
129. Primavera A, Bo GP, Venturi S. Aphasic status epilepticus. Eur Neurol 1988;28:255-257.
130. Wells CR, Labar DR, Solomon GE. Aphasia as the sole manifestation of simple partial status epilepticus. Epilepsia 1992;33:84-87.
131. Murchison JT, Sellar RJ, Steers AJ. Status epilepticus presenting as progressive dysphasia. Neuroradiology 1995;37:438-439.
132. Grimes DA, Guberman A. De novo aphasic status epilepticus. Epilepsia 1997;38:945-949.
133. Ueki Y, Terada K, Otsuka A, Kanda M, Akiguchi I. [A case of non-convulsive status epilepticus worsened Wernicke's aphasia reversely]. Rinsho Shinkeigaku 2000;40:339-343.
134. DeToledo JC, Minagar A, Lowe MR. Persisting aphasia as the sole manifestation of partial status epilepticus. Clin Neurol Neurosurg 2000;102:144-148.
135. Chung PW, Seo DW, Kwon JC, Kim H, Na DL. Nonconvulsive status epilepticus presenting as a subacute progressive aphasia. Seizure 2002;11:449-454.
136. Trinka E, Unterberger I, Spiegel M, Niedermuller U, Benke T, Berger T, Bauer G. De novo aphasic status epilepticus as presenting symptom of multiple sclerosis. J Neurol 2002;249:782-783.
137. Pinol-Ripoll G, Perez-Lazaro C, Beltran-Marin I, Lopez del Val LJ, Pascual-Millan LF, Mostacero-Miguel E. [Aphasia as the sole symptom of partial status epilepticus]. Rev Neurol 2004;39:1096-1097.
138. Hasegawa T, Shiga Y, Narikawa K, Jin K, Fujihara K, Takeda A, Itoyama Y. Periodic episodes of aphasia as an unusual manifestation of partial status epilepticus. J Clin Neurosci 2005;12:820-822.
139. Kirshner HS, Hughes T, Fakhoury T, Abou-Khalil B. Aphasia secondary to partial status epilepticus of the basal temporal language area. Neurology 1995;45:1616-1618.
140. Ozkaya G, Kurne A, Unal S, Oguz KK, Karabudak R, Saygi S. Aphasic status epilepticus with periodic lateralized epileptiform discharges in a bilingual patient as a presenting sign of "AIDS-toxoplasmosis complex." Epilepsy Behav 2006;9:193-196.
141. Slater E, Beard AW. The schizophrenia-like psychoses of epilepsy. Br J Psychiatry 1963;109:95-150.

142. Liporace JD, Sperling MR. Simple autonomic seizures. In: Engel JJ, Pedley TA, eds. Epilepsy: a Comprehensive Textbook. Philadelphia, PA: Lippincott-Raven Publishers; 1997:549-555.
143. Devinsky O, Price BH, Cohen SI. Cardiac manifestations of complex partial seizures. Am J Med 1986;80:195-202.
144. Wessels T, Blaes F, Rottger C, Hugens M, Huge S, Jauss M. [Cortical amaurosis and status epilepticus with acute porphyria]. Nervenarzt 2005;76:992-995, 997-998.
145. Treiman D, Delgado-Escueta AV. Complex partial status epilepticus. In: Delgado-Escueta AV, Wasterlain C, Treiman D, Porter RJ, eds. Status Epilepticus. Adv Neurology. New York, NY: Raven Press; 1983:15-35.
146. Krumholz A. Epidemiology and evidence for morbidity of nonconvulsive status epilepticus. J Clin Neurophysiol 1999;16:314-322; discussion 353.
147. Porter RJ, Penry JK. Petit mal status. In: Delgado-Escueta AV, Wasterlain C, Treiman D, Porter RJ, eds. Status Epilepticus. Adv Neurol New York, NY: Raven Press; 1983:61-67.
148. Hess R, Scollo-Lavizzari G, Wyss FE. Borderline cases of petit mal status. Eur Neurol 1971;5:137-154.
149. Kanemoto K, Tsuji T, Kawasaki J. Reexamination of interictal psychoses based on DSM IV psychosis classification and international epilepsy classification. Epilepsia 2001;42:98-103.
150. Tombini M, Koch G, Placidi F, Sancesario G, Marciani MG, Bernardi G. Temporal lobe epileptic activity mimicking dementia: a case report. Eur J Neurol 2005;12:805-806.
151. Espay AJ, Kumar V, Sarpel G. Anti-Hu-associated paraneoplastic limbic encephalitis presenting as rapidly progressive non-convulsive status epilepticus. J Neurol Sci 2006;246:149-152.
152. Fernandez-Torre JL, Solar DM, Astudillo A, Cereceda R, Acebes A, Calatayud MT. Creutzfeldt-Jakob disease and non-convulsive status epilepticus: a clinical and electroencephalographic follow-up study. Clin Neurophysiol 2004;115:316-319.
153. Cohen D, Kutluay E, Edwards J, Peltier A, Beydoun A. Sporadic Creutzfeldt-Jakob disease presenting with nonconvulsive status epilepticus. Epilepsy Behav 2004;5:792-796.
154. Wieser HG, Schindler K, Zumsteg D. Reply to "Nonconvulsive status epilepticus in Creutzfeldt-Jakob disease." Clin Neurophysiol 2006;117:1881.
155. Papavasiliou A, Vassilaki N, Paraskevoulakos E, Kotsalis C, Bazigou H, Bardani I. Psychogenic status epilepticus in children. Epilepsy Behav 2004;5:539-546.
156. Dworetzky BA, Mortati KA, Rossetti AO, Vaccaro B, Nelson A, Bromfield EB. Clinical characteristics of psychogenic nonepileptic seizure status in the long-term monitoring unit. Epilepsy Behav 2006;9:335-338.
157. Blitshteyn S, Jaeckle KA. Nonconvulsive status epilepticus in metastatic CNS disease. Neurology 2006;66:1261-1263.
158. Tay SK, Hirsch LJ, Leary L, Jette N, Wittman J, Akman CI. Nonconvulsive status epilepticus in children: clinical and EEG characteristics. Epilepsia 2006;47:1504-1509.
159. Wieser HG, Chauvel P. Simple partial status epilepticus and epilepsia partialis continua of Kozhhevnikov. In: Jerome Engel Jr , Pedley TA, eds. Epilepsy: a Comprehensive Textbook, 2nd ed. Philadelphia, PA: Lippincott Williams and Wilkins; 2008:705-726.

CHAPTER 11

# OCCIPITAL LOBE NONCONVULSIVE STATUS EPILEPTICUS

Barbara C. Jobst, David W. Roberts, and Peter D. Williamson

Nonconvulsive status epilepticus (NCSE) includes generalized status epilepticus and focal or localization-related status epilepticus. The classic form of generalized NCSE is absence status epilepticus, which is usually associated with primary generalized epilepsy, whereas focal or localization-related NCSE includes simple and complex partial status epilepticus (1). Gastaut, in 1983, defined complex partial status epilepticus as either recurrent complex partial seizures with psychomotor manifestations without interictal recovery or a prolonged state of ictal confusion accompanied by automatisms (2). Continued seizure activity with preserved consciousness is considered simple partial status epilepticus; the typical example is persistent focal motor activity, epilepsia partialis continua. Subjective seizures, such as somatosensory symptoms or epileptic visual hallucinations, can also represent a subtle form of status epilepticus. For occipital NCSE, Gastaut used the term *elementary visual status epilepticus* (3). In the proposed classification scheme of 2001, these events were termed *aura continua* (4). More recent classifications of status epilepticus use the term *occipital lobe simple partial status with visual features, with or without nystagmus* (5).

There is no definite agreement about the duration of nonconvulsive seizure activity to represent status epilepticus. Nonconvulsive seizure activity for more than 30 minutes is definitely considered status epilepticus (6), but persistent seizure activity lasting a shorter time (10 minutes or more) has also been proposed (7).

In a depth electrode study, Williamson and colleagues described 8 patients with complex partial status epilepticus and found that NCSE is more likely to be associated with extratemporal epilepsy; 1 patient had an occipital seizure origin (8). Subsequent studies found a high incidence of NCSE in localization-related frontal lobe epilepsy (9). In parieto-occipital epilepsy, NCSE is less common.

Localization-related occipital lobe epilepsy is less common than other localization-related epilepsies but is well described (10,11). Studying the occipital lobes with intracranial electrodes can be challenging, and there is a risk of subsequent visual field deficits after resective surgery. In this chapter, we describe a case of NCSE of occipital origin, confirmed by intracranial electroencephalographic (EEG) recordings and subsequent resection. General clinical characteristics of occipital lobe epilepsy and the occurrence of NCSE in symptomatic occipital lobe epilepsy and in idiopathic occipital syndromes of childhood are discussed.

## CASE STUDY

A 42-year-old previously healthy man developed mycoplasma meningoencephalitis. He presented with headache, visual field deficit, and confusion. Imaging studies at initial presentation showed a right occipital lesion. Final diagnosis was established by brain biopsy. Three months after the initial event, he had a generalized tonic-clonic convulsion and developed intractable epilepsy. He described 2 seizure types: visual hallucinations of seeing yellow, red, and blue spots lasting for 60 to 90 minutes, followed by nausea and generalized tonic-clonic seizure activity, and seizures with an epigastric aura, followed by depersonalization and altered consciousness. At the time of presentation to our epilepsy center 10 years after the meningo-encephalitis, he had at least 1 seizure per week and a generalized convulsion every other month. With increasing duration of his epilepsy, his memory became increasingly impaired, impeding employment. On physical examination, he had a left homonymous hemianopsia that had been present since the meningo-encephalitis. A magnetic resonance imaging (MRI) scan showed the lesion in the right temporo-occipital area and mesial temporal sclerosis (Figure 11.1). Mesial temporal sclerosis was clearly not present on an MRI scan done on initial presentation 10 years earlier.

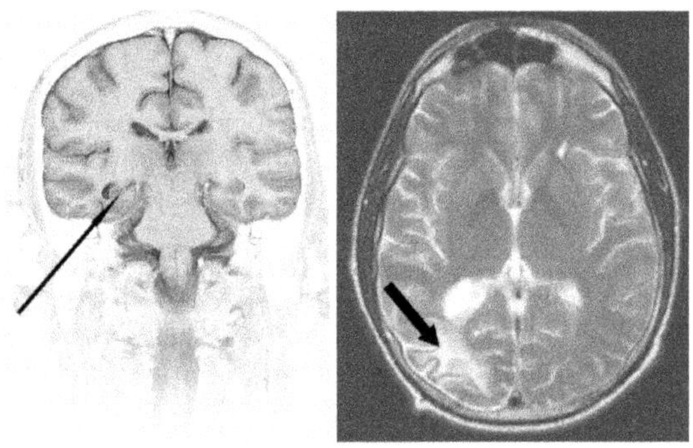

**Figure 11.1** Magnetic resonance imaging findings. Left: Hippocampal atrophy on the right on inversion recovery imaging (arrow). Right: Hyperintense occipital lesion on T2-weighted imaging (arrow).

During scalp EEG monitoring, the patient's interictal EEG showed occasional right posterior occipital spikes. He had several seizures recorded. These were characterized by his report of flickering yellow spots in his left visual field. He had no impairment of consciousness and was completely interactive throughout the visual hallucinations. All seizures recorded during wakefulness lasted between 25 and 46 minutes and were terminated by an intravenously administered injection of lorazepam or by a generalized tonic-clonic convulsion. Ictal scalp EEG showed subtle, right posterior occipital, rhythmic, theta and sharp-wave activity (Figure 11.2). An ictal single-photon emission computed tomographic scan showed clear hyperperfusion in the right occipital area (Figure 11.3).

An intracranial EEG study was performed covering the medial, lateral, and inferior occipital surface with grid electrodes and the hippocampus with an occipito-hippocampal depth electrode (Figure 11.4). The patient had only 1 spontaneous seizure recorded despite intracranial monitoring for 21 days (Figure 11.5). This seizure lasted 39 minutes and again represented NCSE with preserved consciousness. Two similar seizures were induced during functional mapping. Clinically, the patient reported a visual aura, followed by nausea and intermittent vomiting. Later, nystagmus and forced eye deviation to the left were noted. He was fully responsive at all times throughout the event, despite significant epileptiform activity on EEG monitoring (Figure 11.5). The seizure originated in the lateral occipital neocortex (Figure 11.5, arrow) and was confined to the lateral neocortex during initial visual hallucinations. During the increasing nausea and vomiting, epileptiform activity spread to the hippocampus (Figure 11.5). The anterior hippocampus

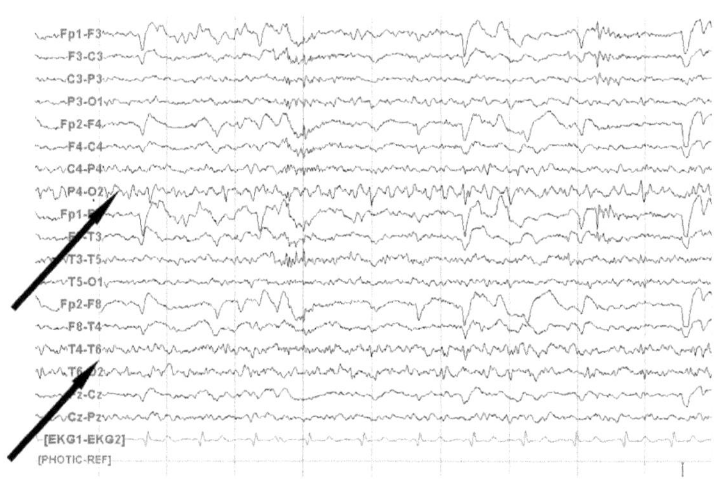


**Figure 11.2** Scalp electroencephalogram changes during nonconvulsive status epilepticus with visual hallucinations. There is subtle right occipital sharp theta activity. Symptoms had started 17 minutes before this recording.

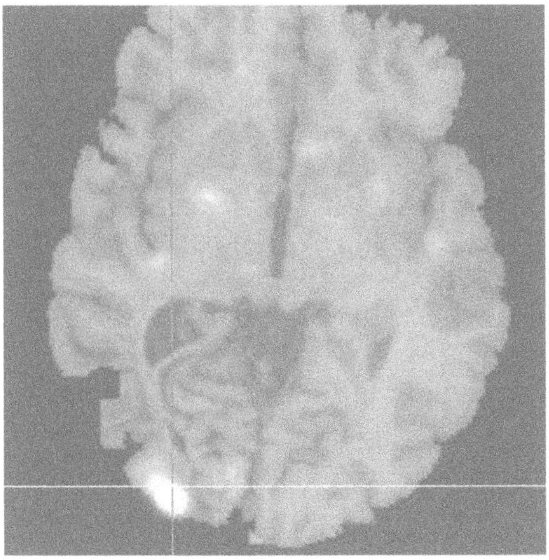

**Figure 11.3** Ictal single photon emission computed tomographic injection while the patient was having visual hallucinations during scalp electroencephalogram recording.

became involved at 7 minutes into the seizure. Epileptiform activity waxed and waned in the hippocampus, but visual symptoms persisted. When nystagmus and eye deviation were present, all cortical surfaces of the occipital lobe were involved, but visual hallucinations had ceased (Figure 11.5). The event was terminated by lorazepam, with resolution of the epileptiform activity.

A resection of the posterior occipital lobe and hippocampus was performed. The patient has remained seizure free during the follow-up period of 6 months after surgery. Pathology showed severe mesial temporal sclerosis with loss of neurons in large portions of the hippocampus and encephalomalacia with gliosis of the resected occipital tissue.

There are several important points to be made regarding this case. The patient exhibited nonconvulsive occipital lobe status epilepticus with primary visual hallucinations and epileptic nystagmus. Whenever he had a typical seizure, he had, in essence, occipital NCSE. None of his seizures was shorter than 20 minutes during video-EEG monitoring, which was consistent with reports of his usual seizures as an outpatient. Despite significant involvement of the entire posterior occipital region and the hippocampus, there was no impairment of consciousness.

Another interesting finding was the patient's extensive mesial temporal sclerosis, definitely not demonstrated by MRI at the time of the meningo-encephalitis. Neuronal loss in the hippocampus was severe at the time of epilepsy surgery. The hippocampus was not the primary site of seizure onset, as demonstrated by the intracranial study. It could be hypothesized that repeated NCSE of occipital origin led to mesial temporal sclerosis. Hippocampal damage seemed to become more relevant over time, as demonstrated clinically by increasing memory difficulties. The relationship between repeated nonconvulsive occipital status epilepticus and hippocampal sclerosis, however, needs to be examined in larger studies.

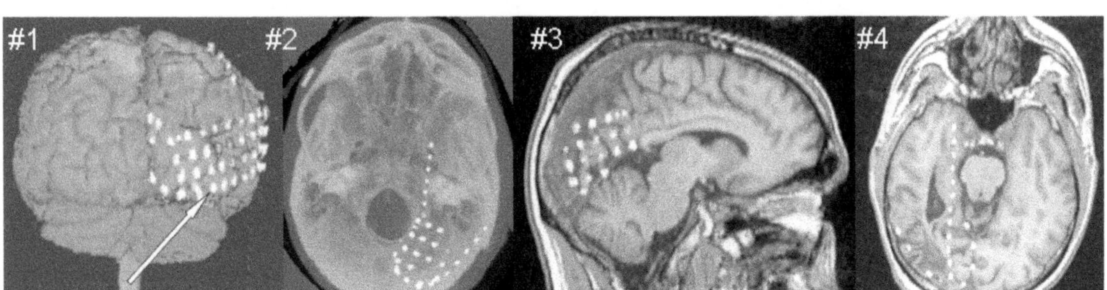


**Figure 11.4** Intracranial study with subdural grid electrodes implanted over the lateral occipito-temporal surface (#1), the inferior occipital surface (#2), and the medial occipital surface (#3) and an occipito-hippocampal depth electrode (#4). The arrow points to the electrical seizure onset.

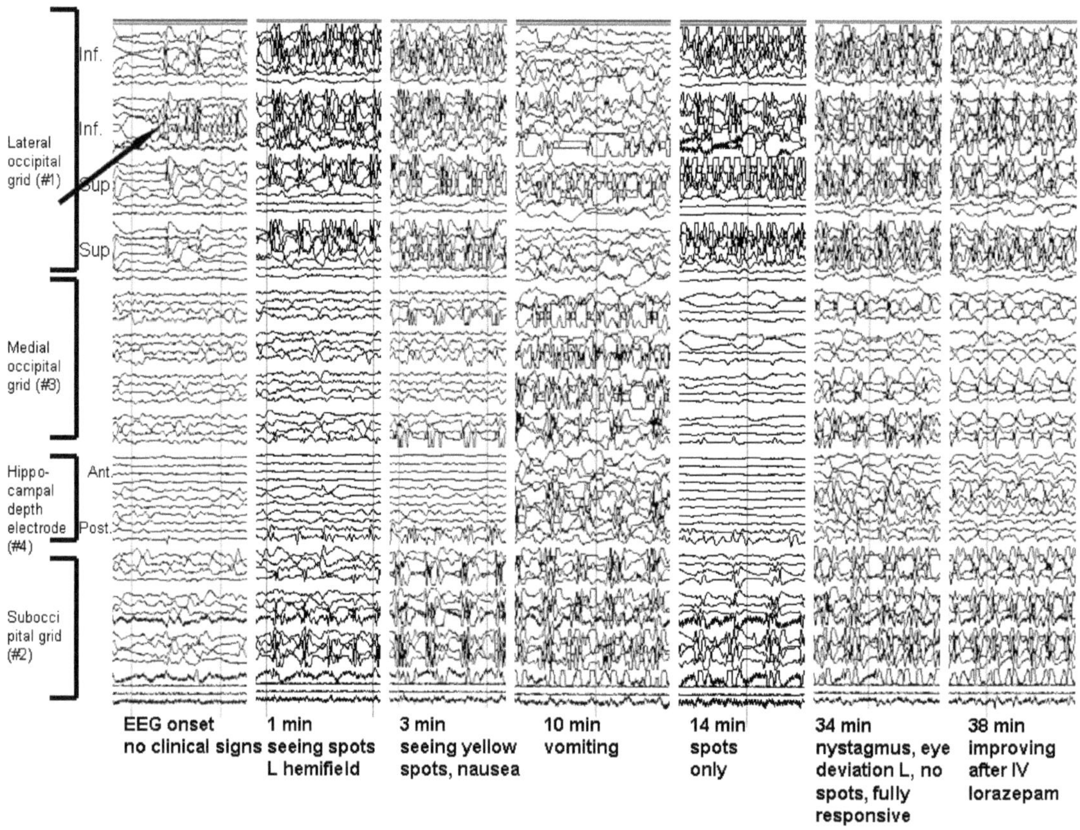


**Figure 11.5** Evolution of intracranial electroencephalogram changes during an episode of nonconvulsive status epilepticus without any impairment of consciousness. Seizure onset was confined to the lateral inferior occipital grid (arrow). At 1 minute, the patient had visual hallucinations and epileptiform activity that was confined to the lateral occipital grid and the lateral suboccipital region. With increasing nausea at 3 minutes, the patient had more involvement of the suboccipital region and of the medial occipital region with persistent epileptiforn activity in the lateral occipital cortex. Ten minutes after seizure onset, the symptoms consisted primarily of vomiting, there was less involvement of the lateral occipital grid, and most epileptiform activity was confined to the medial occipital region, the hippocampus, and the suboccipital region. After the nausea and vomiting ceased at 14 minutes, the patient had purely visual hallucinations; epileptiform activity was confined to the lateral occipital grid and the lateral suboccipital region. At 34 minutes, nearly all implanted electrodes showed epileptiform activity, and the patient was fully awake but had eye deviation and nystagmus, which improved after intravenous administration of lorazepam at 38 minutes. Numbers in brackets refer to electrode placement in Figure 11.4. Abbreviations: sup, superior; inf, inferior; ant, anterior hippocampus; post, posterior hippocampus.

## GENERAL CLINICAL CHARACTERISTICS OF OCCIPITAL LOBE EPILEPSY

Several series have described the clinical manifestations of symptomatic occipital lobe epilepsy. Occipital lobe seizures can present with a variety of clinical manifestations (Table 11.1)(10,12-20). Visual alterations are thought to be the hallmark of occipital lobe epilepsy but occur in just 47% to 85% of patients (Table 11.1) (10,12-20). Visual alterations include elementary visual hallucinations, complex visual hallucinations, visual illusions, and ictal amaurosis (17).

Elementary visual hallucinations consist of unformed (frequently colored) shapes, lines, or flashes that are stationary or moving. They usually occur in the contralateral visual field. Elementary visual hallucinations are the most commonly observed visual alterations in most reported series (Table 11.1). However, they not only are associated with occipital seizure onset, but are also reported with occipito-temporal and antero-medial temporal seizure onset (17). Complex visual hallucinations may consist of seeing people, animals, or scenes. In a study of visual auras, complex visual hallucinations were found exclusively with occipito-temporal and mesial temporal seizure onset but not with seizure onset confined to the occipital lobe (17).

Visual illusions include micropsia (objects appearing smaller), macropsia (objects appearing larger), achromatopsia (loss of color vision), metamorphopsia (distortion of images), or kinetopsia (stationary objects that seem to move). Complex visual hallucinations and visual illusions are far less common than elementary visual hallucinations (Table 11.1) and are thought to involve the temporo-occipital visual association cortex (17,20).

Ictal amaurosis is another common clinical manifestation of occipital lobe seizures, and it can be prolonged (Table 11.1). It can be difficult, however, to determine whether prolonged amaurosis is ictal or postictal. Epileptic nystagmus has been associated with seizure onset in the temporo-parietal-occipital junction (21). It is noted in fewer than 15% of patients with occipital lobe epilepsy (Table 11.1). Eye blinking seems more common. Eye deviation is frequent as the seizure progresses. More often, eye deviation is contralateral to the seizure-onset site (Table 11.1) but is not a reliably lateralizing finding (10,15). Two series report a subjective eye-pulling sensation without objective eye movement (10,11).

Due to ictal propagation, occipital lobe seizures can be indistinguishable from typical temporal lobe seizures with automatisms or typical frontal lobe seizures with tonic posturing and clonic activity (10,13,22). Occipital ictal discharges can propagate to the anterior neocortex in various ways. This was described very well by Ajmone-Marsan in 1957 in his book The Epileptic Seizure (22) (Figure 11.6). Seizure activity can propagate into the hippocampus or lateral temporal neocortex. If so, visual alterations evolve into typical, mesial temporal lobe seizures with altered consciousness, oroalimentary automatisms, ipsilateral manual automatisms, and contralateral dystonia. Other routes of propagation include spread to the mesial fronto-parietal region via the medial interhemispheric neocortex and to the frontal neocortex via suprasylvian pathways. Subsequently, occipital seizures present as tonic seizures, clonic seizures, or typical frontal lobe hyperactive seizures (10,23,24). Occipital lobe seizures that spread rapidly to the contralateral hemisphere can be "false lateralizing" (22,24).

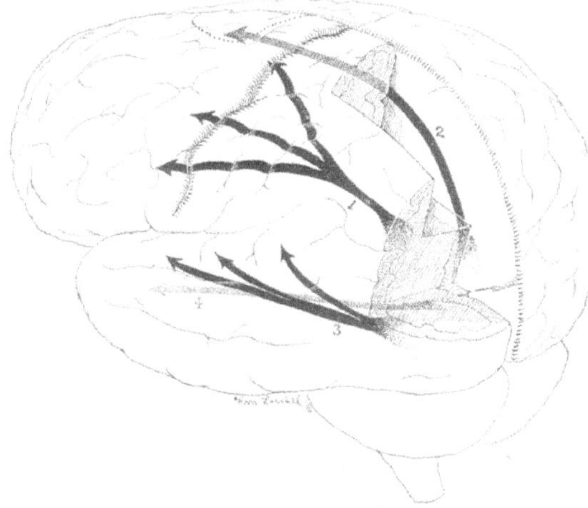

**Figure 11.6** Spread patterns of occipital lobe seizures. Reprinted with permission from Charles C. Thomas Publishers. Ajmone-Marasan and Ralston, The Epileptic Seizure, 1957; 214.

Because patients often do not recall their preceding visual auras, occipital lobe seizures may be easily misdiagnosed as being seizures that arise from other areas of the brain. In some cases, patients present initially with a visual aura that disappears with increasing duration of epilepsy (10,14). This emphasizes the importance of a comprehensive history.

In symptomatic occipital lobe epilepsy, ictal headache and vomiting occur in a minority of patients. Postictal headaches are more com-

**TABLE 11.1** CLINICAL CHARACTERISTICS OF OCCIPITAL LOBE SEIZURES IN SEVERAL REPORTED SERIES OF SYMPTOMATIC OCCIPITAL EPILEPSY

| Series | Patients with visual auras | Elementary visual hallu-cinations | Comple × visual hallu-cinations | Amaurosis | Eye-pulling sensation | Blinking | Nystagmus | Eye deviation | Visual field deficit | Spread patterns: Temporal Frontal | Status epilept icus | GTC |
|---|---|---|---|---|---|---|---|---|---|---|---|---|
| Ludwig, 1974 (13) n = 55 | 26 (47) | NR | NR | NR | NR | NR | 5 (9) | 16 (29) | 11 (20) | NR | NR | 18 (33) |
| Williamson, 5 1992 (10) n = 2 | 19 (77) | 15 (60) | 3 (12) | 10 (40) | 4 (16) | 14 (56) | 1 (4) | C:13 (52)<br>I: 3 (12) | 14 (56) | T:11 (44)<br>F: 3 (12)<br>B:11 (44) | 2 (8)[a] | NR |
| Salanova 1992 (14) n = 42 | 31 (73) | 31 (73) | 4 (9) | 12 (29) | NR | 8 (19) | 3 (7) | C: 5 (11) | 25 (59) | T:21 (50)<br>F:16 (38) | [b] | NR |
| Palmini 1993 (15) n = 8 | 6 (80) | 2 (25) | 2 (25) | 3 (37) | 1 (12) | NR | 1 (12) | C: 3 (37) | 2 (25) | T:6 (75)<br>F:2 (25) | NR | 8 (100) |
| Aykut-Bingol 1998 (16) n=35 | 26 (74) | 20 (57) | 4 (11) | 4 (11) | NR | 11 (31) | NR | C:10 (28)<br>I: 7 (20) | 16 (45) | T:12 (34)<br>F: 8 (22)<br>B:10 (28) | NR | 23 (65) |
| Panayiotopoulos 1999 (17) n = 18 | 18 (100)[c] | 18 (100) | 2 (11) | 2 (11) | NR | NR | NR | C: 4 (22) | 3 (16) | T:7 (38)<br>F: 6 (33) | 3 (16) | 16 (88) |
| Bien 2000 (18) n = 10 | 10 (100)[c] | 6 (60) | 1 (10) | 5 (50) | NR | NR | NR | NR | NR | NR | NR | NR |
| Lee 2005 (19) n=26 | 16 (62) | 9 (34) | 7 (26) | 4 (15) | NR | 4 (15) | NR | NR | 8 (30) | NR | NR | 21 (80) |
| Dalmagro 2005 (20) n = 15 | 9 (60) | 5 (55) | 2 (13) | 2 (13) | NR | NR | NR | NR | NR | T: 2 ( 13) | NR | NR |
| Blume 2005 (21) n = 41 | 35 (85) | 31 (75) | 19 (46) | NR | NR | NR | NR | NR | 11 (27) | NR | NR | NR |

*Data are presented as number (%). Numbers in parentheses after authors are reference numbers.*

***Abbreviations:*** *GTC, generalized tonic-clonic; NR, not reported; C, contralateral; I, ipsilateral; T, temporal spread (oroalimentary automatisms, oral and manual automatisms); F, frontal spread (clonic and tonic activity); B, frontal and temporal spread.*

[a]*During intracranial recordings*

[b]*Salanova reports prolonged ictal blindness if it occurred*

[c]*Visual auras represented inclusion criteria for the study.*

mon, as are postictal nausea and vomiting (16,25). Secondary generalization is frequent (Table 11.1).

Based on clinical seizure characteristics alone, it does not seem possible to differentiate medial occipital from lateral occipital seizure onset (15,20). An earlier, permanent visual field deficit is associated with medial rather than lateral occipital seizure onset (15,20).

EEG during occipital lobe seizures rarely demonstrates epileptiform activity confined purely to the occipital lobes. Most commonly, interictal and ictal EEG shows epileptiform activity in the posterior temporal region (10).

The etiologies of symptomatic occipital lobe epilepsy include tumors, vascular malformations, disorders of cortical development, neurocutaneous disorders, encephalomalacia, and infectious processes (10,15). Disorders of cortical development include cortical dysplasia, occipital periventricular heterotopia, subcortical band heterotopia, polymicrogyria, and ulegyria (26). Intractable symptomatic occipital lobe epilepsy is amenable to epilepsy surgery, with good seizure control but with a significant risk of additional visual field deficits (10,13,15,18,19).

## SYMPTOMATIC OCCIPITAL LOBE EPILEPSY AND NONCONVULSIVE STATUS EPILEPTICUS

A small number of case series of symptomatic occipital lobe epilepsy report the occurrence of status epilepticus and, especially, simple partial NCSE with prolonged visual alterations (Table 11.1). Two of 25 patients had status epilepticus during intracranial monitoring in 1 series (10). Another report comments that ictal amaurosis was prolonged (13). All of the above-mentioned clinical manifestations of occipital lobe epilepsy can be prolonged and represent forms of NCSE.

Most reports of occipital NCSE are case reports (Table 11.2) (27-34). Gowers published the first case report of occipital NCSE in *The Lancet* in 1879 (35). He described the case of Alfred S, who developed initial attacks of altered visual perception, followed by 3 days of persistent "flickering of light, like a gold serpent in the eye." The patient's attacks ceased with the administration of bromide and belladonna. When the patient died, he was found to have a right occipital tumor at autopsy. Gowers correctly identified those attacks as epileptic phenomena originating in the visual areas of the brain.

Barry and colleagues reported the largest series of occipital NCSE (33). Five patients had ictal blindness or status epilepticus amauroticus. The blindness lasted between 2 and 4 days in 4 of the 5 patients and resolved completely in all cases. Two patients had hemianopsia only. In 3 patients, the etiology was a previous stroke.

In his suggested classification of status epilepticus, Gastaut mentioned 2 cases of occipital lobe status with ictal EEG discharges and 5 without definite EEG discharges, but he did not provide any more details (2). Other case reports have described various clinical manifestations of occipital status epilepticus (ictal amaurosis, visual hallucinations) due to various etiologies such as lupus, cavernomas, or pregnancy (27,28). In conclusion, no specific underlying pathology has been associated with a higher incidence of occipital status epilepticus in symptomatic occipital lobe epilepsy.

Celiac disease has been associated with occipital calcifications and occipital lobe seizures (36,37). The incidence of NCSE has not been reported in this syndrome, but epileptic encephalopathy can develop despite appropriate treatment (38).

## OCCIPITAL LOBE EPILEPSY AND HIPPOCAMPAL ATROPHY

The relationship between occipital-parietal epilepsy and hippocampal atrophy has been examined previously in a larger study using MRI (39). The authors concluded that associated mesial temporal sclerosis in occipital-parietal epilepsy is not a result of seizure propagation into the hippocampus. They proposed that hippocampal atrophy is part of an underlying pathologic developmental disorder. In the case reported here, however, there did not

**TABLE 11.2** CASE REPORTS AND SERIES OF OCCIPITAL NONCONVULSIVE STATUS EPILEPTICUS

| Author | Symptoms | Duration | Etiology | EEG | Treatment |
|---|---|---|---|---|---|
| Kawai 2006 (27) | Palinopsia, macropsia, elementary visual hallucinations, hemianopsia | 5 min to hours | Cavernoma | NR | TPM-resolved |
| Fernandez-Torre 2003 (28) | Blurred vision, visual distortions, head and eye deviation, confusion | Minutes to hours | Lupus erythromatodes | Paroxysmal fast, repetitive spike and spike wave discharges unilateral occipito-parieto-temporal | LTG-resolved |
| Spatt 2000 (29) | Elementary visual hallucinations | Every few minutes | Stroke | Unilateral occipital rhythmic slow intermixed with spikes | DZP and CBZ-resolved No treatment |
| Sheth 1999 (30) | Subclinical | 2 years | Unknown | Continous unilateral occipital rhythmic activity | |
| Sawchuk 1997 (31) | Amaurosis | > 4 hours | In the setting of cardiac bypass surgery | Unilateral periodic occipital sharp waves with intermittent seizures | PTH-resolved |
| Thomas 1991 (32) | Eye-deviation, nystagmus, elementary and complex visual hallucinations, hemianopsia | 36 hours | Pregnancy, no history of seizures | NR | Unresponsive to PTH, DZP, PB; resolved after C-section |
| Barry 1985 (33) 5 patients | Amaurosis or hemianopsia | Between minutes up to 2-4 days in 3 patients | Metastasis, stoke, idiopathic | Occipital slowing and rhythmic seizure discharges unilateral and bilateral | PTH resolved |
| Aldrich 1989 (34) | Elementary visual hallucinations | > 45 min up to several days | Unclear | Bilateral and unilateral occipital repetitive spikes and rhythmic sharp waves | CBZ, PHT, PB, DZP Persistent seizures despite multiple AEDS |

*Numbers in parentheses after authors are reference numbers.*

***Abbreviations:*** *NR refers to not reported; TPM, topiramate; DZP, diazepam; CBZ, carbamazepine; PTH, phenytoin; PB, phenobarbital, AEDs, antiepileptic drugs.*

appear to be an underlying developmental disorder. Hippocampal atrophy clearly developed after the encephalitis. Simmons and colleagues reported a similar case with obvious secondary development of hippocampal atrophy after repeated visual NCSE (40). The relationship between occipital epilepsy, and especially the relationship of prolonged occipital NCSE, and mesial temporal sclerosis needs further investigation in larger prospective studies.

## IDIOPATHIC OCCIPITAL EPILEPSY SYNDROMES OF CHILDHOOD AND NONCONVULSIVE STATUS EPILEPTICUS

Gastaut first described benign childhood epilepsies of occipital origin (41). Currently, 3 distinct syndromes of idiopathic childhood epilepsies with occipital paroxysms are recognized (Table 11.3). These include early-onset benign childhood occipital epilepsy (Panayiotopoulos type or benign childhood seizure susceptibility syndrome) (42), late-onset childhood occipital epilepsy (Gastaut type) (41), and idiopathic photosensitive occipital lobe epilepsy (4,43).

Early-onset benign childhood occipital epilepsy (Panayiotopoulos syndrome; susceptibility to early-onset benign childhood seizures with mainly autonomic symptoms) presents in early childhood (mean onset, 4.7 years) with a lack of visual symptoms but with gaze deviation, ictal vomiting, and autonomic symptoms such as pallor and sweating (26, 42). Seizures can progress to hemiconvulsions or generalized convulsions. Visual symptoms are rare. Seizures are mainly nocturnal. EEG shows bilateral high-amplitude, rhythmic, sharp-and-slow-wave activity over the posterior regions with fixation-off sensitivity (44). The average duration of seizures is 9 minutes, and 44% to 46% of patients have NCSE, with seizures lasting more than 30 minutes (45,46). Despite the high incidence of NCSE, the prognosis is excellent, and seizures usually remit spontaneously after 1 to 2 years (46).

Late-onset occipital lobe epilepsy (Gastaut type) has a peak onset age of 7 to 9 years. Seizures are characterized by visual hallucinations followed by postictal headache, nausea, and vomiting (47). Ictal amaurosis occurred in 65% of Gastaut's initial series (47). Consciousness is seldom impaired unless seizures progress to hemiconvulsions, tonic-clonic seizures, or

**TABLE 11.3** CHARACTERISTICS, PROGNOSIS, AND INCIDENCE OF NONCONVULSIVE STATUS EPILEPTICUS IN THE MOST COMMON OCCIPITAL LOBE EPILEPSIES

| Type of epilepsy | Age of onset | Seizure characteristics | Nonconvulsive status | Prognosis |
|---|---|---|---|---|
| Localization-related occipital lobe | Variable, depending on etiology | Visual hallucinations and illusions, amaurosis, nystagmus, eye deviation | Variable | Depending on etiology |
| Early-onset benign childhood occipital (Panayiotopoulos type) | 3-6 y | Gaze deviation, ictal vomiting, headaches, autonomic symptoms | Common, 44%-46% | Remits - spontaneously |
| Late-onset childhood occipital (Gastaut type) | 7-9 y | Visual hallucinations, amaurosis | Uncommon | Good |
| Idiopathic photosensitive occipital | 12 y | Visual hallucinations, head and eye deviation | Possible | Responds well to AEDs |

*AEDs refers to antiepileptic drugs.*

temporal lobe–type seizures (47). Seizures are more commonly diurnal (45). Seizures are typically brief, and NCSE is exceptional (44). EEG is characterized by runs of bilateral occipital spikes and spike-wave complexes occurring with eye closure. Seizures commonly respond to antiepileptic medications. Prognosis is still good, with a high spontaneous remission rate, but the prognosis is not as good as in Panayiotopoulos syndrome.

Idiopathic photosensitive occipital epilepsy is a distinct syndrome, occurring more commonly in girls than in boys (43,48). Diagnosis requires that all seizures are induced by a visual stimulation such as videogames, television, or other sources of flickering lights. The peak age of onset is in early teenage years (43). Seizures consist of visual hallucinations followed by head and eye deviation and, possibly, unresponsiveness. Removal of the visual stimulus does not result in abortion of seizure activity (26). By definition, seizures are mainly diurnal, as they are stimulus-induced, but nocturnal generalized tonic-clonic seizures can occur (49). Duration of seizures is variable, and NCSE occurred in 20% of the initial series (43). EEG shows occipital spike and spike-wave discharges that may become generalized with photic stimulation and increase with eye closure (48). Prognosis is usually good. There is some overlap of this syndrome with juvenile myoclonic epilepsy (48).

## DIFFERENTIAL DIAGNOSIS, TREATMENT, AND PROGNOSIS OF OCCIPITAL NONCONVULSIVE STATUS EPILEPTICUS

Because occipital lobe NCSE can be subtle, without loss of consciousness, there is a broad differential diagnosis. Visual hallucinations associated with migraine are very distinct. Migraine auras consist of black and white zigzag lines, in contrast to the usually colored visual hallucinations that occur with occipital lobe seizures (50). In addition, other clinical manifestations, such as eye deviation and ictal nystagmus, are lacking in migraine or basilar migraine. Primary ophthalmologic disorders such as retinal diseases can present with visual phenomena, but these are not usually transient.

The prognosis of NCSE is generally good, considering the high incidence of benign idiopathic occipital epilepsies of childhood. Standard antiepileptic medications are usually effective in treating occipital NCSE (Table 11.2).

## CONCLUSION

In localization-related occipital lobe epilepsy, NCSE is not uncommon. In idiopathic occipital lobe epilepsy of childhood (Panayiotopoulos type), NCSE seems to occur in nearly half the patients and carries a good prognosis. Nevertheless, systematic large-scale studies, especially of occipital localization-related NCSE, are lacking. The pathophysiology, EEG spread patterns, and secondary consequences such as secondary mesial temporal sclerosis warrant further investigation.

## REFERENCES

1. Kaplan PW. Behavioral manifestations of nonconvulsive status epilepticus. Epilepsy Behav 2002;3:122-139.
2. Gastaut H. Classification of status epilepticus. Adv Neurol 1983;34:15-35.
3. Gastaut H. Classification of status epilepticus. In: Delgado-Escueta AV, Wasterlain CG, Treiman DM, Porter RJ, eds. Status Epilepticus: Mechanisms of Brain Damage and Treatment. New York, NY: Raven Press; 1983:15-35.
4. Engel J Jr. A proposed diagnostic scheme for people with epileptic seizures and with epilepsy: report of the ILAE Task Force on Classification and Terminology. Epilepsia 2001;42:796-803.
5. Kaplan PW. The clinical features, diagnosis, and prognosis of nonconvulsive status epilepticus. Neurologist 2005;11:348-361.
6. Walker M, Cross H, Smith S, Young C, Aicardi j, Appleton R, Aylett S, Besag F, Cock H, DeLorenzo R, Drislane F, Duncan J, Ferrie C, Fujikawa D, Gray W, Kaplan P, Koutroumanidis M, O'Regan M, Plouin P, sander J, Scott R, Shorvon S, Treiman D, Wasterlain C, Wiesh-

mann U. Nonconvulsive status epilepticus: Epilepsy Research Foundation workshop reports. Epileptic Disord 2005;7:253-296.

7. Lowenstein DH, Bleck T, Macdonald RL. It's time to revise the definition of status epilepticus. Epilepsia 1999;40:120-122.
8. Williamson PD, Spencer DD, Spencer SS, Novelly RA, Mattson RH. Complex partial status epilepticus: a depth-electrode study. Ann Neurol 1985;18:647-654.
9. Jobst BC, Siegel AM, Thadani VM, Roberts DW, Williamson PD. Intractable seizures of frontal lobe origin. Epilepsia 2000;41:1139-1152.
10. Williamson PD, Thadani VM, Darcey TM, Spencer DD, Spencer SS, Mattson RH. Occipital lobe epilepsy: clinical characteristics, seizure spread patterns and results of surgery. Ann Neurol 1992;31:3-13.
11. Palmini A, Quesney LF, Olivier A, Andermann F, Gloor P. Clinical and EEG findings in occipital lobe epilepsy: a depth electrode study [abstract]. Epilepsia 1990;31:638.
12. Ludwig BI, Ajmone-Marsan C. Clinical ictal patterns in epileptic patients with occipital electroencephalographic foci. Neurology 1975;25:463-471.
13. Salanova V, Andermann F, Olivier A, Rasmussen T, Quesney LF. Occipital lobe epilepsy: electroclinical manifestations, electrocorticography, cortical stimulation and outcome in 42 patients treated between 1930 and 1991. Surgery of occipital lobe epilepsy. Brain 1992;115(Pt 6):1655-1680.
14. Palmini A, Andermann F, Dubeau F, Gloor P, Olivier A, Quesney LF, Salanova V. Occipitotemporal epilepsies: evaluation of selected patients requiring depth electrodes studies and rationale for surgical approaches. Epilepsia 1993;34:84-96.
15. Aykut-Bingol C, Bronen RA, Kim JH, Spencer DD, Spencer SS. Surgical outcome in occipital lobe epilepsy: implications for pathophysiology. Ann Neurol 1998;44:60-69.
16. Panayiotopoulos CP. Visual phenomena and headache in occipital epilepsy: a review, a systematic study and differentiation from migraine. Epileptic Disord 1999;1:205-216.
17. Bien CG, Benninger FO, Urbach H, Schramm J, Kurthen M, Elger CE. Localizing value of epileptic visual auras. Brain 2000;123(Pt 2):244-253.
18. Kun Lee S, Young Lee S, Kim DW, Soo Lee D, Chung CK. Occipital lobe epilepsy: clinical characteristics, surgical outcome, and role of diagnostic modalities. Epilepsia 2005;46:688-695.
19. Dalmagro CL, Bianchin MM, Velasco TR, Alexandre V, Walz R, Terra-Bustamante VC, Inuzuka LM, Wichert-Ana L, Araujo D, Serafini LN, Carlotti CG, Assirati J A, Machado HR, Santos AC, Sakamoto AC. Clinical features of patients with posterior cortex epilepsies and predictors of surgical outcome. Epilepsia 2005;46:1442-1449.
20. Blume WT, Wiebe S, Tapsell LM. Occipital epilepsy: lateral versus mesial. Brain 2005;128:1209-1225.
21. Kaplan PW, Tusa RJ. Neurophysiologic and clinical correlations of epileptic nystagmus. Neurology 1993;43:2508-2514.
22. Ajmone-Marsan C, Ralston BL. The Epileptic Seizure. Its Functional Morphology and Diagnostic Significance. Springfield, IL: Charles C. Thomas; 1957.
23. Ajmone-Marsan C. Clinical-electrographic correlations of partial seizures. In: Wada JA, ed. Modern Perspectives in Epilepsy, Proceedings of the Inaugural Symposium of the Canadian League Against Epilepsy. Montreal, Canada: Eden Press; 1978:76-98.
24. Fava M, Blume W. Propagation patterns of occipital seizure recorded subdurally [abstract]. Epilepsia 2002;43(Suppl 7)53.
25. Gilliam F, Wyllie E. Ictal amaurosis: MRI, EEG, and clinical features. Neurology 1995;45:1619-1621.
26. Taylor I, Scheffer IE, Berkovic SF. Occipital epilepsies: identification of specific and newly recognized syndromes. Brain 2003;126:753-769.
27. Kawai M, Cherches IM, Goldsmith IL. Visual illusory and hallucinatory phenomena in a patient with left occipital seizures. Neurology 2006;67:1457.
28. Fernandez-Torre JL, Sanchez JM, Gonzalez C, Fernandez-Guinea O. Complex partial status epilepticus of extratemporal origin in a patient with systemic lupus erythematosus. Seizure 2003;12:245-248.
29. Spatt J, Mamoli B. Ictal visual hallucinations and post-ictal hemianopia with anosognosia. Seizure 2000;9:502-504.
30. Sheth RD, Riggs JE. Persistent occipital electrographic status epilepticus. J Child Neurol 1999;14:334-336.
31. Sawchuk KS, Churchill S, Feldman E, Drury I. Status epilepticus amauroticus. Neurology 1997;49:1467-1469.

32. Thomas P, Barres P, Chatel M. Complex partial status epilepticus of extratemporal origin: report of a case. Neurology 1991;41:1147-1149.
33. Barry E, Sussman NM, Bosley TM, Harner RN. Ictal blindness and status epilepticus amauroticus. Epilepsia 1985;26:577-584.
34. Aldrich MS, Vanderzant CW, Alessi AG, Abou-Khali B, Sackellares JC. Ictal cortical blindness with permanent visual loss. Epilepsia 1989;30:116-120.
35. Gowers W. Cases of cerebral tumour illustrating diagnosis and localization. The Lancet 1879:363-365.
36. Bernasconi A, Bernasconi N, Andermann F, Bernasconi A, Bernasconi N, Andermann F, Dubeau F, Guberman A, Gobbi G, Olivier A. Celiac disease, bilateral occipital calcifications and intractable epilepsy: mechanisms of seizure origin. Epilepsia 1998;39:300-306.
37. Gobbi G, Bouquet F, Greco L, Lambertini A, Tassinari CA, Ventura A, Zaniboni MG. Coeliac disease, epilepsy, and cerebral calcifications. The Italian Working Group on Coeliac Disease and Epilepsy. Lancet 1992;340:439-443.
38. Gobbi G, Sorrenti G, Santucci M, Rossi PG, Ambrosetto P, Michelucci R, Tassinari CA. Epilepsy with bilateral occipital calcifications: a benign onset with progressive severity. Neurology 1988;38:913-920.
39. Lawn N, Londono A, Sawrie S, Morawetz R, Martin R, Gilliam F, Faught E, Kuzniecky R. Occipitoparietal epilepsy, hippocampal atrophy, and congenital developmental abnormalities. Epilepsia 2000;41:1546-1553.
40. Simons PJ, Van Paesschen W, Palmini A, Dupont P, Van Driel G, Van Laere K. The development of hippocampal sclerosis in a patient with occipital lobe epilepsy and migraine. Neurology 2004;62:1024-1025.
41. Gastaut H. Benign epilepsy of childhood with occipital paroxysms. In: Roger J, Dravet C, Bureau M, Dreifuss FE, Wolf P, eds. Epileptic syndromes in infancy, childhood, and adolescence. London, England: John Libbey Eurotext; 1985:159-170.
42. Panayiotopoulos CP. Benign childhood epilepsy with occipital paroxysms: a 15-year prospective study. Ann Neurol 1989;26:51-56.
43. Guerrini R, Dravet C, Genton P, Bureau M, Bonanni P, Ferrari AR, Roger J. Idiopathic photosensitive occipital lobe epilepsy. Epilepsia 1995;36:883-891.
44. Ferrie CD, Beaumanoir A, Guerrini R, Kivity S, Vigevano F, Takaishi Y, Watanabe K, Mira L, Capizzi G, Costa P, Valseriati D, Grioni D, Lerman P, Ricci S, Vigliano P, Goumas-Kartalas A, Hashimoto K, Robinson RO, Panayiotopoulos CP. Early-onset benign occipital seizure susceptibility syndrome. Epilepsia 1997;38:285-293.
45. Ferrie C, Caraballo R, Covanis A, Demirbilek V, Dervent A, Kivity S, Koutroumanidis M, Martinovic Z, Oguni H, Verrotti A, Vigevano F, Watanabe K, Yalcin D, Yoshinaga H. Panayiotopoulos syndrome: a consensus view. Dev Med Child Neurol 2006;48:236-240.
46. Lada C, Skiadas K, Theodorou V, Loli N, Covanis A. A study of 43 patients with Panayiotopoulos syndrome, a common and benign childhood seizure susceptibility. Epilepsia 2003;44:81-88.
47. Gastaut H. A new type of epilepsy: benign partial epilepsy of childhood with occipital spike-waves. Clin Electroencephalogr 1982;13:13-22.
48. Taylor I, Marini C, Johnson MR, Turner S, Berkovic SF, Scheffer IE. Juvenile myoclonic epilepsy and idiopathic photosensitive occipital lobe epilepsy: is there overlap? Brain 2004;127:1878-1886.
49. Yalcin AD, Kaymaz A, Forta H. Reflex occipital lobe epilepsy. Seizure 2000;9:436-441.
50. Panayiotopoulos CP. Elementary visual hallucinations in migraine and epilepsy. J Neurol Neurosurg Psychiatry 1994;57:1371-1374.

PART III

# GENERALIZED/ABSENCE (NONCONVULSIVE) STATUS EPILEPTICUS

CHAPTER 12

# ABSENCE STATUS EPILEPTICUS

MICHAEL KOUTROUMANIDIS

The diagnosis and classification of epileptic seizures and syndromes are made initially by clinical and electroencephalographic (EEG) criteria. Typical absences (TA) in idiopathic generalized epilepsy (IGE), for example, may share some principal clinical features with limbic complex partial seizures, such as unresponsiveness and automatisms, and one must turn to either their onset (presence or absence of aura) or termination (presence or absence of depression and confusion) and, of course, to the interictal EEG to differentiate them. Even so, the rate of misdiagnosis is high (1,2). The diagnosis and classification of nonconvulsive status epilepticus (NCSE) follows similar principles. In patients with ongoing nonconvulsive status, the yield from clinical clues diminishes, and the role of EEG becomes essential for diagnosis. Not surprisingly, it is also an essential tool for nosologic taxonomy (Table 12.1).

This chapter will address the 2 forms of NCSE in IGE, namely the more common absence status epilepticus (ASE), and the less common myoclonic status epilepticus (MSE). There is a partial overlap between these 2 types, insofar as ASE in predominantly myoclonic IGE syndromes such as juvenile myoclonic epilepsy (JME) or eyelid myoclonia with absences (EMA) may be associated with a clinically prominent myoclonic component—axial, arm, or regional facial. We shall also refer to forms of NCSE from which idiopathic ASE should be differentiated, including those encountered in various cryptogenic generalized epilepsies, idiopathic focal epilepsies, symptomatic or cryptogenic focal epilepsies, and nonepileptic episodes (Table 1).

Although the first description of ASE using EEG by Putman and Merritt in 1941(3) and by Lennox in 1945 (4) predated that of Gastaut and Roger on complex partial status epilepticus (CPSE) by many years (5), ASE has received considerably less attention. Most large studies on NCSE before the 1989 International League Against Epilepsy (ILAE) epilepsy syndrome classification (6) included mainly or exclusively patients with CPSE, without cues to discern those with possible ASE. Thus, our knowledge on ASE is still limited and relies on a few relatively small series (7-10) and case reports.

## CLASSIFICATION AND TERMINOLOGY

The classification of NCSE is discussed in Chapter 2. The following terminology and its rationale may serve as framework for the present chapter.

## IDIOPATHIC ABSENCE STATUS EPILEPTICUS

The concept of idiopathic ASE (or simply ASE) is firmly attached to that of IGE, a subgroup of epilepsies that are genetically determined, unrelated to any structural brain pathology, and associated with normal neurologic and neuropsychological status. Typically, there are other seizure types and symptoms in various combinations, including TA (hence it has also been called typical ASE), myoclonic seizures (MS), and generalized tonic-clonic seizures (GTCS). The EEG shows interictal generalized spike-wave (GSW) activity at 3 to 4 Hz (but also nonlocalizing focal spikes)(11) and, during the status, usually shows continuous regular

**TABLE 12.1** DIFFERENTIATING CLINICAL AND EEG FEATURES OF IGE (IDIOPATHIC ASE AND MSE) AND OTHER EPILEPSIES AND EPILEPTIC STATES THAT CAN BE MANIFESTED AS GENERALIZED NONCONVULSIVE STATUS EPILEPTICUS

| | **IGE** | **Generalized cryptogenic / symptomatic** | **Focal symptomatic / cryptogenic** | **Focal idiopathic** | **De novo absence-like status** |
|---|---|---|---|---|---|
| Epilepsy syndromes and conditions | Absence syndromes<br>CAE<br>JAE<br>Phantom TAl<br>Myoclonic syndromes<br>JME<br>EMA / PMA<br>GTCS only<br>Mixed / unclassified | Chromosomal disorders<br>Angelman syndrome<br>Ring 20 syndrome<br>Dravet syndrome<br>Myoclonic astatic epilepsy<br>Lennox-Gastaut syndrome<br>Syndrome of myoclonic absences<br>Nonprogressive encephalopathies<br>Cortical dysplasias<br>Early hypoxia | Various syndromes of lobar (mainly frontal and temporal lobe) epilepsies | RE<br>Opercular status (rare)<br>GSWS (rare)<br>Absence status (rare)<br>PS<br>Autonomic status (≈ 50%)<br>GSWS (rare)<br>Absence status (rare) (21)<br>EEG with GSWS, including Landau-Kleffner syndrome | None |
| Types of NCSE | Mainly ASE, with added regional myoclonic element in myoclonic syndromes. MSE is rare even in JME | Variable, mostly mixed absence- myoclonic status | Complex partial status epilepticus | RE: Opercular status. Buccofacial apraxia, drooling and speech arrest, responsive<br>PS: Autonomic status. Autonomic symptoms and signs with gradual unresponsiveness<br>EEG: GSWS during sleep. Absence and myoclonic status with negative myoclonus. | Absence-like |
| Other seizures types | Typical absences<br>Myoclonic Seizures<br>GTCS<br>Rarely tonic | Atypical absences, tonic, clonic, myoclonic, negative myoclonus<br>Complex partial, GTCS<br><br>Syndrome-specific seizures:<br>Myoclonic-astatic<br>Myoclonic absences | Simple or complex partial with semiology reflecting the lobe of origin or propagation | Rolandic seizures in RE<br>Autonomic seizures with or without eye deviation and motor symptoms in PS<br><br>Rolandic and autonomic seizures may coexist in mixed phenotypes | None |

| | | | | | |
|---|---|---|---|---|---|
| Interictal EEG | Normal background, GSW > 2.5 Hz, nonlocalizing focal | Normal or diffusely slow background. Slow, < 2.5-Hz GSW, multifocal spikes; characteristic monomorphic 2-Hz SW in Angelman syndrome | Focal slowing / spikes, but may be normal or show secondary bilateral synchrony | Normal background, multifocal, rolandic or occipital spikes, GSW | Normal or nonspecific slow. Epileptiform activity not expected |
| Ictal EEG (in status) | GSW at > 2.5 Hz, continuous or discontinuous, rhythmic or arrhythmic, slower in late stages<br>Can be slow or arrhythmic when precipitated by inappropriate AED | Generally irregular, slow (< 2.5-Hz) GSW, mixed with bilateral synchronous bursts of slow activity<br>Occasionally, fast GSW may look like idiopathic ASE | Frontal onset, unilateral or bilateral, may evolve to diffuse absence-like GSW<br>Temporal onset in TLE, initially clusters of CPS, then continuous | Focal onset evolving to bilateral diffuse | GSW at variable frequencies |
| Induction by AED | AEDs inappropriate for IGE may induce ASE and MSE (with positive and negative myoclonus) | Occasionally by CBZ, PHT, DZP, LTG, LEV (93,94) | Never reported | Rarely ASE in RE and PS by CBZ<br>Possible aggravation of EEG with GSWS by CBZ | No. Typically, induced by BZP withdrawal. |
| Response to treatment | Usually rapid and full to IV BZP and VPA (but also see Figure 12.1) | Notoriously resistant to IV BZP and VPA, steroids may be useful. | Gradual, IV PHT more effective than BZP | Rapid and full to IV BZP in both opercular and autonomic status | Rapid EEG normalization but variably delayed clinical recovery especially in the elderly. |
| Brain MRI | Normal | Normal or abnormal | Normal or abnormal | Normal | Normal or abnormal (nonspecific) |

***Abbreviations:*** *AED, antiepileptic drugs; ASE, absence status epilepticus; BZP, benzodiazepines CAE, childhood absence epilepsy; CBZ, carbamazepine; CPS, complex partial seizures; EE, epileptic encephalopathy; EEG, electroencephalography; EMA, eyelid myoclonia with absences; IGE, idiopathic generalized epilepsy; IV, intravenously administered; ; GTCS, generalized tonic clonic seizures; GSW, generalized spike wave; GSWS, generalized spike-wave during slow sleep; JAE, juvenile absence epilepsy; JME, juvenile myoclonic epilepsy; LEV, levetiracetam; LTG, lamotrigine; MRI, magnetic resonance imaging; MSE, myoclonic status epilepticus; NCSE, nonconvulsive status epilepticus; PHT, phenytoin; PMA, perioral myoclonia with absences; PS, Panayiotopoulos syndrome; RE, benign rolandic epilepsy; SW, slow wave; TA, typical absences; TLE, temporal lobe epilepsy; VPA, valproate.*

GSW at 3 to 4 Hz with a frontal maximum but also irregular bilateral synchronous discharges at equivalent frequencies. Because similarly diffuse and bilateral synchronous ictal epileptiform activity may occur during other types of NCSE (including CPSE of frontal lobe, de novo absence-like status, and even in nonepileptic encephalopathies), the term *idiopathic ASE* (or simply ASE) requires an established IGE diagnosis and will not be used here as a simple descriptive term.

## NONIDIOPATHIC ABSENCE STATUS EPILEPTICUS

This term *nonidiopathic ASE* denotes continuous or subcontinuous atypical absences (hence it is also called *atypical ASE*) that occur only in the context of mainly severe symptomatic or cryptogenic epilepsies of children with neuropsychological delay and frequent other seizures types, including tonic, atonic, and myoclonic or myoclonic-atonic seizures such as Lennox-Gastaut syndrome (LGS) and in most patients with myoclonic astatic epilepsy (MAE). As opposed to the TA of IGE, in atypical absences (and consequently in nonidiopathic ASE), onset and offset may be gradual and clinically difficult to define, impairment of consciousness is usually mild to moderate and sometimes difficult to ascertain, and ictal changes of tone are usually more pronounced. The ictal GSW discharge is typically slower (< 2.5 Hz) and irregular and may include other paroxysmal activity, especially during sleep. Interictally, slow GSW or consistent multifocal abnormalities with or without evidence of secondary bilateral synchrony (12) may occur, and background activity is usually abnormal.

## MYOCLONIC STATUS EPILEPTICUS

This general term designates long episodes of continuous bilateral rhythmic or arrhythmic myoclonus of varying topographic distribution that can occur in idiopathic and cryptogenic or symptomatic generalized epilepsies. MSE was initially classified into "primary" and "secondary" forms with reference to underlying etiology (13), terms that have now been replaced by the terms *idiopathic* and *cryptogenic*, or *symptomatic (nonidiopathic)*, respectively. Idiopathic MSE occurs in patients with predominantly myoclonic IGE syndromes and conditions. In the archetypal paradigm of JME, MSE usually occurs as an ongoing sequence of bilateral synchronous muscle contractions without impairment of consciousness, ie, as a purely motor state and therefore a distinct type of convulsive status (14,15). The reason that different types of MSE are discussed in this chapter is that such pure motor forms are rare. Patients with severe forms of JME may describe that their concentration and trains of thoughts are disrupted during prolonged and violent volleys of jerks (16). Besides, ASE is more frequent than MSE, even in JME (in which it is usually associated with minor jerks) (8,10,17). Prominent bilateral regional facial myoclonus may feature in ASE of patients with IGE syndromes, in which absence seizures are also associated with bilateral regional myoclonus, such as eyelid or perioral myoclonia (8,9). This partial phenotypic mixture between myoclonic and ASE in myoclonic forms of IGE becomes almost the rule in cryptogenic or symptomatic generalized epilepsies, in which impairment of consciousness dominates the clinical picture and, frequently, cryptogenic MSE can be considered as modified atypical absence status (13). Myoclonic states in association with toxic, metabolic, or anoxic encephalopathies (18) are not included here (19) but are discussed in Chapter 13.

**Important Note:** The terms *idiopathic* and *nonidiopathic*, as designated above, refer to the etiology in accordance with the current terminology of the ILAE (6). Similarly, the terms *typical* or *atypical* characterize the absences in idiopathic and cryptogenic generalized epilepsies, as typical and atypical absences, respectively. The terms *typical* and *atypical*, however, have also been (and are being) used in both daily clinical practice and the literature to indicate whether the presentation of a given clinical or EEG phenomenon is usual or common, as opposed to unusual or uncommon (see, for example, references 10, 20, and 21 of this chapter, all within the context of idiopathic epilepsies). To avoid confusion, we shall restrict the terms *typical* and *atypical* to absences in IGE and cryptogenic or symptomatic generalized epilepsies, respectively, and characterize absence and myoclonic epileptic states as idiopathic or nonidiopathic (cryptogenic or symptomatic).

In this taxonomic frame, the well-delineated, de novo, absence status, an epileptic state with an electroclinical picture similar to that of ASE (occurring usually as an acute reactive event in patients without epilepsy), is not considered as a subtype of idiopathic or of cryptogenic ASE but is examined separately in a subsequent section in this chapter under the name de novo absence-like status.

The term *generalized NCSE* presupposes lack of lateralized or focal ictal clinical semiology and EEG phenomena but does not specify the type of epilepsy. Nonconvulsive epileptic states with "generalized" EEG features include idiopathic and nonidiopathic ASE or MSE, de novo absence-like status, and even some forms of CPSE (for example frontal lobe status); therefore, the term *generalized NCSE* is not synonymous with any of those. It is a purely descriptive term, and its clinical use can be justified only so far as the diagnosis of the type of epilepsy (or the lack of it, as in de novo absence-like status) remains uncertain.

The term *dialeptic* refers exclusively to ictal semiology and denotes an alteration of consciousness as a main ictal feature without significant positive motor signs (22-24). The term *possible dialeptic status epilepticus* expresses the clinical suspicion that a patient with a suggestive clinical presentation may be in a nonconvulsive epileptic state (either focal or generalized) *before* an EEG is performed and while other diagnoses are still being considered. These may include nonepileptic states of psychogenic or toxic etiology. The term *dialeptic status epilepticus* is applicable to cases in which the diagnosis of epilepsy is ascertained but the EEG is inconclusive as to whether the status is focal or generalized (23).

## THE ILAE DEFINITION OF STATUS EPILEPTICUS AND THE PARTICULAR INTERPRETIVE DIFFICULTIES IN THE CASE OF IDIOPATHIC ASE AND MSE

The recent ILAE definition of status epilepticus as "a seizure that shows no clinical signs of arresting after a duration encompassing the great majority of seizures of that type in most patients or recurrent seizures without interictal resumption of baseline central nervous system function" (25) is in line with the original dictum that there are as many types of epileptic status as there are types of epileptic seizure (13) and, essentially, recognizes that the minimum duration of such an epileptic event to be considered as status varies according to the seizure type (26). Because most self-limited seizures last no more than few minutes (27), the time frame for most types of status is now much shorter than 30 minutes, probably between 5 and 20 minutes, with shorter times applying to convulsive states, to foster swift medical intervention.

This operational definition (and time frame) may appear problematic when applied to idiopathic ASE. Typical absences are very brief seizures, only occasionally exceeding 20 to 25 seconds in duration, and tend to become briefer and milder with age (28,29). The classic form of idiopathic ASE is a prolonged absence associated with a more or less continuous spike-wave discharge (Figure 12.1, upper trace, and Figure 12.2), but forms with intermittent discharges of variable duration repeated at short intervals as clusters of absences and with little tendency to cease spontaneously are well known to exist (Figures 12.3 and 12.4) (7,8,10). Typical absences are devoid of postictal depression (somatic, mental, or electrographic), and, therefore, when they occur sequentially, even in quick succession, interictal recovery is prompt and complete, at variance with the ILAE definition. When such EEG patterns persist, however, surrounding reality is perceived not in its entirety and continuity but in brief fragments of variable duration resulting in an impaired awareness and concentration that is imperceptible to bystanders.

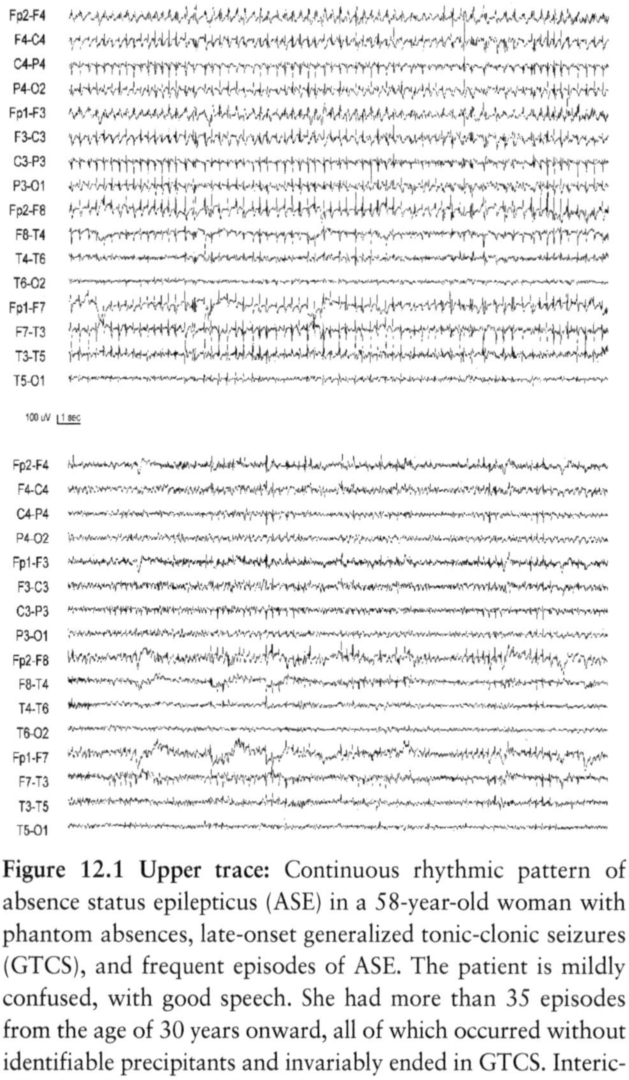


**Figure 12.1 Upper trace:** Continuous rhythmic pattern of absence status epilepticus (ASE) in a 58-year-old woman with phantom absences, late-onset generalized tonic-clonic seizures (GTCS), and frequent episodes of ASE. The patient is mildly confused, with good speech. She had more than 35 episodes from the age of 30 years onward, all of which occurred without identifiable precipitants and invariably ended in GTCS. Interictal video electroencephalography on other recordings confirmed brief absences, of which he and her family were unaware. **Lower trace:** Treatment with 5 mg of intravenously administrered diazepam abolished slow-wave (SW) discharges immediately and completely, but transiently; 3 minutes later, they reappeared, first as abortive generalized discharges, then in duplets and triplets, and becoming denser until the full continuous unabated pattern of the upper trace was reestablished. Another 5 mg of intravenously administered diazepam produced exactly the same response, although SW discharges reappeared a bit later (5 minutes). The lower trace depicts the return of the ASE shortly before it became fully continuous again. Final resolution was achieved much later after valproate was administered intravenously, although spontaneous termination mechanisms might have also been involved.

There is another clinical reason to attempt some modification of the proposed ILAE definition: the increased risk of a GTCS that accompanies the continuous form of ASE and the various discontinuous forms with sequential absences and dense subcontinuous GSW discharges (30). Similar considerations apply to MSE, which can be either almost continuous or take the form of sequential volleys at intervals of several seconds. Such dense clustering of TA, MS, and GSW discharges that disrupts perceptiveness and predisposes for GTCS implies a common pathophysiologic mechanism that facilitates and perpetuates a momentum despite an apparent resumption of the electroclinical baseline, a nonfortuitous "fixed and lasting" condition, according to Gastaut (14).

## DEFINITION OF IDIOPATHIC ABSENCE STATUS EPILEPTICUS

Idiopathic ASE represents a state of variably altered consciousness, observable or subjectively perceived, that occurs in patients with IGE and is associated with continuous or intermittent 2.5-Hz or faster GSW EEG activity. This may occur irrespective of whether there is complete regression of the ictal EEG to an interictal electroclinical state in between individual absences or EEG paroxysms. The minimum duration matters less than in convulsive status, but probably is not longer than a few minutes.

## PATHOPHYSIOLOGIC CONSIDERATIONS AND SOME CLINICAL CORRELATIONS

The regular 3- to 4-Hz GSW, which is the hallmark of IGE and the building block of the typical absence and absence status, is the scalp EEG expression of alternating cycles of excitatory (spike)

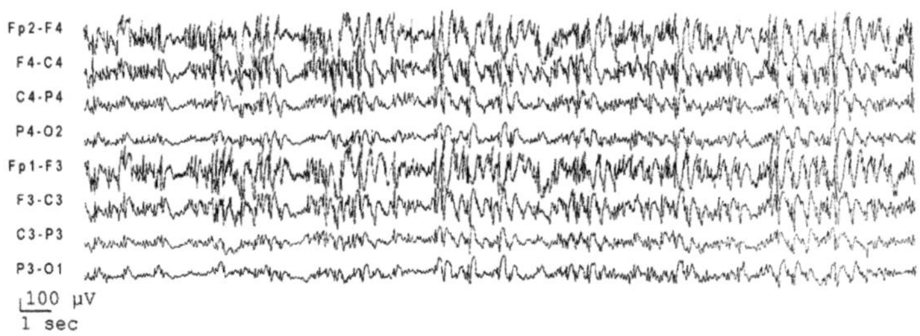


**Figure 12.2** Continuous arrhythmic pattern of absence status epilepticus (ASE) in a 23-year-old woman with frequent absences associated with perioral myoclonia and generalized tonic-clonic seizures (GTCS) since the age of 11 years. She had 4 episodes of ASE and was on carbamazepine on referral. She is mildly confused with continuous twitching around her mouth. On valproate and lamotrigine, she had no further episodes of ASE, but her compliance was poor, and she has continued with rare absences. (HFF 70 Hz, TC 0.3 s) From reference 8 and reproduced with permission of the editor of *Epilepsia*.

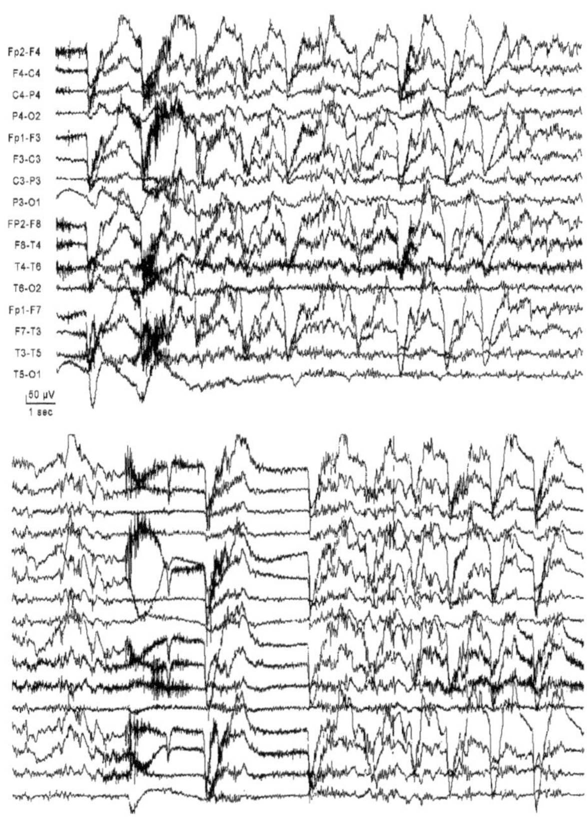


**Figure 12.3** Discontinuous pattern recorded during absence status epilepticus (ASE) in a 40-year-old man with untreated eyelid myoclonia with absences (video-electroencephalography [EEG]). Typical absences started at age 12 years; his eyes "... would flicker may times per day and there were days when eyelid flickering would be almost continuous, would feel unwell, might drop things and would have to go and lie down somewhere quietly to make them stop." In this video-EEG, on awakening, the patient seems fresh from sleep, but when the patients is interrogated by the EEG technologist to assess his consciousness, he is unable to concentrate, his speech is hesitant, and he gives inappropriate answers, especially during the generalized spike-and-wave (GSW) and generalized poly-spike-and-wave (GPSW) bursts. These bursts tended to occur on eye closure and were accompanied by repetitive eyelid myoclonia with retropulsion of the eyes, and occasional jerks of the whole body and head. Note that the eye-closure artifact lasts only 1 second, and there were no features suggesting self-induction. The technologist recognized the clinical significance of the pattern and called the on-call neurologist who only recommended a tablet of valproate. The patient had a generalized tonic-clonic seizure (GTCS) 30 minutes later (HFF 70 Hz, TC 0.3 s).

and inhibitory (slow-wave) phasic activities, mediated through the same thalamocortical network that regulates the normal sleep-spindle oscillation. In the phenomenon of sleep spindles, physiologic brief bursts of synchronized activity in the thalamocortical neurons arouse a sequence of alternating excitatory (EPSPs) and inhibitory (IPSPs) postsynaptic potentials at the thalamic reticular nucleus that is rich in GABAergic interneurons. Experimental work has shown that these IPSPs are mediated through $GABA_A$ receptors and are brief, accounting for the fast frequency of the spindles (~ 10 Hz). In the epileptic 3- to 4-Hz GSW, an abnormal longer burst (possibly from increased regional, but not steadily localized, cortical firing) (31) results in a 3-times-longer IPSP that is now mediated through $GABA_B$ receptors (although again at the level of the thalamic reticular nucleus), effectively setting the frequency of the GSW oscillation down to the familiar 3 Hz (32). The rhythmic 3-Hz GSW oscillations depend on calcium channels that initially deactivate during the slow depolarization of the thalamocortical cells (EPSP) and then reactivate by the hyperpolarization of these neurons (during the IPSP) and open up, producing low-threshold calcium spikes that will trigger a burst of action potentials and lead to the next cycle of the thalamocortical oscillation (31). The slow depolarization of the thalamocortical cells is generated through the activation of a specialized ionic current (h current; *h* for hyperpolarization activated).

The mechanisms responsible for the termination of the 3-Hz GSW discharge of the typical absence are uncertain. It has been hypothesized that repetitive oscillation results in increased intracellular calcium that leads to increased intracellular cyclic adenosine monophosphate (cAMP). The abundant cAMP then binds directly to the h channels, promoting their open state and, thereby, the depolarization of the thalamocortical cells. This blocks their ability to hyperpolarize and reactivate the calcium channels and, in consequence, to generate calcium spikes and bursts of action potentials, finally aborting the slow-wave oscillation (33). The slight depolarization of thalamic neurons (rather than their depression or hyperpolarization) may explain the lack of postictal cognitive deficits (34).

Even less is known (or can be speculated) about the mechanisms that lead to long absences (therefore ASE). Relevant literature is scarce, and extrapolation from animal models (cats and mice) seems problematic. Apart from their role in the initiation of the thalamocortical oscillations, environmental and circadian factors and treatment with GABAergic drugs, such as vigabatrin and tiagabine, may also contribute to reduced inhibition. Finally, what can be operationally defined as ASE (sequential absences or showers of GSW activity that can cloud the sensorium and end in a GTCS) is not necessarily due to a defective termination mechanism; it can also be due to extreme cortical firing that may take a long time to abate. A typical example is a patient with eyelid myoclonia with absences on awakening (Figure 12.3).

Although some debate exists on whether CPSE can induce brain damage (see also Chapters 7, 10, and 22), in ASE there appears to exist no clinical evidence of ensuing morbidity no matter the number and length of episodes in the individual patient. This dictum is shared by most authorities (7,35-37) but is based on clinical impression and not actual neuropsychological measurements. Certainly, no biologic marker of brain injury has been so far identified, and a recent study on 2 patients with frequent episodes of nonidiopathic (cryptogenic and ring chromosome 20-related) ASE found normal cerebrospinal fluid levels of neuronal-specific enolase (an enzyme released by dying neurons) (38).

## PREVALENCE

ASE is not rare. Andermann and Robb (7) found ASE in 10% of their adult patients with TA, whereas, in 1998, we diagnosed ASE in 25% of our adults with TA (15.5% of IGE), using video-EEG (8). ASE has occurred in 56 of 222 patients with IGE (25%), consecutively diagnosed and followed-up in St Thomas' Adult Epilepsy Clinic to date, and its prevalence seems to be syndrome related (Figure 12.5). Interestingly, ASE can also occur in patients with IGE with GTCS only (7 of 36 patients, 19.5%), indicating that specific inquiry for ASE is also needed in IGE patients without clinical or EEG evidence of typical absences.

## AGE AT ONSET

The first episode of ASE usually occurs well after the onset of TA and GTCS (mean onset of ASE: 29.5 years; TA: 9 years; GTCS: 21 years), but it may be the first-ever overt clinical manifestation of IGE in up to one third of patients (8). Reports on ASE in children younger than 10 years of age are scarce (9,39).

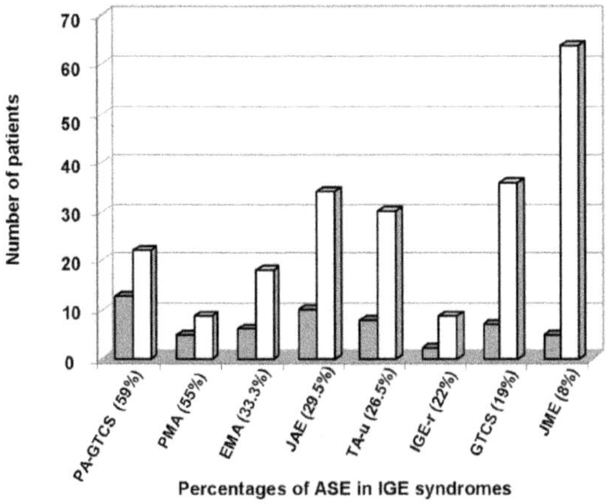


**Figure 12.5** Distribution of absence status epilepticus (ASE) in different syndromes and subtypes of idiopathic generalized epilepsies (IGE) in 222 consecutive patients who were diagnosed and had clinical and electroencephalographic (EEG) follow-up in the epilepsy clinic of St Thomas' Hospital London. The diagnosis of generalized tonic-clonic seizures (GTCS) refers to IGE with GTCS only and is based on the absence of any historical and EEG (using sleep video recordings after partial sleep deprivation with activation with overbreathing and breath counting on awakening) evidence of minor seizures (typical absences or myoclonic seizures) (11). PA-GTCS refers to the syndrome of phantom absences with late onset GTCS and frequent ASE; PMA, perioral myoclonia with absences; EMA, eyelid myoclonia with absences; JAE, juvenile absence epilepsy; TA-u, unclassified absence epilepsy; IGEr, IGE with predominantly reflex (mainly photically induced) seizures; GTCS, IGE with GTCS only, JME: juvenile myoclonic epilepsy.

It seems that ASE tends to occur at an age period when the severity of TA has lessened, accounting perhaps for the relatively mild impairment of responsiveness, memory, and speech during the prolonged state, in contrast with the profound disturbance of awareness of the "archetypical" absences of CAE and JAE in the first 2 decades of life.

## SEX RATIO

Women may be slightly more affected (7); 30 of 54 ASE patients in our epilepsy clinic database are women (54.5%).

## PRECIPITANTS AND RECURRENCE

Precipitating factors for ASE are similar to those for other seizure types in IGE and include sleep deprivation, alcohol, fatigue, stress or relaxation, withdrawal of (or noncompliance with) appropriate antiepileptic drugs (AEDs) (valproate, ethosuximide, lamotrigine) or administration of AEDs that are inappropriate for IGE (vigabatrin [40], carbamazepine [10,41-43], oxcarbazepine [44], tiagabine [45], phenytoin [10,43]), concurrent use of proseizure medications (such as some antidepressants), febrile illness or surgery, menstruation (46,47), hyperventilation, and photic stimulation. Triggers, however, may be absent in up to 30% of patients (8). ASE recurs in 50% (9) to 85% of patients (8), sometimes exceeding 100 times (9). Recurrence may be spontaneous (8).

## CLINICAL FEATURES

### *Duration*

Duration varies, and patients with long episodes lasting several days are included in most large series (7-9). An exceptionally long ASE was documented in a 66-year-old man, in whom subtherapeutic levels of valproate (due to comedication with phenytoin) and chronic white matter ischemic changes were thought to sustain the state (48). Because ASE usually responds well to appropriate treatment (see Treatment and Outcome below), long duration usually reflects underdiagnosis or misdiagnosis.

### *Timing and relation to generalized tonic-clonic seizures*

Being essentially a seizure type or symptom of IGE, ASE tends to occur on awakening (49,50). In some women, it may also relate to menstruation (46,47). ASE is frequently followed, initiated, or punctuated by GTCS; in up to 50% of patients, it consistently terminates with GTCS (8), and this relationship has significant diagnostic and therapeutic implications (see the section Diagnosis).

*Seizure semiology*

The fundamental disturbance in ASE is *clouding of consciousness*, the degree of which appears to regulate the extent of impairment of other cognitive functions. This can vary from a mild, almost exclusively subjective, perception of feeling unwell and not up to the usual personal mental level (a state imperceptible to bystanders and even to family members and physicians) to that of a clinically overt confusional state and, less frequently, to severe psychomotor retardation or stupor. The level of consciousness may fluctuate according to how absences or GSW discharges may cluster (see ILAE definition and interpretation difficulties in ASE above), while gradual deterioration has been reported in up 20% of patients (8). Relevant descriptions of patients with mild clouding include: "My mind slows down ... I am able to understand but takes longer to formulate answers", "... I become slow but can communicate verbally with others...," "I slow down in my behavior ... muddling with words." "I feel confused, like in a trance ... missing pieces of conversation." "I could hear what the other people were saying but had to struggle to find the meaning." There seems to be no direct correlation between the severity of impairment of consciousness during typical absences and that observed during ASE. For example, patients with brief imperceptible absences (such as in the syndrome of phantom absences with late-onset GTCS [51]) may have more severely affected consciousness during ASE than those with JAE and the characteristic long and profound absences (8).

Being dependent on the level of consciousness (ie, subject to the degree of corticothalamic involvement), speech in ASE is usually reasonably preserved, in contrast with the marked dysphasia of CPSE, which is due to direct ictal invasion of speech centers. It may vary from mild slowness and poverty of speech to perseveration and monosyllabic speech. Amnesia is also variable and usually patchy and only occasionally total (7,8,52).

In general, behavior slows down, and patients become withdrawn and quiet and appear bewildered and disorientated or in trance-like state, with a staring gaze. Positive behavioral and affective changes, however, such as agitation, irritability, or aggression, can occasionally occur (7,52). One of our patients reported that she would turn extremely snappy for a couple of hours before a GTCS, whereas another with catamenial episodes of ASE described that she would become confused and aggressive for a couple of days around her menstrual period. Inappropriate behavior may occur when confusion is not severe. Examples from our clinic include putting trousers over pajamas, arranging sugar in the refrigerator, and making coffee twice (8). Similar cases have been reported in other series (7).

Motor phenomena include bilateral regional (mainly facial) myoclonus, automatisms, and pseudo-ataxic or hesitant gait. The distribution of the former is usually similar to the regional (eyelid, perioral, or limb) myoclonus associated with the typical absences of the given patient, conforming thus to the profile of the specific subsyndrome or condition (for example, eyelid or perioral myoclonia or JME) (Figures 12.2 and 12.3) (8,9). Such regional myoclonus does not occur in CPSE, and, therefore, its identification is an important differential diagnostic clue. Because automatisms in individual absences are more likely with longer discharges (28), it is hardly surprising that gestural and ambulatory automatic motor behavior and fugue-like states are reported in ASE, especially in those with more severe impairment of consciousness. True fugue occurred in 2 of our patients with severe confusion (8). Unusual motor features that include complex automatisms or lateralized motor manifestations, such as version or stereotypes, may occur when ASE is precipitated by the use of inappropriate AEDs (10).

Other "focal" symptoms such as experiential phenomena and complex visual hallucinations or illusions are not infrequent (7-9) and may cause diagnostic confusion with CPSE, particularly in the absence of ictal or interictal EEG recordings showing GSW activity (53). Descriptions include "... sensation of viewing the world through a different medium, and a feeling of not being in the same world as everyone else," "I go into a dreamy state," "a feeling of closeness or detachment," "a strange feeling of not being myself," and "my eyes were continuously jerking" (8).

### *Interictal and ictal electroencephalographic and video electroencephalographic findings*

By showing 3-Hz GSW activity against a normal background, interictal (preferably video) EEG can consolidate the diagnosis of IGE and, optimally used (11), may refine the syndromic classification that is important for long-term patient management and definition of outcome. Interictal EEG recordings should be taken after the first ASE, and reports of older EEGs (and actual traces if possible!) are worth pursuing because they may contain important diagnostic clues that are no longer present.

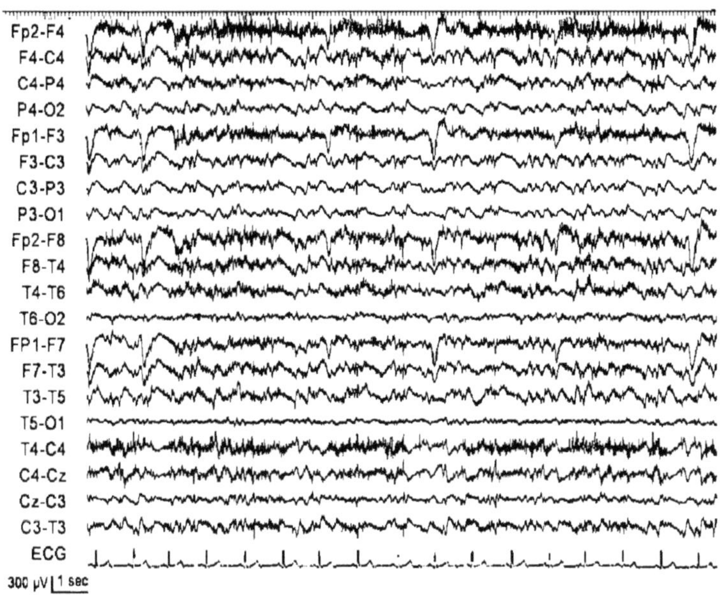


**Figure 12.6** Late stages of absence status epilepticus (ASE) in a 59-year-old woman with generalized tonic-clonic seizures (GTCS) and confusional episodes since the age of 23 years (video-electroencephalography, August 2005). On phenytoin since the beginning, she had more than 100 of these episodes that would almost always end in GTCS. She became seizure free when switched to valproate in 2000, but, because of tremor, she was changed to carbamazepine by her general practitioner, and her seizures started again. She has had no more episodes of ASE after she was put on levetiracetam and a small dose of valproate. Note the slow repetition rate and the irregularity of the generalized spike-wave activity that is intermixed with synchronous bursts of delta activity (HFF 70 Hz, TC 0.3 s).

Ictal video EEG recordings confirm the diagnosis of ASE and guide acute treatment and short-term management (see Treatment and Outcome below). There is usually a rapid clinical and EEG response following intravenous administration of AEDs, whereas a more gradual improvement would suggest another cause with a similar EEG picture, such as focal (frontal lobe) status (54).

Ictal EEG patterns consistent with the diagnosis of ASE may include any continuous (Figures 12.1 and 12.2) or discontinuous (Figure 12.3 and 12.4) and rhythmic or arrhythmic pattern at the equivalent frequency of around 3-Hz GSW activity. Slower repetition rates interspersed with slow waves may occur in late stages of the state (48) when discharges also become increasingly irregular (Figure 12.6), and have also been reported in some patients with ASE precipitated by inappropriate AED treatment (10).

Patterns of ongoing discontinuous pseudo-rhythmic or arrhythmic GSW with brief interspersed epochs of normal background are widely accepted as compatible with ASE (8-10) (Figures 12.3 and 12.4) and must not be ignored in the absence of overt signs of impairment of consciousness. The type of the ictal discharge bears no predictive value with regard to spontaneous termination or culmination in GTCS.

## DIAGNOSIS

All major studies agree that there is a high rate of misdiagnosis and underdiagnosis (7-10). Agathonikou and colleagues (8) reported that ASE was clinically suspected in only 4 of their 21 patients (20%), whereas the diagnosis of NCSE was altogether missed in 15 (71.5%). Misdiagnosis or diagnostic delay of up to 40 years was reported by Baykan and colleagues in all of their 8 patients (9), whereas all 14 patients of Thomas and colleagues with AED-induced ASE had been erroneously diagnosed as having cryptogenic focal or generalized epilepsies (10).

This substantial diagnostic failure is certainly due to the considerable clinical overlap between CPSE and ASE (see Differential Diagnosis later in this chapter) but arguably reflects the perennial bias toward complex partial seizures and temporal lobe epilepsy. Characteristically, there are several papers on the misdiagnosis of IGE as partial epilepsy (2,11,55-58), but none on the reverse. Clinical manifestations are subtle in a possibly substantial number of patients or ASE episodes. Relatives may not volunteer a suggestive history, particularly when symptoms and signs are mild, and physicians may not specifically inquire because awareness of ASE seems to be inadequate even among general neurologists.

Diagnosis is frequently missed when symptoms are mild and mainly subjective because patients' relatively composed appearance may deceive relatives and physicians alike. One of our patients with recurrent episodes once attended the emergency room claiming that he was in ASE, was not believed, and was sent away, so he made his way to our department, where a video-EEG confirmed his own diagnosis. The first episode of ASE was missed in another patient of ours, not only by her general practitioner who was called out, but also by her own daughter. Similar examples are presented by Baykan and colleagues (9). Particular attention is needed when the EEG is discontinuous (Figure 12.3 and 12.4).

Diagnosis of ASE is possible on clinical grounds when a clear history of a prolonged confusional state is available in a patient with clinical and EEG evidence of IGE (7). ASE may be the first manifestation of the IGE, however, and full clinical and video-EEG investigation is necessary *after* the resolution of the status for correct diagnosis and, if possible, for syndromic classification. The most important step toward recognition of such episodes is always to seek suggestive evidence of altered behavior or subjective symptomatology around (and particularly a few hours before) a GTCS, primarily when these seizures tend to occur late morning or in the afternoon. Showers of brief absences may start after awakening. There may be mild symptoms compatible with the ability to carry out everyday tasks, but which are associated with a feeling of strangeness. Patients may not volunteer this unless specifically asked. A 27-year-old patient of ours drove around London for most of New Year's Eve, paying visits to his in-laws but offering the wrong Christmas presents to the wrong persons. He had been feeling "tired, unable to compute his words and slow in mind" since he woke that morning. At 4:00 p.m. he drove to a friend's house with his wife. She described that he appeared "slow and very quiet", and "could hardly say a word", but made no driving errors and had no abnormal movements. He had a GTCS while driving and fortunately a serious accident was avoided. A video EEG a month later showed brief absences, appreciated only by brief hesitations on breath counting, and he was diagnosed with the syndrome of phantom absences with late onset GTCS and ASE.

## DIFFERENTIAL DIAGNOSIS

As all types of NCSE, ASE must be differentiated from nonepileptic conditions that include toxic or metabolic states, post-traumatic or transient amnestic states, psychiatric disorders (depression, schizophrenia or conversion), and epileptic syndromes and states that are listed in Table 1. As ASE may also follow a GTCS, any prolonged "postictal confusion" should raise suspicions and prompt an EEG recording (52). In the next section, we shall discuss the main aspects of the differential diagnosis between CPSE and ASE, leaving the rest of the epileptic syndromes of Table 1 for the end of this chapter.

## FOCAL NONCONVULSIVE STATUS EPILEPTICUS (CONVULSIVE STATUS EPILEPTICUS), INCLUDING TRANSIENT EPILEPTIC AMNESIA

There is a considerable clinical overlap between CPSE and ASE: differences are mainly quantitative, and phenotypes vary a lot across a wide range in both types, making it almost impossible to be certain of the diagnosis on clinical grounds only. In general, impairment of consciousness is milder in ASE than in CPSE and usually lacks the characteristic cycling changes between unresponsiveness and partial responsiveness that occur in CPSE (19), but fluctuations of behavior and mental state may also occur in ASE due to varying clustering of individual absences and the brief interspersed periods of normal state. Speech and memory are also less disturbed in ASE (19,36). Automatic behavior, including wandering about and fumbling with clothes, and experiential phenomena may occur in both forms. Abnormal motor phenomena may provide more distinctive clinical cues, as for example regional bilateral (eyelid, perioral, or upper limb) myoclonus in ASE as opposed to the lateralized or focal patterns in focal NCSE. Such signs may not be present, however, and some inappropriately treated patients with IGE may show lateralized motor behavior during ASE (10). History and EEG provide more valuable clues: the former may disclose complex partial seizures, but, again, differentiation from TA on clinical grounds only may not be straightforward (59). Ictal EEG findings are usually lateralized or focal in focal NCSE (depending on the stage of the episode [19]), but may be diffuse with GSW discharges, especially in frontal lobe NCSE and even in temporal lobe epilepsy (60), mimicking IGE. Interictal EEG and imaging findings may also differ markedly, and response to acute treatment is usually more gradual in focal NCSE, in which phenytoin is more effective than benzodiazepines, including in frontal lobe NCSE (54) (Table 1).

The different forms of focal NCSE are discussed in Chapters 8 to 11, but transient epileptic amnesia, merits a brief comment. Transient epileptic amnesia is a rare and not widely appreciated seizure type of temporal lobe epilepsy that manifests by predominant or exclusive transient amnesia without significant impairment of other cognitive functions (61,62). Characteristically, patients in transient epileptic amnesia remain composed and aware of self and environment and are able to communicate and to deduce missing links from their surroundings through logical thinking. Retention of new memories, however, is severely deranged, there may be some retrograde amnesia, and there are amnesic gaps interrupted by thoughts during the event. In contrast with transient global amnesia, transient epileptic amnesia affects younger people, with recurrent episodes, which are shorter (minutes to an hour) and may be associated with other temporal lobe seizures or symptoms, and there is no impairment of new learning after the offset of the attack. Interictal EEG may show temporal lobe abnormalities, although, in our experience, the electroclinical profile of transient epileptic amnesia is frequently subtle. In ASE, amnesia is never so selectively (and seldom so severely) affected, and the degree is usually proportional to the associated confusion; interictal and ictal EEG and seizure history are also different.

Transient epileptic amnesia is exemplified by a 39-year-old patient of ours who had a brief déjà vu sensation and dizziness as he was exiting an Internet café in Australia, following which he kept wandering and asking himself "Where am I?" and "Where have I just come from?" until he saw a newsagent selling Australian press. He was then helped to his hotel (he had the address and telephone number with the key in his pocket), where he recovered an hour later without significant postictal symptoms. He had 10 similar episodes in the last 6 months and isolated déjà vu symptoms since his late teens. His EEG showed temporal sharp waves, and he has had no other attacks since he was started on carbamazepine.

## THE SYNDROME OF DE NOVO ABSENCE-LIKE STATUS OF LATE ONSET

This condition was reported by Schwartz and Scott in 1971 (63), and the concept was further developed to include nonepileptic patients who experience for the first time in middle or old age a state that bears electroclinical resemblance to idiopathic ASE (64,65). Such episodes of status are usually triggered by acute withdrawal of chronic psychotropic medication (mainly benzodiazepines [65,66], but also tricyclic antidepressants [67], major neuroleptics, and lithium) and in acute brain injuries; during electroconvulsive therapy (68-70), angiography (71) and metrizamide myelography (72, 73); in acute or chronic alcoholism and metabolic imbalance; and with exposure to toxic or other pharmacologic agents (65).

Distinction from idiopathic ASE is clinically important because biologic substrates, and by implication management and prognosis, are different. Patients with ASE have only IGE and need appropriate maintenance treatment with AED. For those with de novo absence-like status, removal of the offending factor may suffice, and the overall prognosis is excellent, with little risk for recurrence (65). Such differentiation may not always be easy or immediately possible. Elderly individuals with a history of IGE can also present with ASE, sometimes under circumstances that may initially appear similar to those that can trigger de novo episodes, including alcohol consumption (but not acute intoxication or withdrawal) and sudden AED changes (discontinuation of therapeutic AEDs, including benzodiazepines, or introduction of a potentially pro-absence drug) as part of their treatment. A history of episodes of ASE, unrelated to toxic or metabolic dysfunction, benzodiazepine withdrawal, and intake of other psychotropic drugs, can be elicited in most patients with IGE, pushing the diagnosis toward that direction. Seven of our 8 patients with a history of alcohol-associated episodes of ASE (8) had several other absence states clearly unrelated to alcohol. Another difficulty may be that a previous history of epilepsy, including past episodes of ASE, may not be readily available or may not exist. This is by no means confirmatory of the diagnosis of de novo absence-like status, and full clinical video-EEG investigations after the resolution of the status are mandatory. ASE was the first ever epilepsy manifestation in adulthood in 5 of our 21 patients (24%, median age 30, average 32, range 18-56 years) (8). Comprehensive video-EEG studies after the first ASE and subsequent clinical follow-up showed that 4 had phantom absences (51) and 1 had JAE.

Finally, caution is needed when using age as major diagnostic criterion (74). Although de novo absence-like status tends to occur in late adult life (7), such late onset is by no means distinctive because it may be observed in patients with IGE either as a delayed event after long remission of seizures (65) or as the first overt epilepsy manifestation (8).

De novo absence-like status is a well-delineated condition with most of the reported patients falling into a relatively homogeneous pattern, with the following distinctive characteristics: (1) no evidence of IGE by virtue of history, clinical examination, video-EEG evaluation, and follow-up after the resolution of status epilepticus, (2) unequivocal evidence of an exogenous trigger or precipitant, mainly drug withdrawal and acute metabolic or toxic insults; and (3) a strong tendency for nonrecurrence if responsible triggers are identified and removed and despite the absence of treatment with AEDs. The underlying pathophysiology is uncertain, and, therefore, its nosologic taxonomy has been controversial. It appears that the triggering or facilitating potential of these factors becomes particularly effective when acting upon brains already compromised by vascular or degenerative processes, as is more frequently the case in elderly people. A contribution of a genetically determined liability cannot be excluded. The condition is reminiscent of (and possibly analogous to) the usually on-off occipital seizures triggered by photic stimuli in nonepileptic alcoholic or migrainous adults (75) although, here, trigger and electroclinical response are specific.

## TREATMENT AND OUTCOME

ASE is not truly a medical emergency because it does not appear to bear any acute or lasting morbidity. Acute treatment is seldom ineffective because most patients appear to respond to any benzodiazepine given intravenously or even orally (76). Intense intravenously administered treatment with benzodiazepine carries a (relatively small) risk for hypotension and respiratory suppression, and it should be administered in an intensive care unit setting under EEG monitoring. In view of the generally mild clinical expression of ASE, such potential morbidity would make a rigorous protocol with intravenously administered benzodiazepine, as in convulsive status, inadvisable (77). On the other hand, the high rates of recurrence, the usually long duration, and the typical termination with a GTCS pose life-threatening risks (ie, the patient driving during ASE) and suggest the need for a standardized approach and comprehensive management. Casual management with agents given orally until patients feel better, followed by a hasty discharge and an outpatient appointment, may be encouraged by patients' (frequently deceptively) "collected" appearance, especially when associated with a discontinuous EEG pattern (Figure 12.3 and 12.4), but are clearly insufficient and no longer acceptable, at least when the first episode of ASE is concerned.

Currently there are no data on the risk of early recurrence (some patients suffer GTCS shortly after the "resolution" of ASE). Clinical features may be deceptive, and there are no EEG criteria to unequivocally define the offset of the episode (reducing the density of GSW discharges may not be enough, particularly in the absence of a baseline interictal recording) (Figure 12.1). Adequate time for full assessment and EEG availability are important, and a brief admission on suspicion is deemed necessary to foster full differential diagnosis and ensure clinical and EEG clearance despite its cost. Besides, not all cases are simple (10,43,48), drug changes may be necessary, and blood levels of appropriate drugs may need to be increased. Benzodiazepines may be used, either intravenously (lorazepam as longer acting), or (perhaps first) orally in the EEG department. Intravenously administered clonazepam (not available in the US) may have a place if there is prominent myoclonus (9). More detailed information on treatment can be found in Chapter 20.

Once the diagnosis of IGE, appropriate treatment, and good compliance are secured, outcome is favorable in most patients (8-10,43). Further information on *outcomes* in NCSE can be found in Chapters 21 and 22.

## OTHER EPILEPTIC SYNDROMES AND CONDITIONS THAT ARE ASSOCIATED WITH NONCONVULSIVE STATUS EPILEPTICUS WITH ASPECTS OF DIFFERENTIAL DIAGNOSIS FROM ABSENCE STATUS EPILEPTICUS

### CRYPTOGENIC GENERALIZED EPILEPTIC SYNDROMES AND ENCEPHALOPATHIES WITH ABSENCE / MYOCLONIC STATUS (NONIDIOPATHIC ABSENCE STATUS EPILEPTICUS AND MYOCLONIC STATUS EPILEPTICUS)

In this group of epilepsies the clinical phenotype is most frequently mixed, with impairment of consciousness and coexistent myoclonus of varying topography and intensity. Either component may predominate, and episodes are usually associated with *irregular* and rather mixed (spike-wave, sharp and slow rhythms) generalized EEG activity. Other common characteristics that distinguish these conditions from IGE may include multiple seizure types, frequent developmental delay, variably abnormal EEG background, and a general reluctance to respond to acute treatment with benzodiazepines (78) (Table 12.1). See also Chapters 16, 17, and 19.

### CHROMOSOMAL DISORDERS

For specific chapters on these entities, refer to Chapters 16, 17, and 19.

#### *Angelman syndrome*

Angelman syndrome (partial monosomy 15q) is a severe neurodevelopmental disorder related to absence of maternal contribution to chromosome 15q11-q13. The interictal EEG shows rather characteristic large monomorphic slow spike-wave activity at 2 Hz over the posterior areas that becomes diffuse symmetrical, bilateral, and synchronous.

Nonidiopathic ASE appears to be frequent. Prolonged and recurrent states of reduced responsiveness associated with continuous or intermittent diffuse spike-wave activity at 2 to 3 Hz and variably with myoclonias and rhythmic eye blinking have been described in 4 of 8 sporadic cases (79) and in 1 of 3 siblings (80) with early onset; episodes of nonidiopathic MSE seem also frequent (81).

### *Ring chromosome 20 syndrome*

Ring chromosome 20 syndrome is a rare chromosomal syndrome characterized by variable psychomotor delay and behavioral disturbance and frequent episodes of NCSE, but there are no dysmorphisms, and this may delay the diagnosis. The NCSE in ring chromosome 20 is probably best described as mainly an absence state with an associated myoclonic component. Episodes take the form of prolonged confusional and variably amnesic or twilight states, with facial or limb myoclonias, ambulatory or persevering automatisms, or even complete arrest and muteness. They last more than 20 to 30 minutes and may recur several times in the same day. The EEG during the status shows mainly diffuse high-voltage, rhythmic, 2- to 4-Hz, slow wave with variably intermixed spike-wave activity that predominate frontally, but forms with either regular spike-wave or rhythmic slow waves only may also occur (82). The condition may be misdiagnosed in middle-aged patients as de novo absence-like status if previous episodes are not identified, and frontal lobe status should be also considered in view of the affective and autonomic symptomatology.

### *Severe myoclonic epilepsy in infancy*

First described by Dravet in 1978 (83), the severe myoclonic epilepsy in infancy (Dravet syndrome) is a genetic channelopathy (84) and a syndromic phenotype that can occur within the frame of generalized epilepsies with febrile seizures plus (GEFS+) (85). Generalized myoclonic seizures typically appear in the second or third year, followed by atypical absences that may be simple or accompanied by a myoclonic component merging into a mixed phenotype. Focal and tonic seizures also occur.

Absence status may occur any time between the second year of life and late teens in at least 30% to 40% of cases and is clinically associated with variably impaired and fluctuating consciousness and erratic myoclonus in the limbs and face. The EEG shows a continuous generalized arrhythmic mixed activity consisting of slow waves, spike-wave activity, and diffuse sharp waves, which is maximal frontocentrally. Typically, there is no relationship between spikes and segmental myoclonus. Episodes can be initiated by, punctuated by, or end in GTCS and persist for hours and even days (obtundation status), maintained by environmental visual stimuli or eye closure (photosensitivity occurs in up to 42% of children and may persist [86]). During status, differentiating electroclinical features include the segmental erratic myoclonias, the never-rhythmic 3-Hz slow-wave activity, and the poor response to diazepam.

## OTHER NONPROGRESSIVE SYMPTOMATIC ENCEPHALOPATHIES

Recurrent episodes of myoclonic status can occur in other nonprogressive symptomatic encephalopathies that relate to cortical dysplasias (probably genetically determined) and early anoxic or hypoxic injuries (87).

## CRYPTOGENIC GENERALIZED EPILEPSIES

### *Myoclonic astatic epilepsy (37, 88)*

Myoclonic astatic epilepsy is a genetically determined (some patients may fall into the spectrum of GEFS+) nonlesional generalized epilepsy that affects previously normal children between 2 and 5 years but has a variable course, ranging from good responsiveness to treatment with normal cognitive functions and even remission to a nonprogressive epileptic encephalopathy with seizure intractability and cognitive impairment (37,88). Episodes of absence or myoclonic status occur in most children and are characterized by depressed consciousness and responsiveness, multifocal arrhythmic twitching in limbs and face, and a very chaotic EEG with asynchronous spike-wave discharges that resemble hypsarrhythmia. Myoclonic astatic epilepsy shares many clinical features with cryptogenic Lennox-Gastaut syndrome, particularly its myoclonic form (89).

*The syndrome of myoclonic absences*

This rare type of cryptogenic generalized epilepsy was described by Tassinari (90,91) and is characterized by myoclonic absences that are associated with 3-Hz regular GSW activity, similar to the typical absences in childhood or juvenile absence epilepsies, but also with bilateral myoclonic jerks of the arms and legs that are time locked to the spike component of the ictal discharge and have a superimposed tonic contraction resulting in a characteristic stepwise upward abduction of the arms. Absence status without myoclonus has been reported in 17% of patients, but myoclonic absence status is rare.

*Nonconvulsive epileptic states in idiopathic focal epilepsies of childhood and related syndromes*

Benign rolandic epilepsy with centrotemporal spikes and Panayiotopoulos syndrome are the 2 major representatives of this group of disorders and are detailed in Chapter 17. They are only briefly described in Table 12.1 here because both may present with prolonged NCSE that, despite their "focal" character, can manifest with bilateral or diffuse symptoms, distinctly different from the focal semiology of the symptomatic focal epilepsies (92). Apart from the the autonomic status that may occur in about half of the children with Panayiotopoulos syndrome, all the other forms of NCSE in idiopathic focal epilepsies (Table 12.1) are rare and occur in atypical evolution of rolandic epilepsy and Panayiotopoulos syndrome.

## ACKNOWLEDGMENT

We would like to express our gratitude for the generous moral support and the charitable donation kindly bestowed to us by Mrs. Ellis Stewart in honor of the memory of her belated son Stewart; her support encourages us to continue our research on epilepsies. We are also grateful to Chrysostomos P. Panayiotopoulos for his expert review of the manuscript and helpful comments.

## REFERENCES

1. Panayiotopoulos CP, Chroni E, Daskalopoulos C, Baker A, Rowlinson S, Walsh P. Typical absence seizures in adults: clinical, EEG, video-EEG findings and diagnostic/syndromic considerations. J Neurol Neurosurg Psychiatry 1992;55:1002-1008.
2, Usui N, Kotagal P, Matsumoto R, Kellinghaus C, Luders HO. Focal semiologic and electroencephalographic features in patients with juvenile myoclonic epilepsy. Epilepsia 2005;46:1668-1676.
3. Putman TJ, Merritt HH. Dullness as an epileptic equivalent. Arch Neurol Psychiatry 1941;45:797-813.
4. Lennox WG. The petit mal epilepsies: their treatment with tridione. JAMA 1945;129:1069-1074.
5. Gastaut H, Roger J, Roger A. [The significance of certain epileptic fugues; concerning a clinical and electrical observation of temporal status epilepticus.] Rev Neurol (Paris) 1956;94:298-301.
6. Commission on Classification and Terminology of the International League Against Epilepsy. Proposal for revised classification of epilepsies and epileptic syndromes. Epilepsia 1989;30:389-399.
7. Andermann F, Robb JP. Absence status. A reappraisal following review of thirty-eight patients. Epilepsia 1972;13:177-187.
8. Agathonikou A, Panayiotopoulos CP, Giannakodimos S, Koutroumanidis M. Typical absence status in adults: diagnostic and syndromic considerations. Epilepsia 1998;39:1265-1276.
9. Baykan B, Golkyigit A, Gurses C, Eraksoy M. Recurrent absence status epilepticus: clinical

and EEG characteristics. Seizure 2002;11:310-319.
10. Thomas P, Valton L, Genton P. Absence and myoclonic status epilepticus precipitated by antiepileptic drugs in idiopathic generalized epilepsy. Brain 2006;129:1281-1292.
11. Koutroumanidis M, Smith S. Use and abuse of EEG in the diagnosis of idiopathic generalized epilepsies. Epilepsia 2005;46(Suppl 9):96-107.
12. Blume WT, Pillay N. Electrographic and clinical correlates of secondary bilateral synchrony. Epilepsia 1985;26:636-641.
13. Gastaut H. Classification of status epilepticus. Adv Neurol 1983;34:15-35.
14. Gastaut H. Clinical and electroencephalographical classification of epileptic seizures. Epilepsia 1970;11:102-113.
15. Panayiotopoulos CP, Obeid T, Tahan AR. Juvenile myoclonic epilepsy: a 5-year prospective study. Epilepsia 1994;35:285-296.
16. Panayiotopoulos CP. Idiopathic generalised epilepsies. In: Panayiotopoulos CP, ed. The Epilepsies: Seizures, Syndromes and Management. Oxford, UK: Bladon Medical Publishing, 2005:271-348.
17. Dziewas R, Kellinghaus C, Ludemann P. Nonconvulsion status epilepticus in patients with juvenile myoclonic epilepsy: types and frequencies. Seizure 2002;11:335-339.
18. Drislane FW, Schomer DL. Clinical implications of generalized electrographic status epilepticus. Epilepsy Res 1994;19:111-121.
19. Treiman DM. Electroclinical features of status epilepticus. J Clin Neurophysiol 1995;12:343-362.
20. Fejerman N, Caraballo R, Tenembaum SN. Atypical evolutions of benign localization-related epilepsies in children: are they predictable? Epilepsia 2000;41:380-390.
21. Ferrie CD, Koutroumanidis M, Rowlinson S, Sanders S, Panayiotopoulos CP. Atypical evolution of Panayiotopoulos syndrome: a case report [published with video- sequences]. Epileptic Disord 2002;4:35-42.
22. Noachtar S, Desudchit T, Lueders H. Dialeptic seizures. In: Lüders HO, Noachtar S, eds. Epileptic seizures. Pathophysiology and Clinical Semiology. New York, NY: Churchill Livingstone; 2000:361-376.
23. Rona S, Rosenow F, Arnold S, Carreño M, Diehl B, Ebner A, Fritsch B, Hamer HM, Holthausen H, Knake S, Kruse B, Noachtar S, Pieper T, Tuxhorn I, Lüders HO. A semiological classification of status epilepticus. Epileptic Disord 2005;7:5-12.
24. Engel J Jr, Berg A, Andermann F, Avanzini G, Berkovic S, Blume W, Dulac O, van Emde Boas W, Fejerman N, Plouin P, Scheffer I, Seino M, Williamson P, Wolf P. Are epilepsy classifications based on epileptic syndromes and seizure types outdated? Epileptic Disord 2006;8:159-160.
25. Blume WT, Lűders HO, Mizrahi E, Tassinari C, van Emde BW, Engel J, Jr. Glossary of descriptive terminology for ictal semiology: report of the ILAE task force on classification and terminology. Epilepsia 2001;42:1212-1218.
26. Lowenstein DH, Bleck T, Macdonald RL. It's time to revise the definition of status epilepticus. Epilepsia 1999;40:120-122.
27. Theodore WH, Porter RJ, Albert P, Kelley K, Bromfield E, Devinsky O, Sato S. The secondarily generalized tonic-clonic seizure: a videotape analysis. Neurology 1994;44:1403-1407.
28. Penry JK, Porter RJ, Dreifuss RE. Simultaneous recording of absence seizures with video tape and electroencephalography. A study of 374 seizures in 48 patients. Brain 1975;98:427-440.
29. Panayiotopoulos CP, Obeid T, Waheed G. Differentiation of typical absence seizures in epileptic syndromes. A video EEG study of 224 seizures in 20 patients. Brain 1989;112:1039-1056.
30. Mirsky AF, Duncan CC, Levav LM. Neuropsychological and psychophysiological aspects of absence epilepsy. In: Duncan JS, Panayiotopoulos CP, eds. Typical Absences and Related Epileptic Syndromes. London, UK: Churchill Communications Europe; 1995:112-121.
31. Blumenfeld H. Cellular and network mechanisms of spike-wave seizures. Epilepsia 2005;46(Suppl 9):21-33.
32. Kostopoulos GK. Spike-and-wave discharges of absence seizures as a transformation of sleep spindles: the continuing development of a hypothesis. Clin Neurophysiol 2000;111(Suppl 2):S27-S38.
33. Luthi A, McCormick DA. Modulation of a pacemaker current through Ca(2+)-induced stimulation of cAMP production. Nat Neurosci 1999;2:634-641.
34. McCormick DA. Cortical and subcortical generators of normal and abnormal rhythmicity. Int Rev Neurobiol 2002;49:99-114.
35. Niedermeyer E, Khalifeh R. Petit mal status ("spike-wave stupor"). An electro-clinical appraisal. Epilepsia 1965;6:250-262.

36. Shorvon SD. Status epilepticus: its clinical features and treatment in children and adults. Cambridge. UK: Cambridge University Press; 1994.
37. Panayiotopoulos CP. The epilepsies: seizures, syndromes and management. Oxford, UK: Bladon Medical Publishing; 2005.
38. Shirasaka Y. Lack of neuronal damage in atypical absence status epilepticus. Epilepsia 2002;43:1498-1501.
39. Panayiotopoulos CP, Ferrie CD, Koutroumanidis M, Rowlinson S, Sanders S. Idiopathic generalised epilepsy with phantom absences and absence status in a child. Epileptic Disord 2001;3:63-66.
40. Panayiotopoulos CP, Agathonikou A, Sharoqi IA, Parker AP. Vigabatrin aggravates absences and absence status. Neurology 1997;49:1467.
41. Callahan DJ, Noetzel MJ. Prolonged absence status epilepticus associated with carbamazepine therapy, increased intracranial pressure, and transient MRI abnormalities. Neurology 1992;42:2198-2201.
42. Genton P, Gelisse P, Thomas P, Dravet C. Do carbamazepine and phenytoin aggravate juvenile myoclonic epilepsy? Neurology 2000;55:1106-1109.
43. Osorio I, Reed RC, Peltzer JN. Refractory idiopathic absence status epilepticus: A probable paradoxical effect of phenytoin and carbamazepine. Epilepsia 2000;41:887-894.
44. Gelisse P, Genton P, Kuate D, Pesenti A, Baldy-Moulinier M, Crespel A. Worsening of seizures by oxcarbazepine in juvenile idiopathic generalized epilepsies. Epilepsia 2004;45:1282-1288.
45. Jette N, Cappell J, VanPassel L, Akman CI. Tiagabine-induced nonconvulsive status epilepticus in an adolescent without epilepsy. Neurology 2006;67:1514-1515.
46. Agathonikou A, Koutroumanidis M, Panayiotopoulos CP. Fixation-off-sensitive epilepsy with absences and absence status: video-EEG documentation. Neurology 1997;48:231-234.
47. Ming X, Kaplan PW. Fixation-off and eyes closed catamenial generalized nonconvulsive status epilepticus with eyelid myoclonic jerks. Epilepsia 1998;39:664-668.
48. D'Agostino MD, Andermann F, Dubeau F, Fedi M, Bastos A. Exceptionally long absence status: multifactorial etiology, drug interactions and complications. Epileptic Disord 1999;1:229-232.
49. Janz D. 'Aufwach'-epilepsien (als ausdruckeinerden 'nacht'-oder 'schlaf'-epilepsien gegenűberzustellenden verlaufsform epileptischer erkrankungen). Arch Z Neurol 1953;73-98.
50. Janz D. Epilepsy with grand mal on awakening and sleep-waking cycle. Clin Neurophysiol 2000;111(Suppl 2):S103-S110.
51. Panayiotopoulos CP, Koutroumanidis M, Giannakodimos S, Agathonikou A. Idiopathic generalised epilepsy in adults manifested by phantom absences, generalised tonic-clonic seizures, and frequent absence status. J Neurol Neurosurg Psychiatry 1997;63:622-627.
52. Kaplan PW. Behavioral manifestations of nonconvulsive status epilepticus. Epilepsy Behav 2002;3:122-139.
53. Ferner RE, Panayiotopoulos CP. 'Phantom' typical absences, absence status and experiential phenomena. Seizure 1993;2:253-256.
54. Thomas P, Zifkin B, Migneco O, Lebrun C, Darcourt J, Andermann F. Nonconvulsive status epilepticus of frontal origin. Neurology 1999 12;52:1174-1183.
55. So EL, King DW, Murvin AJ. Misdiagnosis of complex absence seizures. Arch Neurol 1984;41:640-641.
56. Panayiotopoulos CP, Tahan R, Obeid T. Juvenile myoclonic epilepsy: factors of error involved in the diagnosis and treatment. Epilepsia 1991;32:672-676.
57. Lancman ME, Asconape JJ, Golimstok A. Circling seizures in a case of juvenile myoclonic epilepsy. Epilepsia 1994;35:317-318.
58. Benbadis SR, Tatum WO, Gieron M. Idiopathic generalized epilepsy and choice of antiepileptic drugs. Neurology 2003;61:1793-1795.
59. Koutroumanidis M, Bourvari G, Tan SV. Idiopathic generalized epilepsies: clinical and electroencephalogram diagnosis and treatment. Expert Rev Neurother 2005;5:753-767.
60. Shorvon S, Walker M. Status epilepticus in idiopathic generalized epilepsy. Epilepsia 2005;46(Suppl 9):73-79.
61. Zeman AZ, Boniface SJ, Hodges JR. Transient epileptic amnesia: a description of the clinical and neuropsychological features in 10 cases and a review of the literature. J Neurol Neurosurg Psychiatry 1998;64:435-443.
62. Gallassi R. Epileptic amnesic syndrome: an update and further considerations. Epilepsia 2006;47(Suppl 2):103-105.

63. Schwartz MS, Scott DF. Isolated petit-mal status presenting de novo in middle age. Lancet 1971;2:1399-1401.
64. Thomas P, Beaumanoir A, Genton P, Dolisi C, Chatel M. 'De novo' absence status of late onset: report of 11 cases. Neurology 1992;42:104-110.
65. Thomas P, Andermann F. Late-onset absence status epilepticus is most often situation-related. In: Malafosse A, Genton P, Hirsch E, Marescaux C, Broglin D, Bernasconi R, eds. Idiopathic Generalized Epilepsies. London, UK: John Libbey & Company Ltd; 1994:95-109.
66. Dunne JW, Summers QA, Stewart-Wynne EG. Non-convulsive status epilepticus: a prospective study in an adult general hospital. Q J Med 1987;62:117-126.
67. Bourrat C, Garde P, Boucher M, Fournet A. [Prolonged absence states in aged patients without epileptic antecedents]. Rev Neurologique 1986;142:696-702.
68. Varma NK, Lee SI. Nonconvulsive status epilepticus following electroconvulsive therapy. Neurology 1992;42:263-264.
69. Grogan R, Wagner DR, Sullivan T, Labar D. Generalized nonconvulsive status epilepticus after electroconvulsive therapy. Convuls Ther 1995;11:51-56.
70. Dean CE, Borchardt CM. Nonconvulsive status epilepticus after electroconvulsive therapy: an additional case and risk factor. J ECT 2004; 20:54-55.
71. Vickrey BG, Bahls FH. Nonconvulsive status epilepticus following cerebral angiography. Ann Neurol 1989;25:199-201.
72. Pritchard PB, III, O'Neal DB. Nonconvulsive status epilepticus following metrizamide myelography. Ann Neurol 1984;16:252-254.
73. Obeid T, Yaqub B, Panayiotopoulos C, al-Jasser S, Shabaan A, Hawass NE. Absence status epilepticus with computed tomographic brain changes following metrizamide myelography. Ann Neurol 1988;24:582-584.
74) Fernandez-Torre JL, Diaz-Castroverde AG. Non-convulsive status epilepticus in elderly individuals: report of four representative cases. Age Ageing 2004;33:78-81.
75) Naquet R, Fegersten L, Bert J. Seizure discharges localised to the posterior cerebral regions in man, provoked by intermittent photic stimulation. Electroencephalogr clin Neurophysiol 1960;12:305-316.
76) Berkovic SF, Andermann F, Guberman A, Hipola D, Bladin PF. Valproate prevents the recurrence of absence status. Neurology 1989;39:1294-1297.
77. Kaplan PW. Prognosis in nonconvulsive status epilepticus. Epileptic Disord 2000;2:185-193.
78. Dulac O, Plouin P, Shewmon A. Myoclonus and epilepsy in childhood: 1996 Royaumont meeting. Epilepsy Res 1998;30:91-106.
79. Matsumoto A, Kumagai T, Miura K, Miyazaki S, Hayakawa C, Yamanaka T. Epilepsy in Angelman syndrome associated with chromosome 15q deletion. Epilepsia 1992;33:1083-1090.
80. Sugimoto T, Yasuhara A, Ohta T, Nishida N, Saitoh S, Hamabe J, Niikawa N. Angelman syndrome in three siblings: characteristic epileptic seizures and EEG abnormalities. Epilepsia 1992;33:1078-1082.
81. Viani F, Romeo A, Viri M, et al. Seizure and EEG patterns in Angelman's syndrome. J Child Neurol 1995;10:467-471.
82. Inoue Y, Fujiwara T, Matsuda K, Kubota H, Tanaka M, Yagi K, Yamamori K, Takahashi Y. Ring chromosome 20 and nonconvulsive status epilepticus. A new epileptic syndrome. Brain 1997;120(Pt 6):939-953.
83. Dravet C. Les epilepsies graves de l'enfant. Vie Med 1978;8:543-548.
84. Claes L, Del Favero J, Ceulemans B, Lagae L, Van Broeckhoven C, De Jonghe P. De novo mutations in the sodium-channel gene SCN1A cause severe myoclonic epilepsy of infancy. Am J Hum Genet 2001;68:1327-1332.
85. Scheffer IE, Berkovic SF. Generalized epilepsy with febrile seizures plus. A genetic disorder with heterogeneous clinical phenotypes. Brain 1997;120:479-490.
86. Dravet C, Bureau M, Guerrini R, Giraud N, Roger J. Severe myoclonic epilepsy in infants. In: Roger J, Bureau M, Dravet C, Dreifuss FE, Perret A, Wolf P, eds. Epileptic Syndromes in Infancy, Childhood and Adolescence. London, UK: John Libbey & Company; 92:75-78.
87. Dalla Bernardina B, Fontana E, Darra F. Myoclonic status in nonprogressive encephalopathies. Adv Neurol 2005;95:59-70.
88. Guerrini R, Parmeggiani A, Kaminska A, Dulac O. Myoclonic astatic epilepsy. In: Roger J, Bureau M, Dravet C, Genton P, Tassinari CA, Wolf P, eds. Epileptic syndromes in infancy, childhood and adolescence, 3rd ed. London: John Libbey & Co Ltd, 2002:105-12.
89. Kaminska A, Ickowicz A, Plouin P, Bru MF, Dellatolas G, Dulac O. Delineation of cryptogenic Lennox-Gastaut syndrome and myoclonic asta-

tic epilepsy using multiple correspondence analysis. Epilepsy Res 1999;36:15-29.
90. Tassinari CA, Lyagoubi S, Santos V, Gambarelli G, Roger J, Dravet C, Gastaut H. [Study on spike and wave discharges in man. II. Clinical and electroencephalographic aspects of myoclonic absences]. Rev Neurol (Paris) 1969;121:379-383.
91. Bureau M, Tassinari CA. Myoclonic absences: the seizure and the syndrome. Adv Neurol 2005;95:175-183.
92. Koutroumanidis M. Panayiotopoulos syndrome: an important electroclinical example of benign childhood system epilepsy. Epilepsia 2007;48:1044-1053.
93. Guerrini R, Belmonte A, Parmeggiani L, Perucca E. Myoclonic status epilepticus following high-dosage lamotrigine therapy. Brain Dev 1999;21:420-424.
94. Kroll-Seger J, Mothersill IW, Novak S, Salke-Kellermann RA, Kramer G. Levetiracetam-induced myoclonic status epilepticus in myoclonic-astatic epilepsy: a case report. Epileptic Disord 2006;8:213-218.
95. Koutroumanidis M, Aggelakis K, Panayiotopoulos CP. Idiopathic epilepsy with generalized tonic–clonic seizures only versus idiopathic epilepsy with phantom absences and generalized tonic–clonic seizures: One or two syndromes? Epilepsia 2008 (Published Online: Jul 4 2008 DOI:10.1111/j.1528-1167.2008.01702.x)
96. Genton P, Ferlazzo E, Thomas P. Absence status epilepsy: Delineation of a distinct idiopathic generalized epilepsy syndrome. Epilepsia 2008; 49: 213-218.

CHAPTER 13

# NONCONVULSIVE STATUS EPILEPTICUS IN CRITICALLY ILL AND COMATOSE PATIENTS IN THE INTENSIVE CARE UNIT

JEFFREY JIRSCH, LAWRENCE J. HIRSCH

Over the last 2 decades, continuous electroencephalographic EEG monitoring (CEEG) has become an important tool in neurocritical care, with multiple potential indications (Table 13.1). Its widespread availability has allowed clinicians to recognize that nonconvulsive seizures (NCSzs) and nonconvulsive status epilepticus (NCSE) are common in critically ill patients. Indeed, it is fair to say that physicians taking care of critically ill patients with neurologic problems who are not recognizing NCSzs or NCSE with some frequency are missing the diagnosis. Although NCSzs and NCSE are not rare, most experienced neurologists may be challenged by complexities in clinical and EEG presentation when trying to identify and treat these patients. This chapter highlights selected clinical and EEG aspects in critically ill patients and suggestions for the practicing physician.

## RECOGNITION OF NONCONVULSIVE STATUS EPILEPTICUS IN THE CRITICALLY ILL

Most often, CEEG monitoring is begun in patients with depressed levels of consciousness, either unexplained or in the setting of a known acute brain injury. In some patients, there has been a prior clinical seizure or there are on-going

**TABLE 13.1** POTENTIAL INDICATIONS FOR CONTINUOUS ELECTROENCEPHALOGRAPHIC MONITORING

1. Detection of subclinical seizures
    a) Fluctuating mental status
    b) Unexplained alteration of mental status
    c) Acute supratentorial brain injury with altered mental status
    d) After convulsive status epilepticus
2. Characterization of spells
    a) Episodic posturing, other paroxysmal or repetitive movements
    b) Subtle twitching, nystagmus, eye deviation, chewing
    c) Paroxysmal autonomic spells including tachycardia or hypertension
3. Assessment of level of sedation and following trends
4. Management of burst-suppression in anesthetic coma
5. Detection of ischemia
    a) After subarachnoid hemorrhage
    b) During and after vascular neurosurgical or interventional neuroradiological procedures
    c) In patients with hemodynamic lesions and borderline flow
    d) In other patients at risk for in-hospital acute ischemia
6. Prognostication

*From Hirsch LJ. Continuous EEG monitoring in the intensive care unit: an overview. J Clin Neurophysiol 2004;21:332-40. Reprinted with permission from the American Clinical Neurophysiology Society.*

subtle clinical manifestations raising the possibility of status epilepticus. Estimates of the prevalence of NCSzs and NCSE among critically ill neurologic patients vary. Comparison among studies is partly complicated by lack of a clear definition for NCSzs. For example, subtle movements (eg, facial twitching, eye deviation, nystagmus) are included in the definition of NCSE in some studies (1,2) but not others (3). Moreover, differing CEEG practices (eg, time of initiation, duration, patient selection) and interindividual variability in the diagnosis of ictal activity also complicate the mostly retrospective series.

Even with the most stringent diagnostic criteria, the prevalence of NCSzs and NCSE is high, suggesting that even the most attentive critical care physician would miss the diagnosis without EEG monitoring. Towne and colleagues studied 236 comatose patients in the intensive care unit (ICU) who had no prior clinical seizures or even subtle movements and found that 8% of this population was in NCSE (3). In other series, the overall rate of all types of electrographic seizures varies between 19% and 34% among various large centers using CEEG; NCSzs, defined by subtle or no overt manifestations, occurred in 54% to 92% of seizing patients (2,4,5). Almost any acute structural or toxic central nervous system insult can manifest as NCSzs and NCSE. Some notable subpopulations at risk are those with intracerebral hemorrhage (29% have NCSzs) (6), central nervous system infection (26%) (2), brain tumor (23%) (2), severe head trauma (22%) (7), and subarachnoid hemorrhage (18%) (2,8) or following neurosurgery (23%) (2). The presence of subarachnoid or intraparenchymal blood seems to be a particularly important factor in the development of seizures and is more significant than the size of the stroke. Accordingly, several series have shown that critically ill patients with ischemic stroke have a lower incidence of seizures than do patients with intracerebral hemorrhage (2,6,9). The location of hemorrhage is also important, with lobar bleeds being complicated by seizures more frequently than deep subcortical bleeds in 2 separate studies (7,10).

Aside from the primary diagnosis, there are other clinical and EEG factors that should alert the clinician to the possibility of NCSE. The presence of coma is probably the most important risk factor for seizures in the critically ill because more than half of 97 comatose patients undergoing CEEG had electrographic seizures in 1 study (2). Younger patients (age < 18 years) may be particularly prone to developing all types of seizures, including nonconvulsive events (2,11). In the series by Jette and colleagues (11), 44% of critically ill pediatric patients who had CEEG were in fact seizing, with 75% of these having no overt clinical signs, compared with 19% and 92% of adult patients, respectively (2). Recent generalized tonic-clonic seizures, a history of epilepsy, or a history of a remote symptomatic central nervous system insult (eg, stroke, neurosurgical intervention, or brain tumor) are further important risk factors for electrographic seizures (2,12). Two large series showed that continued electrographic seizure activity is common after the apparent control of generalized tonic-clonic seizures, with 20% having NCSzs in 1 large prospective trial (1) and 14% in NCSE on CEEG in another (13). Indeed, a prolonged "postictal" state following generalized convulsions should alert the physician to the possibility of NCSE.

NCSE and NCSzs in the critically ill are often generalized on EEG by the time of diagnosis and throughout the event. Given the frequent associated structural foci, these are usually considered secondarily generalized seizures, and a precise seizure-onset zone is often absent from the EEG. Some forms of generalized NCSE, also known as "absence status epilepticus," are usually managed outside of the ICU because patients are not comatose and tend to respond well to treatment.

There are a number of electrographic interictal findings that are associated with seizures. The absence of electrographic reactivity to external stimuli is associated with a greater risk of NCSzs in children (11), and periodic patterns such as periodic lateralized epileptiform discharges and generalized periodic epileptiform discharges are associated with NCSz activity on

CEEG (2,10); these periodic patterns are discussed in further detail in Chapter 6.

Young and colleagues (14) wrote that ongoing seizure activity in the ICU should be suspected in the following instances: (1) prolonged encephalopathy following generalized convulsions, an operative procedure, or a neurologic insult; (2) acutely impaired consciousness or fluctuating consciousness interrupted by normal alertness; (3) impaired mentation or consciousness with facial myoclonus or nystagmus; (4) episodic staring, aphasia, or automatisms (eg, limb or facial); or (5) other acutely altered behavior without obvious etiology. To this list must be added that encephalopathic patients with a history of epilepsy or remote symptomatic brain lesions (eg, stroke, brain contusion) should also be considered at high risk for developing electrographic seizures in the ICU, and periodic interictal EEG patterns warrant further attention with more-prolonged EEG monitoring for NCSzs. We now recognize that the variety of clinical signs associated with NCSE includes not only clonic movements of the face or limbs, but also ocular movements (eg, hippus, nystagmus, sustained eye deviation, eyelid blinking), and these last have high specificity for the diagnosis of NCSE in the appropriate clinical context (12).

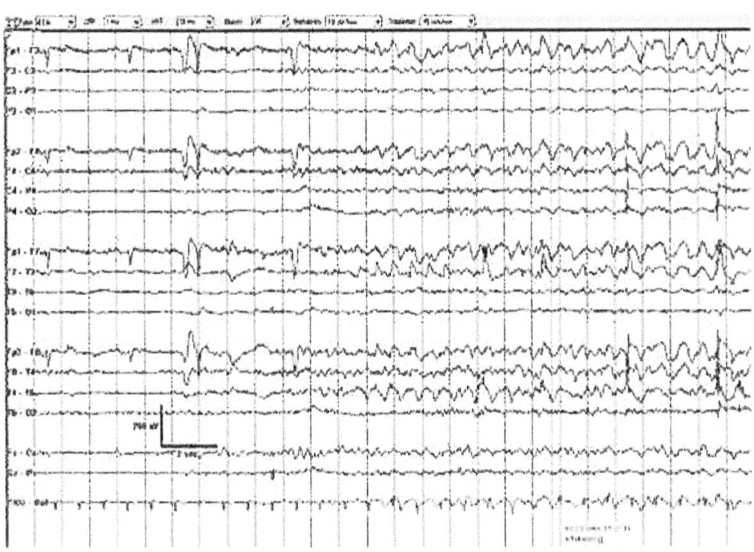

**Figure 13.1** Rhythmic chewing artifact mimicking an electrographic seizure. Reprinted with permission of the American Society of Electroneurodiagnostic Technologists, Inc. (16).

## EEG DETECTION OF NCSZS

### TECHNICAL ASPECTS

CEEG recording requires thorough technical maintenance of the entire recording pathway to ensure high quality. Ideally, electrodes are secured with collodion and inspected at least twice daily because critically ill patients are frequently agitated, being repositioned, or transported for various tests and procedures. Some institutions use magnetic resonance imaging (MRI)-compatible electrodes and cables that can simplify technical maintenance of monitoring (15), although there are no convenient, noninvasive, MRI-compatible, and US Food and Drug Association-approved electrodes available yet. Skull defects (eg, for a catheter or craniotomy) and scalp swelling are often present, and these alterations in recording surface may result in enhancement or blunting of faster frequencies, respectively. Technicians need to judiciously follow this altered scalp topology and concomitant altered placements of electrodes.

An important evolution of CEEG occurred when video recording became used more routinely during recordings. EEGs in the ICU are frequently contaminated by rhythmic artifacts that may mimic electrocerebral activity and even seizures. Some of these artifacts, including pacemaker and chewing patterns, are familiar to all electroencephalographers, but others are more specific for critically ill patients, such as ventilator, intravenous fluid pumps, patting/chest percussion, and vibrating-bed artifacts (Figures 13.1-13.3) (16). Many EEG artifact patterns are challenging for even the most experienced interpreter but become simple to recognize with the use of video recording. Moreover, video and audio can help assess EEG reactivity to external stimuli and aid in the diagnosis of stimulus-induced,

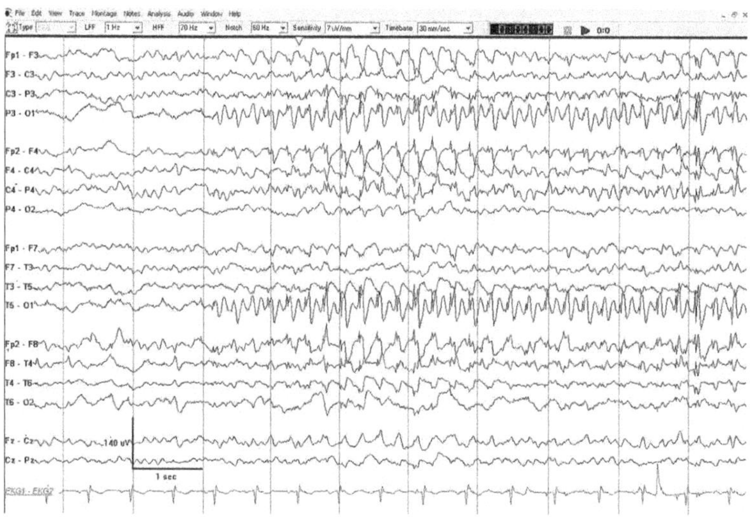

**Figure 13.2** Chest-percussion artifact mimicking an electrographic seizure. Jette N, Hirsch LJ. Continuous electroencephalogram monitoring in critically ill patients. Curr Neurol Neurosci Rep 2005;5:312-321. Reprinted with permission from Current Science, Inc.

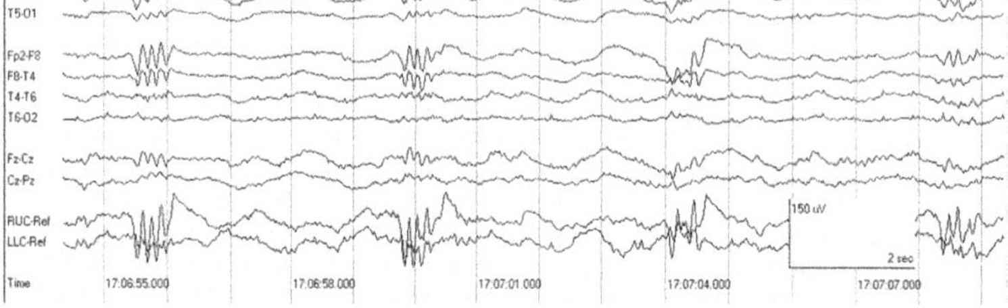

**Figure 13.3** Respirator artifact with frontally dominant rhythmic theta discharges coinciding with triggering of the respirator. From Wittman JJ, Hirsch LJ. Continuous electroencephalogram monitoring in the critically ill. Neurocrit Care 2005;2:330-341. Reprinted with permission of the Neurocritical Care Society.

rhythmic, periodic, or ictal discharges (SIRPIDs) that are quite common in comatose patients but would often be missed without simultaneous audio-visual records (17).

Although simultaneous video can help discriminate artifacts from epileptic EEG patterns, it can also aid in the characterization of spells that we have referred to as "ICU pseudoseizures." It is not uncommon for comatose patients to have episodic posturing, twitching, tremors, chewing, or sudden changes of blood pressure and heart rate without obvious source. These are occasionally diagnosed clinically as seizures at the bedside but are later shown to have no EEG correlate. It is helpful for the electrophysiologist to be able to link the clinical events to the EEG, with clear implications in terms of management.

## DURATION OF EEG RECORDING

In terms of NCSz and NCSE detection, it is clear that the use of only briefer EEGs fails to capture seizures in many patients. Pandian and colleagues recorded routine 30-minute EEGs at the beginning of the vast majority of their 105 critically ill patients undergoing CEEG (median duration 2.9 days) and identified electrographic seizures in 11% of patients with routine EEG, versus 27% with prolonged recording ($P < 0.01$) (5). Similarly, the Columbia series involved 110 patients with seizures detected on CEEG, and only slightly more than half had electrographic seizures in the first hour of recording (2). As for NCSE, 1 study found that a prolonged test was more than 5 times as likely to reveal the diagnosis (18). Thus, a 30- to 60-minute EEG is clearly inadequate in identifying many patients with NCSzs or NCSE.

Although routine 30-minute recordings are clearly inadequate, economic considerations militate against prolonged EEG in all critically ill neurologic patients. The Columbia series determined that, of all patients with seizures on CEEG, 95% of those not in coma had the first

**TABLE 13.2** CRITERIA FOR NONCONVULSIVE SEIZURE

Any pattern lasting at least 10 sec satisfying any 1 of the following 3 primary criteria:

## PRIMARY CRITERIA

- Repetitive generalized or focal spikes, sharp-waves, spike-and-wave complexes at ≥ 3/sc
- Repetitive generalized or focal spikes, sharp waves, spike-and-wave or sharp-and-slow wave complexes at < 3/sec and the secondary criterion
- Sequential rhythmic, periodic, or quasi-periodic waves at ≥ 1/sec and unequivocal evolution in frequency (gradually increasing or decreasing by at least 1/sec, eg, 2 to 3/sec), morphology, or location (gradual spread into or out of a region involving at least 2 electrodes). Evolution in amplitude alone is not sufficient. Change in sharpness without other change in morphology is not enough to satisfy evolution in morphology.

## SECONDARY CRITERION

- Significant improvement in clinical state or appearance of previously absent normal EEG patterns (such as posterior dominant "alpha" rhythm) temporally coupled to acute administration of a rapidly acting antiepileptic drug. Resolution of the "epileptiform" discharges leaving diffuse slowing without clinical improvement and without appearance of previously absent normal EEG patterns would not satisfy the secondary criterion.

*From Chong DJ, Hirsch LJ. Which EEG patterns warrant treatment in the critically ill? Reviewing the evidence for treatment of periodic epileptiform discharges and related patterns. J Clin Neurophysiol 2005;22:79-91. Chong and Hirsch modified the criteria of Young and colleagues (14). Reprinted with the permission or the American Clinical Neurophysiology Society. EEG refers to electroencephalographic.*

**TABLE 13.3** BENZODIAZEPINE TRIAL FOR THE DIAGNOSIS OF NONCONVULSIVE STATUS EPILEPTICUS

**Patients:** Rhythmic or periodic focal or generalized epileptiform discharges on EEG with neurological impairment.

**Monitoring:** EEG, pulse oximetry, blood pressure, ECG, respiratory rate with dedicated nurse.

**Antiepileptic Drug Trial:**

- Sequential small doses of rapidly acting short-duration benzodiazepine such as midazolam at 1 mg/dose.
- Between doses, repeated clinical and EEG assessment.
- Trial is stopped after any of the following:
  - Persistent resolution of the EEG pattern (and exam repeated)
  - Definite clinical improvement
  - Respiratory depression, hypotension, or other adverse effect
  - A maximum dose is reached (such as 0.2 mg/kg midazolam, though higher may be needed if on chronic benzodiazepines)
- Test is considered positive if there is resolution of the potentially ictal EEG pattern AND either an improvement in the clinical state or the appearance of previously absent normal EEG patterns (eg, posterior dominant "alpha" rhythm). If EEG improves but patient does not, the result is equivocal.

*From Jirsch J, Hirsch LJ. Nonconvulsive seizures: developing a rational approach to the diagnosis and management in the critically ill population. Reprinted with permission of the International Federation of Clinical Neurophysiology (53). EEG refers to electroencephalogram; ECG, electrocardiogram.*

seizure detected in the first 24 hours of recording (2). In contrast, comatose patients may require longer recordings to identify seizures because only 80% of comatose patients with seizures have the first seizure detected in the first 24 hours, and 87% in the first 48 hours. In children, half of patients with seizures have the first seizure within the first hour of EEG, and 80% within 24 hours (11). For the detection of NCSzs, it is probably reasonable to monitor critically ill neurologic patients who are not comatose for 24 hours but to continue for at least 48 hours in comatose patients, when periodic discharges are present, or if antiepileptic medication is being withdrawn.

## EEG INTERPRETATION

There are several problems in the EEG and clinical diagnosis of NCSE. Neurophysiologists are far from reaching a consensus, but attempts have been made to develop electrographic criteria for NCSzs (Table 13.2). As part of the diagnosis, many use the clinical and EEG response to benzodiazepines (Table 13.3), but, unfortunately, an equivocal result is not uncommon. A given patient's EEG pattern may fail to fulfill the proposed seizure criteria yet remain suspicious both clinically and electrographically for the presence of ictal activity, and the diagnosis may remain unproven. Beyond the rhythmic and periodic artifacts listed above, electrographic seizures in these patients are usually slower in frequency than those seen in ambulatory patients with epilepsy and usually remain in the delta frequency range (19,20). As a result, traditional adult seizure-detection algorithms used in epilepsy monitoring units are not sufficiently sensitive in the ICU setting (21).

There is a clear need for validation of detection algorithms for this population in order to lighten the burden of analyzing the enormous quantity of data that quickly accumulates. Compressed spectral array using fast Fourier transformation and other quantitative EEG trending tools, such as amplitude-integrated EEG or alpha:delta ratios, are used increasingly at many centers for EEG monitoring. Examples are shown in Figures 13.4 and 13.5.

# MANAGEMENT OF NONCONVULSIVE STATUS EPILEPTICUS IN THE COMA AND IN THE INTENSIVE CARE UNIT

## EVIDENCE FOR THE DELETERIOUS EFFECTS OF NONCONVULSIVE STATUS EPILEPTICUS IN THE CRITICALLY ILL

Permanent dysfunction following prolonged NCSE without any other acute brain insult is rarely reported and has generally involved seizures that were very prolonged, for more than 36 hours (22,23). Moreover, animal models that are commonly cited to argue for the damaging effects of status epilepticus on the brain (24) may not be pertinent in critically ill patients because seizures in those models involve rapid epileptiform discharges that are much different from the slower, less intense discharges usually seen in the ICU. The NCSE seen in comatose patients is similar to the generalized spike-and-wave pattern seen in idiopathic generalized epilepsies, such as absence seizures, and absence status does not cause permanent injury (25).

Nevertheless, there are many observational, epidemiologic, and laboratory findings to bolster the view that NCSE is harmful in these patients. Jaitly and colleagues found that having ictal discharges that persisted after clinical status epilepticus was controlled was associated with a highly significant increase in morbidity and mortality, even after controlling for etiology (26). Young and colleagues examined 49 patients with NCSzs and found that age, ICU length of stay, and etiology all correlated with mortality, but only seizure duration and delay to diagnosis remained significant after multiple logistic regression analysis (14). Also, in a rodent model of NCSzs produced by acute middle cerebral artery occlusion, seizure prevention with antiepileptic drugs resulted in a significant reduction in mortality, with the frequency of NCSz correlating with infarct size (27).

Many also argue that the acute symptomatic brain may be particularly prone to the

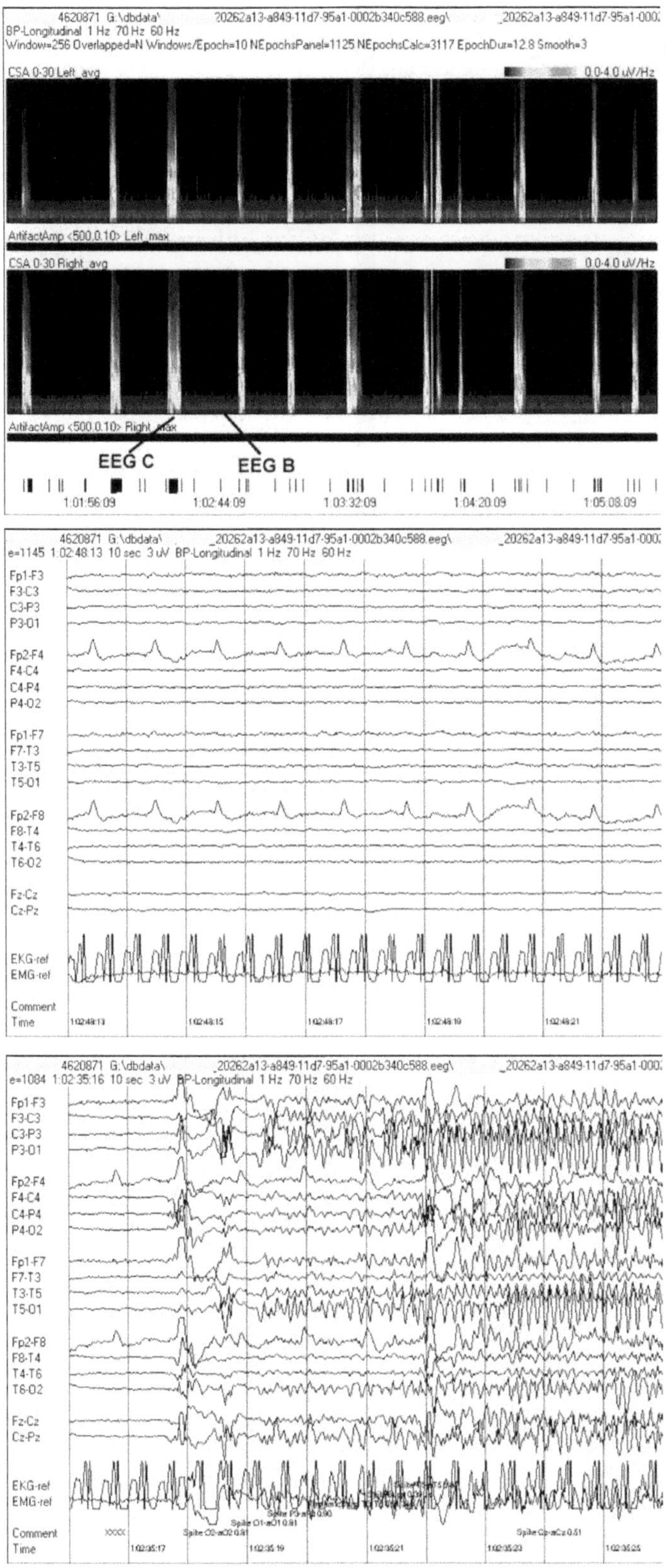


A

B

C

**Figure 13.4** Nonconvulsive status epilepticus from flat background. Utility of compressed spectral array (CSA) in rapid detection of seizures during prolonged monitoring. This 8-year-old child had refractory status epilepticus, treated with barbiturate-induced coma for several weeks, and seizures continued to arise even from complete isoelectric suppression approximately 3 times per hour. (From Jette N, Hirsch LJ. Continuous electroencephalogram monitoring in critically ill patients. Curr Neurol Neurosci Rep 2005;5:312-321. Reprinted with permission of Current Science Reports.) (A) Compressed spectral array showing 4 hours of electroencephalogram (EEG). Each burst of activity on CSA represents a seizure, with the background flat in between. (B) EEG B: EEG between seizures showing complete suppression and Fp2 artifact. Note high gain of 3 uV/mm. (C) EEG C: Subclinical electrographic seizure, bilateral but better developed on the left, arising from the completely suppressed background.

damaging effects of all types of seizures. There are dynamic changes in the neurochemistry of injured brains that likely cause vulnerability to the effects of increased metabolic demand, blood flow, and glutamate release associated with seizure discharges (28,29). Microdialysis recordings from patients with traumatic brain injury show an elevation in parenchymal glutamate to toxic levels in association with seizures (30). The cerebral perfusion pressures that increase along with glutamate levels in these patients with seizures can result in hyperemia and further cell injury in the

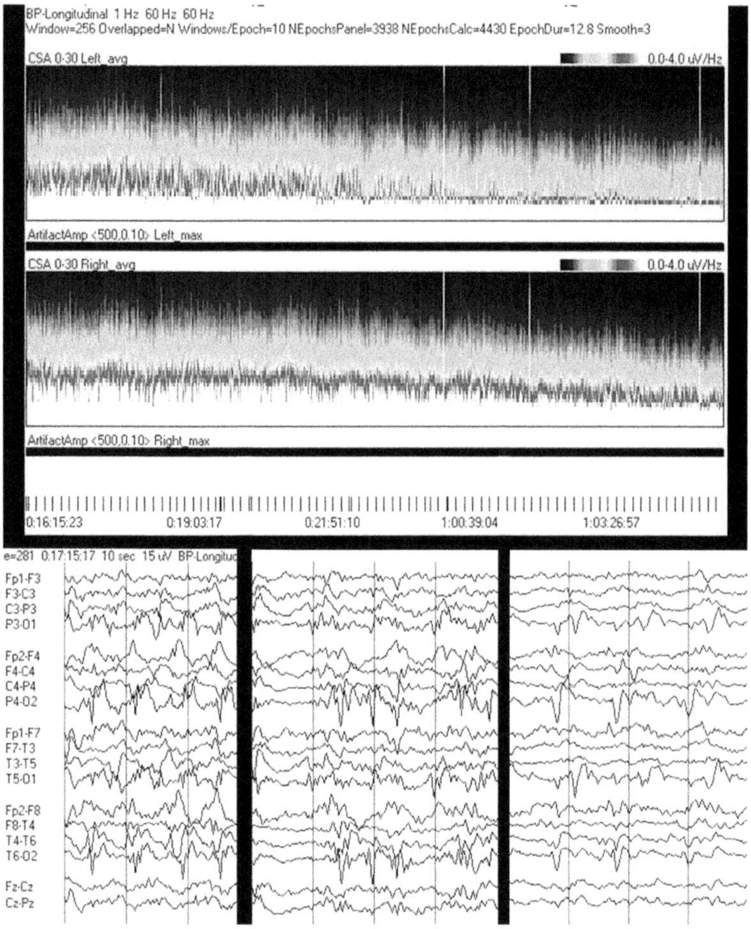


**Figure 13.5** Resolving nonconvulsive status epilepticus (NCSE): compressed spectral array (CSA) and electroencephalogram (EEG). CSA is useful for long-term EEG trends. A spectrogram from 0-30 Hz (frequency on y axis, with 30 at top) is shown for 11 hours with gradual resolution of NCSE. Associated EEG from beginning, middle, and end of the 11-hour period is shown below the spectral figure. (From Wittman JJ, Hirsch LJ. Continuous electroencephalogram monitoring in the critically ill. Neurocritical Care 2005;2:330-341. Reprinted with permission of the Neurocritical Care Society).

setting of disturbed cerebrovascular autoregulation and a damaged blood-brain barrier. In fact, Vespa and colleagues showed that seizures detected by continuous monitoring after intracerebral hemorrhage were associated with a significantly increased midline shift and a trend toward worse outcome, after controlling for hemorrhage location and size (6). The number of patients in the study was small, however, and analysis of convulsive and NCSzs were grouped together. To our knowledge, there has never been a reported case of NCSE or NCSzs alone resulting in brain herniation, and the relationship among seizures, cerebral edema, and progressive midline shift, though plausible, remains unclear.

Further evidence that NCSzs are harmful to the brain involves the biomarker neuron-specific enolase, a key enzyme for energy metabolism and a marker of acute brain and blood-brain barrier injury (31). De Giorgio and colleagues prospectively measured levels of neuron-specific enolase in consecutive patients with status epilepticus and found significant elevations in the rate of complex partial status epilepticus and subclinical generalized status epilepticus, even when there were no other evident causes for acute brain injury beyond seizures (32). Moreover, the study found that absolute levels of neuron-specific enolase correlated with the duration of status epilepticus, again supporting the view that early treatment of NCSzs is beneficial.

## TREATMENT OF NONCONVULSIVE SEIZURES AND STATUS EPILEPTICUS

Although NCSzs may damage the brain, it is not as clearly established that NCSzs or NCSE must be treated as aggressively as the convulsive varieties. Claassen and colleagues performed a systematic review comparing various continuous intravenous infusions of AEDs in patients treated for refractory convulsive and nonconvulsive status epilepticus and found a poor outcome overall (50% mortality), regardless of the agent utilized or the titration goal (ie, seizure suppression or background suppression) (33). Pentobarbital treatment appeared to be more effective than other medications in preventing breakthrough seizures, even in cases of NCSE—which are known to be more refractory than GCSE to treatment (34). Treatment, however, is frequently complicated by hypotension, and ultimate outcome was the same. Although propofol has a shorter half-life than pentobarbital and may be safer than long-acting barbiturates, it has become clear that the propofol infusion syndrome is an important complication. This serious entity is characterized by refractory metabolic acidosis, cardiac failure, rhabdomyolysis, and renal failure; occurs most often with prolonged infusion at more than 5 mg/kg per hour for more than 48 hours; and seems to be most common in patients with traumatic or other acute brain injury (35,36). See also Chapter 20.

Several centers, including ours, have used intravenously administered benzodiazepines (eg, midazolam) in cases of refractory NCSE. These medications can be titrated rapidly because of their short half-lives (similar to propofol), and they may be used synergistically with propofol to lower infused dosages of propofol. They may also result in a lower mortality rate—22% in a study combining clonazepam and propofol (37). In the rodent model of NCSzs after acute middle cerebral artery occlusion, however, benzodiazepines and barbiturates were of no benefit for seizures, and barbiturates led to continuous EEG spiking in some animals (27). Moreover, 1 retrospective human study compared critically ill older patients with NCSE treated aggressively in an ICU setting with intravenously administered benzodiazepines to those with advance directives directing less-intense treatment out of the ICU (38). Use of intravenously administered benzodiazepines was associated with an increased mortality, despite the lack of difference in severity of illness. Aggressive ICU care in these patients prolonged hospitalization but did not lead to improved outcomes. Thus, it is unclear how intensive the treatment of NCSzs should be.

Although the malignancy of NCSzs remains debated, it is clear that poor outcomes in critically ill patients with NCSzs are more affected by other factors. Important factors are the underlying etiology and the length of ICU stay, with its attendant infectious complications (39,40). At our center, a concerted effort is made to diagnose and treat NCSzs as quickly as possible, but with minimal sedation, to avoid prolonging coma and the period of intubation, thereby minimizing ICU complications (41). Non-coma–inducing agents such as intravenously administered fosphenytoin, valproate and, perhaps, intermittent benzodiazepines are the mainstays of therapy. The efficacy and attractive cardiopulmonary side-effect profile of sodium valproate over phenytoin has been recently demonstrated for convulsive status epilepticus, and this needs to be studied in NCSE as well (42,43). Additional adjunct orally administered medications (via nasogastric tube) can be helpful. These include gabapentin, pregabalin, carbamazepine and oxcarbazepine (with a concern for hyponatremia), topiramate, and levetiracetam (44-46). The newer medications have fewer drug interactions and potentially neuroprotective properties (47,48). A potential problem of using enteric medications in the ICU is the irregular gastrointestinal absorption in critically ill patients, but newer intravenously administered preparations are becoming available (eg, levetiracetam).

Often, NCSE must be treated with a continuous intravenous infusion of AED because of the resistance of the seizures to bolus medications. Intravenously administered fluids, vasopressors, or both are frequently required to treat concomitant hypotension resulting from propofol or pentobarbital; midazolam is less problematic in this regard (32). The titration endpoint of an anesthetic drip (ie, seizure cessation vs background suppression) remains debated (49). One argument favoring a burst-suppression goal emphasizes that breakthrough seizures portend NCSE relapse and occur less often with significant EEG suppression (50). The converse opinion stresses that, regardless of the anesthetic or target used, a more-suppressed EEG endpoint has not been associated with an improved patient outcome; it may in fact result in needless oversedation, with all its attendant risks. Tapering an anesthetic drip after 12 to 24 hours of seizure control, while monitoring with CEEG, is likely to be sufficient in most cases, assuming that adequate blood levels of other AEDs (such as phenytoin or valproate) are present. Gradual weaning of AEDs is more important for the short-acting drugs (midazolam and propofol) than for barbiturates (pentobarbital or thiopental sodium). CEEG monitoring is important to monitor for electrographic seizure relapse.

## LOOKING TO THE FUTURE

How best to monitor comatose patients with, or at risk for developing, NCSE and how to diagnose and manage NCSE are unknown. One advance would be researchers' use of common definitions for terms such as *ictal* or *nonconvulsive*, as well as terminologies for various EEG patterns encountered in critically ill patients (51,52). We have much to learn about which EEG patterns reflect ongoing neuronal damage and which patients might benefit from intensive antiseizure treatment. Many of these questions will require large multicenter clinical trials before definitive answers appear.

## REFERENCES

1. Treiman DM, Meyers PD, Walton NY, Collins C, Rowan AJ, Handforth A, Faught E, Calabrese VP, Uthman BM, Ramsay RE, Mamdani MB. A comparison of four treatments for generalized convulsive status epilepticus. Veterans Affairs Status Epilepticus Cooperative Study Group. N Engl J Med 1998;339:792-798.
2. Claassen J, Mayer SA, Kowalski RG, Emerson RG, Hirsch LJ. Detection of electrographic seizures with continuous EEG monitoring in critically ill patients. Neurology 2004;62:1743-1748.
3. Towne AR, Waterhouse EJ, Boggs JG, Garnett LK, Brown AJ, Smith JR, DeLorenzo RJ, Smith JR Jr. Prevalence of nonconvulsive status epilepticus in comatose patients. Neurology 2000;54:340-345.
4. Jordan KG. Continuous EEG and evoked potential monitoring in the neuroscience intensive care unit. J Clin Neurophysiol 1993;10:445-475.
5. Pandian JD, Cascino GD, So EL, Manno E, Fulgham JR. Digital video-electroencephalographic monitoring in the neurological-neurosurgical intensive care unit: clinical features and outcome. Arch Neurol 2004;61:1090-1094.
6. Vespa PM, O'Phelan K, Shah M, Mirabelli J, Starkman S, Kidwell C, Saver J, Nuwer MR, Frazee JG, McArthur DA, Martin NA. Acute seizures after intracerebral hemorrhage: a factor in progressive midline shift and outcome. Neurology 2003;60:1441-1446.
7. Vespa PM, Nuwer MR, Nenov V, Ronne-Engstrom E, Hovda DA, Bergsneider M, Kelly DF, Martin NA, Becker DP. Increased incidence and impact of nonconvulsive and convulsive seizures after traumatic brain injury as detected by continuous electroencephalographic monitoring. J Neurosurg 1999;91:750-760.
8. Dennis LJ, Claassen J, Hirsch LJ, Emerson RG, Connolly ES, Mayer SA. Nonconvulsive status epilepticus after subarachnoid hemorrhage. Neurosurgery 2002;51:1136-1143.
9. Carrera E, Michel P, Despland PA, Maeder-Ingvar M, Ruffieux C, Debatisse D, Ghika J, Devuyst G, Bogousslavsky J. Continuous assessment of electrical epileptic activity in acute stroke. Neurology 2006;67:99-104.
10. Claassen J, Jette N, Chum F, Green R, Schmidt M, Choi H, Jirsch J, Frontera JA, Connolly S, Emerson RG, Mayer SA, Hirsch LJ. Electrographic seizures and periodic discharges after intracerebral hemorrhage. Neurology 2007;69:1356-1365.
11. Jette N, Claassen J, Emerson RG, Hirsch LJ. Frequency and predictors of nonconvulsive seizures during continuous electroencephalographic monitoring in critically ill children. Arch Neurol 2006;63:1750-1755.
12. Husain AM, Horn GJ, Jacobson MP. Non-convulsive status epilepticus: usefulness of clinical features in selecting patients for urgent EEG. J Neurol Neurosurg Psychiatry 2003;74:189-191.

13. DeLorenzo RJ, Waterhouse EJ, Towne AR, Boggs JG, Ko D, DeLorenzo GA, Brown A, Garnett L. Persistent nonconvulsive status epilepticus after the control of convulsive status epilepticus. Epilepsia 1998;39:833-840.
14. Young GB, Jordan KG, Doig GS. An assessment of nonconvulsive seizures in the intensive care unit using continuous EEG monitoring: an investigation of variables associated with mortality. Neurology 1996;47:83-89.
15. Ives JR. New chronic EEG electrode for critical/intensive care unit monitoring. J Clin Neurophysiol 2005;22:119-123.
16. Hirsch LJ, Kull LL. Continuous EEG monitoring in the intensive care unit. Am J Electroneurodiagnostic Technol 2004;44:137-158.
17. Hirsch LJ, Claassen J, Mayer SA, Emerson RG. Stimulus-induced rhythmic, periodic, or ictal discharges (SIRPIDs): a common EEG phenomenon in the critically ill. Epilepsia 2004;45:109-123.
18. Varelas PN, Spanaki MV, Hacein-Bay L, Hether T, Terranova B. Emergent EEG: Indications and diagnostic yield. Neurology 2003;61:702-704.
19. Granner MA, Lee SI. Nonconvulsive status epilepticus: EEG analysis in a large series. Epilepsia 1994;35:42-47.
20. Scheuer ML, Wilson SB. Data analysis for continuous EEG monitoring in the ICU: seeing the forest and the trees. J Clin Neurophysiol 2004;21:353-378.
21. Gotman J. Automatic recognition of epileptic seizures in the EEG. Electroencephalogr Clin Neurophysiol 1982;54:530-540.
22. Engel J Jr, Ludwig BI, Fetell M. Prolonged partial complex status epilepticus: EEG and behavioral observations. Neurology 1978;28:863-869.
23. Krumholz A, Sung GY, Fisher RS, Barry E, Bergey GK, Grattan LM. Complex partial status epilepticus accompanied by serious morbidity and mortality. Neurology 1995;45:1499-1504.
24. Meldrum BS, Brierley JB. Prolonged epileptic seizures in primates: ischemic cell change and its relation to ictal physiological events. Arch Neurol 1973;28:10-17.
25. Shorvon, S, Walker M. Status epilepticus in idiopathic generalized epilepsy. Epilepsia 2005;464(Suppl 9):73-79.
26. Jaitly R, Sgro JA, Towne AR, Ko D, DeLorenzo RJ. Prognostic value of EEG monitoring after status epilepticus: a prospective adult study. J Clin Neurophysiol 1997;14:326-334.
27. Williams AJ, Tortella FC, Lu XM, Moreton JE, Hartings JA. Antiepileptic drug treatment of nonconvulsive seizures induced by experimental focal brain ischemia. J Pharmacol Exp Ther 2004;311:220-227.
28. Bergsneider MA, Hovda DA, Shalmon E, Kelly DF, Vespa PM, Martin NA, Phelps ME, McArthur DL, Caron MJ, Kraus JF, Becker DP. Cerebral hyperglycolysis following severe human traumatic brain injury: a positron emission tomography study. J Neurosurg 1997;86:241-251.
29. Bullock R, Zauner A, Myseros JS, Marmarou A, Woodward JJ, Young HF. Evidence for prolonged release of excitatory amino acids in severe human head trauma: relationship to clinical events. Ann N Y Acad Sci 1995;59:290-297.
30. Vespa P, Prins M, Ronne-Engstrom E, Caron M, Shalmon E., Hoyda DA, Martin NA, Becker DP. Increase in extracellular glutamate caused by reduced cerebral perfusion pressure and seizures after traumatic brain injury: a microdialysis study. J Neurosurg 1998;89:971-982.
31. Correale J, Rabinowicz AL, Heck CN, Smith TD, Loskota WJ, DeGiorgio CM. Status epilepticus increases CSF levels of neuron specific enolase and alters the blood brain barrier. Neurology 1998;50:1388-1391.
32. DeGiorgio CM, Heck CN, Rabinowicz AL, Gott PS, Smith T, Correale J. Serum neuron-specific enolase in the major subtypes of status epilepticus. Neurology 1999;52:746-749.
33. Claassen J, Hirsch LJ, Emerson RG, Bates JE, Thompson TB, Mayer SA. Continuous EEG monitoring and midazolam infusion for refractory status epilepticus. Neurology 2001;57:1036-1042.
34. Mayer SA, Claassen J, Lokin J, Mendelsohn F, Dennis LJ, Fitzsimmons BF. Refractory status epilepticus: frequency risk factors, and impact on outcome. Arch Neurol 2002;59:205-210.
35. Vasile B, Rasulo F, Candiani A, Latronico N. The pathophysiology of propofol infusion syndrome: a simple name for a complex syndrome. Intensive Care Med 2003;29:1417-1425.
36. Cremer OL, Moons KG, Bouman EA, Kruijswijk JE, de Smet AM, Kalkman CJ. Longterm propofol infusion and cardiac failure in adult head injury patients. Lancet 2001;357:117-118.
37. Rossetti AO, Reichart MD, Schaller MD, Despland PA, Bogousslavsky J. Propofol treatment of refractory status epilepticus: a study of 31 episodes. Epilepsia 2004;45:757-763.

38. Litt B, Wityk RJ, Hertz, SH, Mullen PD, Ryan DD, Henry TR. Nonconvulsive status epilepticus in the critically ill elderly. Epilepsia 1998;39:1194-1202.
39. Yaffe K, Lowenstein SH. Prognostic factors of pentobarbital therapy for refractory generalized status epilepticus. Neurology 1993;43:895-900.
40. Krishnamurthy KB, Drislane FW. Relapse and survival after barbiturate anesthetic treatment of refractory stsus epilepticus. Epilepsia 1996;37:863-867.
41. Schweickert WD, Gehlbach BK, Pohlman AS, Hall JB, Kress JP. Daily interruption of sedative infusions and complications of critical illness in mechanically ventilated patients. Crit Care Med 2004;32:1272-1276.
42. Peters CAN, Pohlmann-Eden B. Intravenous valproate as an innovative therapy in seizure emergency situations including status epilepticus—experience in 102 adult patients. Seizure 2005;14:164-169.
43. Misra UK, Kalita J, Patel R. Sodium valproate vs. phenytoin in status epilepticus: A pilot study. Neurology 2005;67:340-342.
44. Rossetti AO, Bromfield EB. Levetiracetam in the treatment of status epilepticus in adults: a study of 13 episodes. Eur Neurol 2005;54:34-38.
45. Towne AR, Garnett LK, Waterhouse EJ, Morton LD, DeLorenzo RJ. The use of topirimate in refractory status epilepticus. Neurology 2003;60:332-334.
46. Rupprecht S, Franke K, Fitzek S, Witte OW, Hagemann G. Levetiracetam as a treatment option in nonconvulsive status epilepticus. Epilepsy Res 2007;73:238-244
47. Hanon E, Klitgaard H. Neuroprotective properties of the novel antiepileptic drug levetiracetam in the rat middle cerebral artery occlusion model of cerebral ischemia. Seizure 2001;10:287-293.
48. Rekling JC. Neuroprotective effects of anticonvulsants in rat hippocampal slice cultures exposed to oxygen/glucose deprivation. Neurosci Lett 2003;335:167-170.
49. Jordan KG, Hirsch LJ. In nonconvulsive status epilepticus (NCSE), treat to burst-suppression: Pro and con. Epilepsia 2006;47:41-45.
50. Claassen J, Hirsch LJ, Emerson RG, Mayer SA. Treatment of refractory status epilepticus with pentobarbital, propofol, or midazolam: a systematic review. Epilepsia 2002;43:146-153.
51. Hirsch LJ, Brenner RP, Drislane FW, So E, Kaplan PW, Jordan KG, Herman ST, LaRoche SM, Young B, Bleck TP, Scheuer ML, Emerson RG. The ACNS Subcommittee on Research Terminology for Continuous EEG Monitoring: proposed standardized terminology for rhythmic and periodic EEG patterns encountered in critically ill patients. J Clin Neurophysiol 2005;22:128-135.
52. Jirsch J, Hirsch LJ. Nonconvulsive seizures: developing a rational approach to the diagnosis and management in the critically ill population. Clin Neurophysiol 2007;117:1660-1670.

# PART IV

# SEMIOLOGY OF NONCONVULSIVE STATUS EPILEPTICUS

CHAPTER 14

# NONCONVULSIVE STATUS EPILEPTICUS: A MIMICKER OF NEUROLOGIC DISORDERS

KRZYSZTOF BUJARSKI, MICHAEL R. SPERLING

At the end of the 19th century, Jonathan Hutchinson nicknamed syphilis "the great imitator" for its propensity to mimic the symptoms of many other diseases, such as tuberculosis, smallpox, and lupus (1). In recent times, HIV and Lyme disease have been granted the same title (2). The significance of imitators lies in their ability to produce clinical signs and symptoms that are usually associated with unrelated disorders. Physicians may be misled and may suggest an incorrect diagnosis. Diseases that mimic other conditions offer a challenge to established medical practice and remind physicians of the occasional lack of direct one-to-one correlation between clinical presentation and pathophysiology.

The title of "the great imitator" in clinical epileptology may be given to nonconvulsive status epilepticus (NCSE) because NCSE may produce neurologic syndromes which have been associated with nonepileptic conditions. NCSE may mimic nonepileptic disease processes because it violates 2 common clinical rules in diagnosing epilepsy: that seizures are discrete episodes with a relatively short time course and that they usually display an evolution of ictal symptoms. For instance, when considering the differential diagnosis for a particular symptom, the diagnosis of epilepsy is generally considered if the symptom duration is shorter than several minutes and if the symptoms evolve or change over that time period. A typical complex partial seizure may start with an epigastric aura, progress to loss of awareness with oral automatisms, and end with a postictal period. The seizure typically lasts 1 to 2 minutes. In contrast, when symptoms last several hours or days and fluctuate only slightly over that time, then the diagnosis of seizure is less apt to be considered. NCSE mimics other disease processes precisely because it can produce a prolonged, relatively fixed and focal neurologic deficit that may not be commonly associated with epileptic disorders. Thus, the prolonged time course of NCSE and a lack of evolution of symptoms may falsely suggest that the symptoms may not be related to seizure activity at all.

Since persistent epileptic discharges may disrupt any region of the cerebral cortex, NCSE can present with a wide variety of symptoms. Persistent seizures can disrupt small regions of the cortex and produce isolated motor, sensory, or linguistic symptoms. If the discharges involve wide-spread neural networks, symptoms mimicking psychosis or encephalopathy may be produced. If large regions of both hemispheres are involved, syndromes resembling akinetic mutism or coma can result. Therefore, NCSE can produce a wide clinical spectrum of symptoms depending on the regions and the relative amount of brain that is made dysfunctional by the persistent epileptic discharge.

NCSE usually mimics other neurologic disorders, not the other way around. For instance, if an elderly patient presents with a clinical history of a subacute confusional state, a physician may think about possible metabolic derangement. It would be unlikely that a physician would consider NCSE as the most likely etiology for the confusion. If the patient turns out to have spike-wave stupor, NCSE would have mimicked a metabolic encephalopathy. The reverse, ie, other neurologic conditions mimicking NCSE, is less often encountered because NCSE is infrequently considered to be the most likely explanation for a given set of symptoms. This view may, in some ways, be justified because NCSE occurs less frequently than do most conditions that it mimics. In addition, because NCSE can produce variable clinical presentations, there is a lack of "typical" features, so NCSE is probably underdiagnosed.

## CLINICAL SYNDROMES

This section will review various clinical syndromes produced by NCSE that are usually associated with other neurologic conditions. In each section, we give the typical clinical findings in each syndrome and descriptions of the behavior and neurologic findings. Next, we summarize the published studies on NCSE causing such a syndrome. Subsequently, we provide the differential diagnosis for the clinical syndrome. And, lastly, we list the clinical features that may guide the physician to consider NCSE.

## SYNDROME OF ALERT UNRESPONSIVENESS

The behavior of patients in NCSE most frequently resembles several conditions in which a striking dissociation exists between the level of arousal and responsiveness. For instance, patients in generalized absence status often appear to be awake, maintain posture, and may attend to certain stimuli but are partially or totally unresponsive (3). Other conditions that may cause a similar clinical picture are listed in Table 14.1. Although the clinical appearance of a patient with one of these syndrome may be similar to that of a patient in NCSE, the neurobehavioral mechanism that causes the dysfunction in each syndrome may be strikingly different.

Akinetic mutism is a neurobehavioral syndrome in which emotionally driven, motivated behavior is lost in the context of preserved alertness and awareness. It is frequently caused by bilateral destructive lesions of the anterior cingulate gyrus (4,5), which functions in assigning motivational content to external and internal stimuli. Patients with akinetic mutism are awake and aware of their environment and may intermittently attend to stimuli. However, they lack purposeful movement and may not follow instructions or respond to questions.

**TABLE 14.1** DIFFERENTIAL SIAGNOSIS OF THE SYNDROME OF ALERT UNRESPONSIVENESS

| | Arousal | Awareness | Posture | Responsiveness | EEG | MRI |
|---|---|---|---|---|---|---|
| NCSE | Full | Not aware or partially aware of surroundings, no memory for event | Maintained | Fully or semi-unresponsive, may have automatisms | Epileptiform discharges | May be normal |
| Akinetic mutism | Full | Aware of surroundings, should have normal cognitive ability other then motivation (difficult to demonstrate) | Maintained | Impoverished but may respond | May be normal. Bifrontal polymorphic delta may be seen. | Lesion in bilateral mesial frontal lobe |
| Locked-in syndrome | Full | Fully preserved | Atonic or spastic tone | May respond by vertical eye movements | Normal | Brain stem lesion |
| MCS and PVS | Full | Not aware of surroundings | Maintained or spastic tone | Variable responsiveness, may react only to basic stimuli | Diffuse slowing | Diffuse cortical injury |

***Abbreviations:*** *NCSE, nonconvulsive status epilepticus; EEG, electroencephalography; MRI, magnetic resonance imaging; MCS: minimally conscious state; PVS persistent vegetative state.*

The diagnosis of akinetic mutism is suggested when, in the context of an appropriate clinical history and examination, a destructive lesion of the mesial frontal lobes is found with brain imaging.

Locked-in syndromes arise when a normal cerebrum is deefferented and disconnected from lower motor neurons of the spinal cord and lower brainstem (6). The condition is typically caused by lesions in the ventral pons, which preserve the ascending reticular formation while destroying descending pyramidal tract fibers, such as central pontine myelinolysis. Locked-in patients are awake and fully aware of their surroundings. Their cognitive abilities are normal. However, they can neither maintain posture nor produce purposeful movements, with the exception of intact vertical eye movements, with which the patient may communicate. The diagnosis of locked-in syndrome is made by establishing the dissociation between normal alertness and cognition (as judged by establishing communication by eye movements) and lack of voluntary movement. The electroencephalogram (EEG) in locked-in syndrome is normal, and imaging will show a lesion in the basis pontis (7). Although it would be distinctly unusual for NCSE to mimic a locked-in syndrome, this diagnosis should be considered in the absence of long tract signs in the neurologic examination.

Minimally conscious state and persistent vegetative state are similar neurobehavioral conditions in which severe widespread damage to the cortex occurs with relative sparing of the projections arising in the brain stem and subcortical structures that mediate arousal (8). Differences between minimally conscious state and persistent vegetative state lie only in the severity of the cognitive deficit. Patients in minimally conscious state and persistent vegetative state are awake but are not aware of their surroundings, due to a widespread disturbance of cognition. They may maintain basic posture and produce some movements. These syndromes occur in patients following traumatic brain injury or cerebral anoxia or as a result of end-stage neurodegenerative disease. Diagnosis is based on history of diffuse cerebral injury with the above examination. EEG in persistent vegetative state may be associated with a variety of patterns and is unlikely to be helpful in making the diagnosis (9). Magnetic resonance imaging scans shows diffuse cortical injury.

## SYNDROME OF CATATONIA

Catatonic syndromes are characterized by disturbances of posture and tone, such as "waxy flexibility"; mutism; resistance or even opposition to instructions or attempts to be moved; extreme negativism; echolalia; and echopraxia (10). Patients in catatonia maintain axial and appendicular posture even if placed is an uncomfortable position. For instance, when the pulse is examined, the arm will sustain the raised posture in which it was placed during the examination. If a supine catatonic patient's pillow is removed, the patient's head may remain elevated, levitating above the bed. Although the catatonic patient neither follows instructions nor responds to questions, he is awake, is aware of his surroundings, and generally recalls details of events that occurred during the period of clinical symptoms.

Ictal catatonia has been described in the medical literature through isolated case reports and limited series (11-13) . Most notably, Primavera (14) described the EEG findings of 29 patients with catatonia of unclear etiology. NCSE was identified to be the primary cause in 4 of 29 patients. The neurologic examination revealed mutism and "lead-pipe rigidity," and the symptoms of catatonia resolved with antiepileptic drug treatment. Lim (15) described 3 patients who presented in a catatonic state and had EEG findings consistent with NCSE. The symptoms were promptly reversed by intravenous administration of phenytoin. Although many of these patients suffering from ictal catatonia had secondary neurologic insult, such as viral encephalitis, at the time of presentation, improvement of symptoms and normalization of the EEG following the administration of antiepileptic drugs clearly established the diagnosis.

Because NCSE can present with a catatonic syndrome, it can mimic catatonia caused by psychiatric or other neurologic diseases. The differential diagnosis is listed in Table 14.2. Catatonia can present in the setting of major depression, bipolar disorder, or schizophrenia (16). In these instances, history of psychopathology is apparent. Structural lesions of the frontal lobes can cause catatonia. For instance, catatonia caused by butterfly glioma of the corpus callosum (17) or traumatic injury to the prefrontal cortex (18) and as sequelae of bacterial meningitis (19) has been described. Catatonia can likewise be seen as part of the neuroleptic malignant and serotonin syndromes and has been reported as a complication of rapid benzodiazepine withdrawal (20).

The evaluation of a patient with catatonia should initially focus on searching for medical conditions. Elevation of body temperature and a finding of an elevated creatine kinase level should prompt discontinuation of neuroleptic or serotonin medications. Prior history of psychiatric disturbances should prompt more aggressive treatment, including possible electroconvulsive therapy. In the situations in which catatonia is not explained, EEG monitoring should be considered to evaluate for possible NCSE. See Chapter 15 for the psychiatric manifestations of NCSE.

**TABLE 14.2** THE DIFFERENTIAL DIAGNOSIS OF CATATONIA

| |
|---|
| **Nonconvulsive status epilepticus** |
| **Psychiatric** |
| 1. Major depression |
| 2. Bipolar disorder |
| 3. Schizophrenia |
| **CNS infections (postinfectious syndromes)** |
| 1. Viral encephalitis |
| 2. Bacterial meningitis |
| **Focal lesions of the orbitofrontal or mesial frontal lobes** |
| 1. Butterfly glioma |
| 2. Bifrontal contusions |
| **Medication** |
| 1. Neuroleptic malignant syndrome |
| 2. Serotonin syndrome |
| 3. Withdrawal from benzodiazepines |
| **Autoimmune or paraneoplastic diseases** |
| 1. Lupus |
| 2. Acute disseminated encephalomyelitis |
| 3. Limbic encephalitis |

***Abbreviation:*** *CNS, central nervous system.*

## SYNDROME OF AMNESIA

Focal seizures that remain restricted to the mesial portions of the temporal lobes in the region of the hippocampal complex may produce anterograde amnesia (21,22). This syndrome, referred to in the literature as epileptic amnesia, is an excellent example of NCSE. Epileptic amnesia can mimic various other acute amnestic conditions that are listed in Table 14.3. A patient with epileptic amnesia has transient difficulty forming new memories during seizures. Once a seizure has ended, memory circuits recover, and the patient is once again able to form new memories. If the seizure repeats, then the patient may have "islands of memory loss" (22). For example, a patient with temporal lobe epilepsy remembered driving to his daughter's wedding but had no recollection of specific events that transpired during the wedding. Thus, epileptic amnesia is caused by recurrent or ongoing dysfunction of the memory structures by repetitive focal seizures.

Transient global amnesia may present in a fashion similar to that of transient epileptic amnesia. Similar to patients with epileptic amnesia, patients with transient global amnesia usually are acutely aware that something is wrong and pose questions. In contrast with epileptic amnesia, the symptoms of transient global amnesia last between 4 to 6 hours, and the attack usually occurs only once. Following recovery from the symptoms, the patient cannot remember anything that occurred during the event, ie, the memory loss is generally complete (23).

Vascular disturbances in the region of the posterior circulation may also present with symptoms of anterograde amnesia. Migraine can cause disturbances of blood flow and can cause transient amnesia as a migraine aura (24,25). The symptoms are generally brief and are usually followed by a typical migraine

**TABLE 14.3** DIFFERENTIAL DIAGNOSIS OF THE SYNDROME OF AMNESIA

| | Clinical course | Type of memory loss | EEG findings | MRI findings | Treatment | Other |
|---|---|---|---|---|---|---|
| TEA (NCSE) | Acute onset, may repeat multiple times | Anterograde amnesia, islands of memory loss | Epileptic discharges | Normal or abnormal depending on cause of seizures | AED | Previous diagnosis of epilepsy is common |
| TGA | Single event lasting several hours | Dense anterograde and variable retrograde during the episode | Normal | Normal | Time. Complete resolution of symptoms within several hours. | No strong risk factors; patients are generally in their 50s |
| Stroke | Acute, persistent mostly anterograde amnesia | Dense anterograde and variable retrograde | Normal | Bilateral stroke in region of hippocampal complex, or mesial dorsal region of thalamus | Antiplatlelet therapy | Vascular risk factors |
| Migraine | Amnesia precedes a headache | Dense anterograde and variable retrograde | Occasional intermittent bitemporal delta | Normal | Multiple agents available | Family history |
| Limbic encephalitis | Subacute onset, progressive | Dense anterograde and variable retrograde | Bi-temporal delta, PLEDs | Bilateral hyperintensity in the mesial temporal lobes | Immunomodulatory treatment, antiviral treatment, search for occult neoplasm | Occult neoplasm |
| Korsakoff psychosis | Acute onset and nonprogressive | Dense anterograde and variable retrograde | Normal | Hemorrhagic lesions in the mammilary bodies or thalamus | None | History of alcohol abuse |
| Psychogenic amnesia | Acute onset, may repeat several times | Dense retrograde with normal anterograde | Normal | Normal | Cognitive therapy focused on stress reduction | Family history of psychiatric diagnosis |

*5 EEG, electroencephalogram; MRI, magnetic resonance imaging; AED, antiepileptic drug; TEA, transient epileptic amnesia; NCSE, nonconvulsive status epilepticus; TGA, transient global amnesia; PLEDs, periodic lateralized epileptiform discharges.*

headache, but acephalgic migraine may occur as well. A posterior circulation stroke in the region of the mesial dorsal nucleus of the thalamus or the mesial temporal structures can present as a syndrome anterograde amnesia (26). The amnesia is complete and does not improve. Patients generally have vascular risk factors. Korsakoff syndrome, or severe anterograde amnesia in the context of alcohol abuse with hemorrhagic necrosis of thalamic nuclei and the mamillary bodies, is a similar syndrome.

Anterograde amnesia can also be produced by limbic encephalitis. This can be secondary to paraneoplastic (anti-Hu or -Ma antibodies), autoimmune (voltage-gated potassium channel antibodies), or infectious (herpes simplex encephalitis) mechanisms. Limbic encephalitis can usually be distinguished on the basis of subacute memory loss, which may be progressive. It can be accompanied by behavior disturbances, such a personality changes, irritability, and aggression. Magnetic resonance imaging scans will show bilateral lesions in the mesial temporal structures. EEG may show bilateral temporal focal delta or sharp waves.

The differential diagnosis of amnestic states likewise includes psychogenic amnesia (27). The typical features of psychogenic amnesia include severe retrograde amnesia with no anterograde amnesia during the period of memory dysfunction. For instance, a patient will work normally throughout the day performing difficult tasks in the office. Later, she will report dense amnesia for the entire period that she worked normally. This is in striking contrast to epileptic amnesia and transient global amnesia, in which the patient cannot function properly during the period of memory loss.

## SYNDROME OF APHASIA

Acute onset of aphasia most frequently is a symptom of acute cortical stroke in the left middle cerebral artery distribution. Less frequently, other structural lesions such as central nervous system neoplasms or an intracerebral hemorrhage, can present with acute aphasia. NCSE that presents solely as periods of prolonged aphasia has been reported (28-32). Clinical characteristics of isolated language disturbances are compared with other conditions in Table 14.4. Aphasia attributable to NCSE has been reported as sudden in onset with a fluctuating level of language disability. In the majority of cases, the aphasia associated with focal seizures is

**TABLE 14.4** DIFFERENTIAL DIAGNOSIS OF THE SYNDROME OF APHASIA

| | History | EEG | MRI |
|---|---|---|---|
| NCSE | Acute onset, may be intermittent, variable course | Epileptiform discharges lesion | May be normal, possible |
| Stroke | Acute onset and persistent | Polymorphic delta | Most frequent, left hemisphere lesion |
| Migraine | Acute onset followed by a headache | Occasional intermittent bitemporal delta | Normal |
| Tumor | Subacute onset | Polymorphic delta. | Most frequent, left hemisphere tumor |
| CJD | Subacute onset | 2-Hz PLEDs | Initially negative, cortical ribbon sign |
| PPA | Chronic and gradual progression of language disturbance | Normal<br>Left temporal delta | Atrophy of perisylvian area |

***Abbreviations:*** *EEG, electroencephalogram; MRI, magnetic resonance imaging; NCSE, nonconvulsive status epilepticus; CJD, Creutzfeldt-Jacob disease; PPA, primary progressive aphasia; PLEDs, periodic lateralized epileptiform discharges.*

global in character, with nonfluent speech and difficulty with comprehension. In addition, it has been associated in all cases with a focal epileptic discharge in the left hemisphere on EEG, usually in the left temporal region. Following treatment with antiepileptic medications, aphasia resolves fully over a period of several days.

Prolonged periods of aphasia have also been associated with migraine. Both paraphasias and word-finding difficulties can occur prior to the headache phase of migraine and may last for many days (33). These should be considered a prolonged migraine aura. During these episodes, a gradual change in the type of language dysfunction may be seen; for instance, paraphasias over time may yield to word-finding difficulties. These are likely related to spreading depression and subsequent recovery of function. In addition to prolonged auras, both sporadic hemiplegic migraine and familial hemiplegic migraine may present with headache followed by periods of aphasia (34).

Subacute onset of aphasia has been reported as the presenting and initial symptom in Creutzfeldt-Jakob disease (35). Several types of language deficits can be appreciated, including transcortical motor and sensory aphasia. EEG may show 1- to 2-Hz periodic sharp-wave complexes limited to the left temporal region, and a mistaken diagnosis of NCSE could be made. However, these patients fail to respond to treatment with antiepileptic drugs, and prolonged EEG monitoring reveals no seizures or ictal evolution of periodic lateralized epileptiform discharge activity (36). The progression of cognitive decline may be very rapid.

Neurodegenerative diseases such as primary progressive aphasia present with disturbances in language processing. The clinical course is typically chronic with a gradual progression. On initial presentation, patients may have disturbances of language, which later progress to behavioral and memory disturbances (37). The EEG is either normal or may show focal slowing over the left temporal region, and magnetic resonance imaging shows atrophy of the left perisylvian cortex.

## SYNDROME OF COMA

Coma is defined as unarousable unresponsiveness and is a sign of diffuse or multifocal cerebral injury (38). Patients in comatose states generally have their eyes closed, do not attend to stimulation, and may require support of cardiopulmonary functions. With current brain imaging and laboratory technology, the underlying etiology for comatose states is frequently known. However, in routine clinical practice, a patient is occasionally encountered who continues to be persistently comatose despite seemingly mild cerebral insult. In these situations of persistent and unexplained coma, the differential diagnosis should include NCSE.

Long-term bedside EEG studies of patients in the intensive care unit have generally revealed that NCSE is common in comatose patients (39). It occurs in a variety of clinical settings, including acute traumatic brain injury (40), subarachnoid hemorrhage, and anoxic or metabolic encephalopathy and as an undiscovered consequence of inadequate or unsuccessful treatment of convulsive status epilepticus (41). A complete discussion of the differential diagnosis of coma is beyond the scope of this chapter, and the reader is referred to Plum and Posner's definitive work on this topic (40). In general, the significance of NCSE in the comatose patient lies in the ability of NCSE to exaggerate the appearance of brain injury through dysfunction of potentially normal and uninjured neuronal networks. Consequently, NCSE can mimic severe brain injury in a less severely injured person.

Physicians involved in the care of comatose patients find it difficult to diagnose NCSE by clinical criteria alone. The uncertainty stems from lack of sensitive or specific clinical signs that can exclude the possibility of nonconvulsive status in a comatose patient. Occasionally, subtle muscle jerks and twitches, variability in the diameter of the pupil, and unprovoked fluctuations of blood pressure may be noticed (42). However, there may be no outward clinical signs of seizures, and the diagnosis might be made only by EEG recording. Therefore, the diagnosis of NCSE in a comatose patient should be considered if it is determined that the patient's level of neurologic deficit is unexplained or if it is out of proportion to the type and severity of any known insult. For instance, if a patient who has undergone a craniotomy to clip a middle cerebral artery aneurysm is persistently unresponsive following surgery, an EEG might be obtained to evaluate for possible NCSE.

## SYNDROME OF PSYCHOSIS

Psychosis is characterized by fixed delusions, auditory or (less commonly) visual hallucinations, disorganized speech and thought, and disorganized behavior (43). This symptom cluster is most frequently seen in idiopathic psychiatric diseases such as schizophrenia. Similar clusters of symptoms can arise secondary to neurologic disturbances, most notably epilepsy. Although NCSE causing ictal behaviors resembling psychosis, such as aggression (44), auditory hallucinations (45), and delusions, may be relatively common, clear case reports of NCSE causing all the features of psychosis have not been published. NCSE can present with bizarre complex hallucinations, but the hallucinations are generally isolated and not perceived as real by the patient. In addition, NCSE may present with disorganized behavior. However, such patients will frequently have a superimposed confusional state. NCSE may present as fixed delusions, such as have been noted by Capgrass (46) or Cottard (47). However, these are isolated delusions and are not associated with other delusional ideation in general. Therefore, although NCSE may present with symptoms that can mimic psychosis, the full syndrome in the context of preserved consciousness (alertness, attention, language, and memory) is probably not seen.

The differential diagnosis of a patient who presents with symptoms of psychosis in the context of epilepsy is listed in Table 14.5. Although true ictal psychosis has not been well described, postictal psychosis has been well documented and is relatively frequently seen in an epilepsy center. The symptoms of postictal psychosis occur 12 to 72 hours following a seizure and, on average, last 70 hours (48), although much longer periods have been reported (49). Patients in postictal psychosis may have fixed persecutory, grandiose, referential, somatic, or religious delusions. Postictal psychosis occurs most frequently in patients who have EEG evidence of bilateral temporal dysfunction and irritability (50).

Another cause of psychosis in epileptic patients that may be mimicked by NCSE is alternative psychosis or forced normalization (51). This phenomenon occurs in patients who develop paranoid delusions and auditory hallucinations following successful treatment of seizures. A defining feature of alternate psychosis is the relative normalization of the EEG during the period of clinical symptoms and the lack of clinical seizures. Symptoms of forced normalization generally occur several weeks following successful treatment of epilepsy with surgery or novel medication. The symptoms may be diverse and are not always consistent with a diagnosis of psychosis. For instance, affective symptoms, anxiety, dissociative states, and affective-somatoform features may characterize forced normalization (51).

In addition to postictal psychosis and forced normalization, some antiepileptic medications may cause psychotic behavior. Psychotic behavior has been associated with the use of ethosuximide (52), phenytoin (53), topiramate (54), and levetiracetam (55). Generally, the psychosis occurs following the initiation of the medication treatment of epilepsy and may be mistaken for the phenomena of forced normalization.

The evaluation of a patient with epilepsy who develops acute psychosis should include a careful history that focuses on the relationship of the psychotic symptoms to seizures. In addition, recent changes in medication should be noted. An EEG should be obtained, preferably a prolonged study to evaluate for possible uncontrolled seizures.

## SYNDROME OF FRONTAL LOBE DISTURBANCE

Lesions that are restricted to the orbitofrontal, frontopolar, or mesial frontal regions can pro-

**TABLE 14.5** DIFFERENTIAL DIAGNOSIS OF PSYCHOSIS AND EPILEPSY

| | History | Examination | EEG | Treatment |
|---|---|---|---|---|
| NCSE | Acute onset, full syndrome may not exist | Confused, preserved insight into hallucinations, isolated delusions | Seizures | AED |
| Postictal psychosis | Recent seizure clusters, tonic clonic seizures | Agitated and paranoid | Bi-temporal sharp waves | Short course of antipsychotics |
| Forced normalization | Recent change in medication, reduction in seizures frequency. | Visual hallucinations, paranoid, mood disturbance | Normal, previously abnormal | Reduce AED dose (?), antipsychotics |
| Medication effects | Levetiracetam, ethosuximide, phenytoin, topiramate | Agitated, rare cases of suicidal ideation | Uncertain | Change medication |
| Primary psychiatric disorder | Onset in early adulthood, family history | Negative symptoms | Normal | Antipsychotics |
| Acute confusional state | Visual hallucinations most common, disruption of sleep-wake cycle | Fluctuations of alertness and attention, autonomic disturbances | Diffuse slowing | Depends on the cause |

***Abbreviations:*** *EEG, electroencephalogram; MRI, magnetic resonance imaging; AED, antiepileptic drug.*

duce unique disturbances of social behavior, planning, and motivation in the absence of a generalized confusional state. Frontal behavioral syndromes arise when incoming information regarding the current social environment is not labeled with the appropriate contextual significance. For instance, in a patient with frontotemporal dementia, the appropriate emotion of embarrassment is not generated as the patient asks inappropriate questions of strangers. A description of the full spectrum of frontal lobe disturbances is beyond the scope of this chapter, and the reader is referred to Mesulam's work on the subject (56).

NCSE may cause frontal lobe syndromes. A study of 10 patients with NCSE of frontal lobe origin revealed disinhibition or abulic symptoms to be the most common syndrome associated with only subtle overt confusion (57). Phenytoin abolished the behavior in 6 out of 10 patients. A structural lesion was thought to be the cause of the NCSE in most patients. Other case reports of NCSE causing repeated prolonged episodes of altered behavior have been published (58). The changes have consisted of poor organizational strategies, impaired set shifting, emotional indifference, reduced motivation, and impairment of emotional decision making. EEG has shown right frontal rhythmic spikes and waves with spread to the homologous left region. Behavioral and EEG abnormalities were successfully reversed with the intravenous administration of diazepam.

The diagnosis of frontal lobe syndrome in a patient may be difficult because of significant variability in frontal lobe function in the normal population. The differential diagnosis includes destructive lesions, neurodegenerative diseases, psychiatric disorders, and NCSE.

## SYNDROME OF VISUAL HALLUCINATIONS

Persistent visual hallucinations and illusions have been reported as the sole manifestation of NCSE (59). The character and complexity of visual hallucinations depend on the region of the cortex from which epileptic discharges arise. Colorful elementary shapes are more likely to be caused by epileptic activation of the primary visual cortex and may be isolated to the contralateral visual field. More complex scenes of objects, places, or people generally occur when seizures arise from association cortex in the temporal and parietal region or the limbic cortex of the temporal or orbitofrontal regions (60). In contrast with activation of the primary visual cortex, these hallucinations generally involve both visual fields. If the visual hallucinations are accompanied by experiential phenomena such as déjà vu or they are an expression of previously encoded memories, then hippocampal or amygdala involvement should be considered.

Persistent visual hallucinations have been described in a diverse range of neurologic conditions that are summarized in Table 14.6. Hypnopompic hallucinations related to cataplexy are generally brief, are associated with transitions from sleep, and should not be mistaken for NCSE. Migraine headaches may be preceded by prolonged visual hallucinations that usually are elementary but have been reported to take on complex forms, such as macropsia and micropsia (Alice in Wonderland syndrome). In addition, complex visual distortions such as mosaic vision, in which images appear fragmented, and cinematographic vision, in which the appearance of motion is lost, may be seen (61). At times, these may occur in the absence of a subsequent headache.

Peduncular hallucinosis is a syndrome described only by case report in which persistent complex visual hallucinations are caused by a destructive lesion to the regions of the mesencephalon and thalamus (62). The hallucinations may be perceived as real to the patient. They are often very complex, involving scenes of animals and people moving in circles. The hallucinations may last several months and are often stereotyped. Because the most frequent etiology is stroke, patients will commonly have cranial nerve abnormalities and cognitive deficits.

Visual hallucinations in the setting of neurodegenerative disease usually are associated with Lewy body disease and Parkinson disease (63). The hallucinations are generally brief, lasting several minutes, but may recur frequently. They may be quite complex and vivid, often with movement of objects or figures. In Parkinson disease, these may be produced or exacerbated by the use of dopaminergic medication.

Charles Bonnet syndrome occurs in elderly individuals who have ocular pathology such as macular degeneration. The hallucinations likely arise from the deafferentation of the visual cortex from upstream retinal and geniculate input. The hallucinations are complex, occur in low-lighting conditions, and generally are not perceived to be threatening.

## CONCLUSION

Observations that epilepsy may be associated with severe interictal behavioral disturbances date back to antiquity. However, it was after the EEG was invented that it became clear that seizures themselves could directly produce abnormal behavioral states in the absence of convulsions. Subsequently, improved techniques such as video-EEG monitoring have clearly established that seizures can cause a persistent and focal cortical disturbance that can lead to focal behavioral syndromes. Such persistent focal syndromes have not been classically associated with epilepsy and may be easily misdiagnosed as unrelated conditions.

To successfully diagnose NCSE, neurologists must maintain a high degree of suspicion in circumstances when seizures are known to occur, as in the intensive care unit. In addition, certain clinical features, such as cyclic alterations in behavior, the presence of stereotyped repetitive behaviors, the presence of occasional obvious seizures, or a past history of seizures, should lead to a heightened suspicion of NCSE.

**TABLE 14.6** DIFFERENTIAL DIAGNOSIS OF PERSISTENT VISUAL HALLUCINATIONS

| | Type | Associated findings | EEG | Treatment |
|---|---|---|---|---|
| NCSE | Simple or complex, may include experiential phenomena | Wax and wane | Seizures of temporal or parietal lobe | AED |
| Migraine | Elementary figures, visual illusions such as micropsia, macropsia, and mosaic vision | Followed by a headache | Intermittent bitemporal delta | Various agents |
| Lewy body disease | Short but may | | | |
| and Parkinson disease | recur frequently, vivid animals and people | Cognitive decline, extrapyramidal features | Normal or diffuse slowing | Atypical antipsychotics, lower dose of dopaminergic medications |
| Peduncular hallucinosis | Very vivid complex scenes of action and movement | Cranial nerve deficits, cognitive disturbances | Uncertain | Possible SSRI? |
| Occipital lesions due to stroke or trauma | Simple or complex, may include images of living things | Visual field defect (lateralized) | Focal slow waves in region of lesion | None |
| Charles Bonnet syndrome | Nonthreatening, dim lighting, vivid | Poor vision | Normal | Improve vision and lighting |

***Abbreviations:*** *EEG, electroencephalogram; AED, antiepileptic drugs; SSRI, selective serotonin reuptake inhibitor.*

Promptly obtaining an EEG, preferably a prolonged study (ie, 24-48 hours), should either permit the accurate diagnosis of NCSE or eliminate that diagnosis from consideration.

## REFERENCES

1. Patterson, L. The Great Imitator. Belleview Literary Rev; 2002;5:18-26.
2. Stechenberg BW. Lyme disease: the latest great imitator. Pediatr Infect Dis J 1988;7:402-409.
3. Kaplan PW. Behavioral manifestations of nonconvulsive status epilepticus. Epilepsy Behav 2002;3:122-139.
4. Mega MS, Cohenour RC. Akinetic mutism: disconnection of frontal-subcortical circuits. Neuropsychiatry Neuropsychol Behav Neurol 1997;10:254-259.
5. Devinsky O, Morrell MJ, Vogt BA. Contributions of anterior cingulate cortex to behaviour. Brain 1995;118:279-306.
6. Virgile RS. Locked-in syndrome. Case and literature review. Clin Neurol Neurosurg 1984;86:275-279.
7. Brenner RP. The interpretation of the EEG in stupor and coma. Neurologist. 2005;11:271-284.
8. Bernat J. Chronic disorders of consciousness. Lancet 2006;367:1181-1192.
9. Kulkarni VP, Lin K, Benbadis SR. EEG findings in Persistent Vegetative State. J Clin Neurophysiol 2007;24:433-437.
10. American Psychiatric Association. Catatonic disorder due to a general medical condition. In: Diagnostic and Statistical Manual of Mental Disorders IV-R. Washington, DC: American Psychiatric Association; 2000:187.
11. Kirubakaran V, Sen S, Wilkinson CB. Catatonic stupor: unusual manifestation of temporal lobe epilepsy. Psychiatr J Univ Ott 1987;12:244-246.

12. Walls MJ, Bowers TC, Dilsaver SC, Swann AC. Catatonia associated with depression secondary to complex partial epilepsy. J Clin Psychiatry 1993;54:73.
13. Drake ME Jr, Coffey CE. Complex partial status epilepticus simulating psychogenic unresponsiveness. Am J Psychiatry 1983;140:800-801.
14. Primavera A. Catatonic seizures. J Neurol Neurosurg Psychiatry 1994;57:1419-1422.
15. Lim J, Yagnik P, Schraeder P, Wheeler S. Ictal catatonia as a manifestation of nonconvulsive status epilepticus. J Neurol Neurosurg Psychiatry 1986; 49(7):833-6.
16. Beng-Choon H, Black D, Andreasen NC. Schizophrenia and other psychotic disorders. In: Hales RE, Yudofsky SG. Textbook of Clinical Psychiatry. Washington, DC: American Psychiatric Publishing; 2003:.
17. Arora M, Praharaj SK. Butterfly glioma of corpus callosum presenting as catatonia. World J Biol Psychiatry 2007;8:54-55.
18. Rommel O, Tegenthoff M, Widdig W, Bräunig P, Malin JP. Organic catatonia following frontal lobe injury: response to clozapine. J Neuropsychiatry Clin Neurosci 1998;10:237-238.
19. Orland RM, Daghestani AN. A case of catatonia induced by bacterial meningoencephalitis. J Clin Psychiatry 1987;48:489-490.
20. Kanemoto K, Miyamoto T, Abe R. Ictal catatonia as a manifestation of de novo absence status epilepticus following benzodiazepine withdrawal. Seizure 1999; 8:364-366.
21. Hawley RJ, Cuenco N, Lastinger L. Pure transient amnesia during nonconvulsive status epilepticus. Neurology 1997;48:1736.
22. Zemani AZ, Boniface SJ, Hodges JR. Transient epileptic amnesia: a description of the clinical and neuropsychological features in 10 cases and a review of the literature. J Neurol Neurosurg Psychiatry 1998;64:435-443 .
23. Zeman AZ, Hodges JR. Transient global amnesia. Br J Hosp Med 1997;58:257-260.
24. Santoro G, Casadei B, Vencoi A. The transient global amnesia-migraine connection. Case report. Funct Neurol 1988;3:353-360.
25. Evans RW, Lewis SL. Transient global amnesia and migraine. Headache 2005;45:1408-1410.
26. Taylor RA, Wu GF, Hursht RW, Kasner SE, Cucchiara BL. Transient global amnesia heralding basilar artery thrombosis. Clin Neurol Neurosurg 2005;108(1):60-2.
27. Brandt J, Van Gorp WG. Functional ("psychogenic") amnesia. Semin Neurol 2006;26:331-340.
28. Chung PW. Seo DW. Kwon JC. Kim H. Na DL. Nonconvulsive status epilepticus presenting as a subacute progressive aphasia. Seizure 2002;11:449-454.
29. Hamilton NG, Matthews T. Aphasia: the sole manifestation of focal status epilepticus. Neurology 1979;29:745-748.
30. Kirshner HS, Hughes T, Fakhoury T. Aphasia secondary to partial status epilepticus of the basal temporal language area. Neurology 1995;45:1616-1618.
31. Knight RT, Cooper J. Status epilepticus manifesting as reversible Wernicke's aphasia. Epilepsia 1986;27:301-304.
32. Wells CR. Aphasia as the sole manifestation of NCSE. Epilepsia 1992; 33: 84-7
33. Cutrer FM, Huerter K. Migraine aura. Neurologist 2007;13:118-125.
34. Gutschalk A, Kollmar R, Mohr A, Henze M, Ille N, Schwaninger M, Hartmann M, Hähnel S, Haberkorn U, Rupp A, Meyding-Lamade U. Multimodal functional imaging of prolonged neurological deficits in a patient suffering from familial hemiplegic migraine. Neurosci Lett 2002;332:115-118.
35. Mandell AM, Alexander MP, Carpenter S. Creutzfeldt-Jakob disease presenting as isolated aphasia. Neurology 1989:39:55-58.
36. Cohen D, Kutluay E, Edwards J, Peltier A, Beydoun A. Sporadic Creutzfeldt-Jakob disease presenting with nonconvulsive status epilepticus, Epilepsy Behav 2004;5:792-796.
37. Mesulam MM. Primary progressive aphasia—differentiation from Alzheimer's disease. Ann Neurol. 1987;22(4):533-4.
38. Plum F, Posner J. The pathological physiology of signs and symptoms of coma. In: Plum F, Posner J, eds. The Diagnosis of Stupor and Coma. Philadelphia, PA: F.A. Davis Company; 1972: 5.
39. Towne AR, Waterhouse EJ, Boggs JG, Garnett LK, Brown AJ, Smith JR Jr, DeLorenzo RJ. Prevalence of nonconvulsive status epilepticus in comatose patients. Neurology 2000;54:340-345.
40. Jordan KG. Nonconvulsive status epilepticus in acute brain injury. J Clin Neurophysiol 1999;16:332-340.
41. DeLorenzo RJ, Waterhouse EJ, Towne AR, Boggs JG, Ko D, DeLorenzo GA, Brown A, Garnett L. Persistent nonconvulsive status epilepticus after the control of convulsive status epilepticus. Epilepsia. 1998;39:833-8340.
42. Brenner RP. Is it status? Epilepsia 2002;43(Suppl 3):103-113.

43. Sadock B, Sadock V. Synopsis of Psychiatry, 10th ed. Philadelphia, PA: Lippincott and Williams; 2007.
44. Sumer MM, Atik L, Unal A, Emre U, Atasoy HT. Frontal lobe epilepsy presented as ictal aggression. Neurol Sci 2007;28:48-51.
45. Florindo I, Bisulli F, Pittau F, Naldi I, Striano P, Striano S, Michelucci R, Testoni S, Baruzzi A, Tinuper P. Lateralizing value of the auditory aura in partial seizures. Epilepsia 2006;47(Suppl 5):68-72.
46. Edelstyn NM, Oyebode F. A review of the phenomenology and cognitive neuropsychological origins of the Capgras syndrome. Int J Geriatr Psychiatry 1999;14:48-59.
47. Mendhekar DN, Gupta N. Recurrent postictal depression with Cotard delusion. Indian J Pediatr 2005;72:529-531.
48. Kanner AM. Psychosis of epilepsy: a neurologist's perspective. Epilepsy Behav 2000;1(4):219-227.
49. Adachi N, Ito M, Kanemoto K et al. Duration of postictal psychotic episodes. Epilepsia 2007;48(8):1531-7.
50. Devinsky O, Abramson H, Alper K, FitzGerald LS, Perrine K, Calderon J, Luciano D. Postictal psychosis: a case control series of 20 patients and 150 controls. Epilepsy Res 1995; 20(3):247-53.
51. Krishnamoorthy, M.R. Trimble. Forced normalization: clinical and therapeutic relevance. Epilepsia 1999;40(10)S57–S64.
52. Yamamoto T, Pipo JR, Akaboshi S, Narai S. Forced normalization induced by ethosuximide therapy in a patient with intractable myoclonic epilepsy. Brain Dev 2001;23:62-64.
53. Gatzonis SD, Angelopoulos E, Sarigiannis P, Mantouvalos V, Ploumbidis D, Siafakas A. Acute psychosis due to treatment with phenytoin in a nonepileptic patient. Epilepsy Behav 2003;4:771-772.
54. Kober D, Gabbard GO. Topiramate-induced psychosis. Am J Psychiatry 2005;162:1542.
55. Kossoff EH, Bergey GK, Freeman JM, Vining EP. Levetiracetam psychosis in children with epilepsy. Epilepsia 2001;42:1611-1613.
56. Mesulam, M. The human frontal lobes: transcending the default mode through contingent encoding. In: Stuss DT, Knight RT, eds. Principles of Frontal Lobe Function. New York, NY: Oxford University Press; 2002:8-30.
57. Thomas P, Zifkin B, Migneco O, Lebrun C, Darcourt J, Andermann F. Nonconvulsive status epilepticus of frontal origin. Neurology 1999;12;52:1174-1183.
58. Bauer G, Dobesberger J, Bauer R, Embacher N, Benke T, Unterberger I, Walser G, Luef G, Trinka E. Prefrontal disturbances as the sole manifestation of simple partial nonconvulsive status epilepticus. Epilepsy Behav 2006;8:331-335.
59. Sowa MV, Pituck S. Prolonged spontaneous complex visual hallucinations and illusions as ictal phenomena. Epilepsia 1989;30:524-6.
60. Bien CG, Benninger FO, Urbach H, Schramm J, Kurthen M, Elger CE. Localizing value of epileptic visual auras. Brain 2000;123:244-253.
61. Sacks O. Migraine aura and classical migraine. In: Sacks O. Migraine. New York, NY: Vintage; 1992:73-81.
62. Benke T. Peduncular hallucinosis: a syndrome of impaired reality monitoring. J Neurol 2006;253:1561-1571.
63. Mosimann UP, Rowan EN, Partington CE et al. Characteristics of visual hallucinations in Parkinson disease dementia and dementia with lewy bodies. Am J Geriatr Psychiatry 2006;14:153-160.

CHAPTER 15

# PSYCHIATRIC MANIFESTATIONS OF NONCONVULSIVE STATUS EPILEPTICUS

ADA V. CHICHARRO, ANDRES M. KANNER

*A 46-year-old man was admitted to the hospital with a 20- year history of complex partial seizures and occasional secondarily generalized tonic-clonic seizures that had failed to remit with multiple trials of antiepileptic drugs (AEDs). He reported periods of marked anxiety of several hours that occurred "out of the blue" without any apparent stressor or trigger. His family commented that during these episodes of anxiety he would become confused and at times fail to respond for several minutes. During one episode, he was brought to the emergency room and admitted to the video-electroencephalographic (EEG) monitoring unit. In the course of a monitoring study, he appeared restless and kept calling the nurse because of feelings of "fear that something bad was going to happen." He had repetitive purposeless movements of the fingers of his right hand, as if he were rolling a pill. These symptoms persisted for 2 hours. Although he appeared to respond to the nurse in a coherent manner, his mother commented that he appeared slower than his normal self and at times would stop talking in midsentence. His mother indicated that he had been displaying these phenomena for the last 5 hours. Concurrent EEG recordings showed an ictal pattern involving bifrontal derivations but that was maximal in the mesial-frontal regions (see Figure 15.1).*

This patient illustrates a case of nonconvulsive status epilepticus (NCSE) in which the most prominent symptoms are psychiatric. It also exemplifies the subtlety of the semiology that often results in the underrecognition or misdiagnosis of NCSE until the patient develops a generalized tonic-clonic seizure. Although the objective confirmation of a diagnosis of NCSE was only possible after the introduction of the EEG in the 1930s, its existence was already suspected in the 19th century, as evidenced by published case reports by Prichard, Wilks, Trousseau, Falret, and Charcot (1). All of these reports included patients with prolonged periods of wandering in a confusional state, often referred to as "somnambulism," as if the patient were in the midst of a dream. For example, Falret described a patient "in an absent-minded state, thought dulled, subject to fits and despair and unprovoked anger with impulses following one after the other at brief intervals; he was forgetful, had complete lapses of memory, headaches and giddiness and noted luminous sparks, frightening

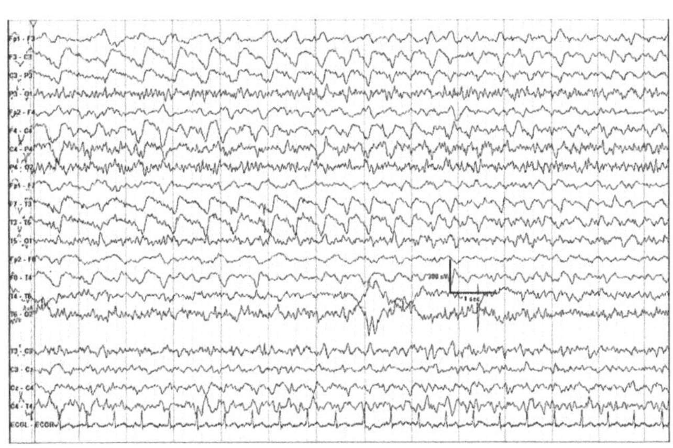

**Figure 15.1** Ictal pattern involving bifrontal derivations.

objects and visions" (2). Falret referred to this as *petit mal intellectuel*. Jackson described a "dreamy state" in seizures thought to be originating in mesial temporal structures, consisting of vivid memory-like hallucinations, the sense of having previously lived throughout the same situation (déjà vu), or both (3).

Behavior and mental-status changes associated with electrographic ictal discharges are the hallmark of NCSE. Typically, NCSE has been divided into 2 main classes: generalized NCSE presenting as absence status (ASE) and lateralization-related NCSE. The latter can be subdivided into simple partial (SPSE) and complex partial status epilepticus (CPSE). Psychiatric phenomena are usually the expression of SPSE and CPSE, although they may also be part of the clinical manifestations of ASE.

The purpose of this chapter is to review (1) the available literature on ictal psychiatric phenomena that have been identified in NCSE; (2) the nature of postictal psychiatric episodes; and (3) paraictal psychiatric phenomena associated with some of the epileptic encephalopathies that present with electrographic status epilepticus, such as acquired epileptic aphasia (Landau-Kleffner syndrome [LKS]) and the syndrome of continuous spike-waves of slow sleep (CSWS).

## PSYCHIATRIC SYMPTOMS IN NONCONVULSIVE STATUS EPILEPTICUS

The psychiatric manifestations of NCSE include the full spectrum of psychiatric semiology. There may be depression, anxiety, panic attacks, delusions, hallucinations (visual and auditory), irritability, impulsive behavior, and thought disorder. The severity can range from overt disruptive symptoms to subtle manifestations that may be recognized only by relatives or friends. The frequent absence of overt confusion, or associated motor ictal phenomena, and the fluctuation of symptoms are factors that contribute to obscuring the diagnosis of NCSE.

## PSYCHIATRIC ICTAL SYMPTOMS AS EXPRESSIONS OF SPSE AND CPSE

These psychiatric manifestations typically occur in NCSE of temporal (psychosensory symptoms, complex visual hallucinations, and illusions), frontal (behavioral manifestations), or occipital (simple visual hallucinations) lobe origin. SPSE is clinically characterized by the presence of somatosensory, visual, auditory, vegetative, psychic, cognitive, affective, or behavior symptoms without impairment of consciousness. *Aura continua* is a term describing prolonged episodes of sensory symptoms identical to a seizure aura, lasting more than 30 minutes and typically ranging from hours to days (5,6). Although this term is not found in some recent glossaries of epilepsy terminology, Seshia and McLachlan have suggested that aura continua represents a subtype of SPSE (5).

SPSE can be difficult to confirm because electrographic recordings with scalp electrodes often fail to detect epileptiform activity. Scalp reflection of seizure activity may occur when the seizure focus activates an area of cortex equivalent to at least 10 cm2. There are well-documented cases manifesting such ictal EEG correlates, eg, patients who have experienced prolonged episodes of intense fear (5-8). Zappoli and colleagues reported a case of woman who had SPSE and CPSE of temporal lobe origin (8). They recognized 2 clinical and electrographic phases. The first phase was characterized by a prolonged feeling of intense fear associated with semirhythmic left temporal epileptiform discharges but without apparent impairment of consciousness. The electroclinical features of the first phase suggested an epileptogenic focus in the left amygdalo-hippocampal complex. In the second phase, the left temporal discharges were followed by generalized discharges resulting in a severe impairment of consciousness. Wieser and colleagues reported on 4 patients with NCSE of temporal lobe origin in which the clinical symptoms accompanying neocortical and mesiobasal limbic discharges consisted of various psychosensory and vegetative signs (7). One patient had associated continuous gustatory auras for several days. Electrographic recordings obtained with depth electrodes in the left hippocampus showed continuous discharges in that region. The events resolved after amygdalohippocampectomy.

Seshia and McLachlan reported on 6 patients who had prolonged symptoms identical to, but less intense than, the aura experienced before their typical complex partial seizures (5). The symptoms occurred intermittently over 2 to 8 years. They were not associated with electrographic seizure activity on scalp and subdural recordings. Indirect clinical evidence supporting the existence of an ongoing focal status epilepticus was the elimination of the aura continua after surgery in 5 patients and transient abolition of symptoms after intravenously administered lorazepam in 1. Scalp recordings of some of the epileptogenic areas better known for the ability to generate ictal psychiatric symptoms (eg, amygdala, insula, or mesial frontal and orbito-frontal regions) may show a lack of interictal epileptiform discharges or evident ictal patterns. In such cases, the epileptic nature of these symptoms may be demonstrated by functional neuroimaging with ictal single-photon emission computed tomography studies.

Hallucinations and illusions can also be an expression of SPSE. Ictal hallucinations may include visual and, less frequently, auditory hallucinations. Although studies of visual hallucinations as an ictal manifestation have shown that they are usually brief and stereotyped, there have been reports of cases with hallucinations of long duration. One patient without a previous history of seizures experienced complex visual hallucinations and illusions lasting weeks after a secondarily generalized tonic-clonic seizure (9). EEGs showed rhythmic right temporal activity that occurred only during the visual hallucinations and illusions, which remitted after treatment with AEDs. The patient described some of them as "puffs of smoke," a "wall filled with water and fish," and "the American flag on a pole, growing larger." Concurrent electrographic recordings showed an ictal pattern in the lateral right temporal derivations. In contrast with patients with primary psychotic disorders, patients with ictal hallucinations are able to recognize the unreal nature of these phenomena.

Patients also have elementary visual hallucinations. A 26-year-old man with SPSE presented with seeing "snowing on TV," "flickering lights," and "rotating colored balls" that continued for several days, appearing in his right upper visual field (10). Magnetoencephalography showed continuous periodic epileptiform discharges over the left posterior superior temporal region, and simultaneous EEG showed rhythmic theta waves and sporadic spikes over the left temporal region. Symptoms disappeared after treatment with AEDs. Transient cortical blindness is also a manifestation of SPSE of occipital origin (11,12).

In contrast with NCSE of temporal lobe origin, status epilepticus of frontal lobe origin frequently occurs without overt confusion (13,14). This entity has been recognized since the early 1970s and different terms have been used, such as *absence status with focal characteristics, prolonged cyclic epileptic seizures, acute prolonged confusion as a frontal-onset ictal state, nonconvulsive confusional frontal status, CPSE of frontal lobe origin*, and *frontal status*. The term *NCSE of frontal lobe origin* is used here because it is a topographic description that does not necessarily denote clinical specificity or the degree of impairment of consciousness. In a series of 60 patients with NCSE, 57.5% suffering from status epilepticus of frontal origin did not have overt confusion (13). Mood changes of euphoria and difficulty in sequential planning were observed most frequently in these patients. Of note, confabulation, an "ironic" appearance, and inappropriate laughter were features seen in NCSE of frontal lobe origin only. Many patients appeared "indifferent."

Thomas and colleagues identified 2 different types of NCSE of frontal origin in a study of 10 patients (14). Type I occurred in 7 patients who had no clear impairment of consciousness; their clinical presentation was characterized by continuous mood and behavior disturbances, either with a mild hypomanic state with affective disinhibition, enhanced word fluency, and familiarity or with a state of affective indifference with blank facial expression, reduced word fluency, and lack of spontaneous activity and emotivity. After the remission of NCSE, most patients could recall events that had occurred during the episode. Simple gestural automatisms such as picking at clothing, rubbing, or scratching movements were common, but oroalimentary or complex bipedal or bimanual automatisms were never seen. All patients showed a strictly unilateral spread of ictal activity that involved either the right or the left frontal areas. Type II occurred in 3 patients and was characterized by a confusional state with temporospatial disorientation, gross behavioral disturbances, and perseveration. Ictal patterns consisted of recurrent epileptiform activity involving frontotemporal regions bilaterally in 2 patients and bilateral frontocentral derivations in 1.

In a study conducted at our center that included 18 consecutive patients, 15 with CPSE and 3 with SPSE, 10 patients with frontal lobe seizure activity displayed psychiatric symptoms. One patient appeared totally uninvolved with her son on the day of his birthday, while still interacting with him. Nine patients appeared withdrawn and confused, with a fluctuating course.

CPSE of frontal lobe origin may also present with severe psychiatric symptoms, as illustrated by 3 patients with ictal catatonia (15). The electrographic recordings of 1 patient demonstrated continuous bilateral pseudoperiodic sharp waves and spike discharges, whereas those of the second patient consisted of spike-and-wave complexes and were seen prominently in the right frontocentral region. The recordings of the third patient showed periodic lateralized epileptiform discharges. The catatonic state remitted following an intravenous infusion of phenytoin.

Amnesia as the only ictal clinical manifestation of NCSE has been reported in patients with either ASE or focal NCSE (16,17). In a recent study, 6 patients who had NCSE in the course of video-EEG monitoring studies as part of their presurgical evaluations underwent neuropsychologic testing during interictal and ictal states, and all had psychiatric features (18). Four patients displayed marked neuropsychologic impairment, and 2 had more limited disturbances. Four patients had epilepsy of frontal lobe origin, and 2 had temporal lobe epilepsy. Patient 1 exhibited a discrete reduction of his

**TABLE 15.1** CLINICAL PRESENTATION OF PATIENTS IN SIMPLE PARTIAL NCSE AND COMPLEX PARTIAL NCSE OF FRONTAL LOBE ORIGIN

| Study | Rohr-Le Floch J 1988 (13) | Thomas 1997 (14) | Thomas 1999 (31) |
|---|---|---|---|
| Patients, no. | 18 | 1 | 10 |
| Overt confusion | 57.5 | No | 30 |
| Fluctuation of symptoms | 31.5 | Yes | 70 |
| Affective disinhibition | 42 | Yes | 50 |
| Affective indifference | 21 | No | NR |
| Decrease in word fluency or spontaneous activity | 36.8 | Yes | 40 |
| Subtle cognitive disturbances | | Yes | 40 |

*Data are provided as percentage of subjects with the specific clinical presentation, unless otherwise indicated. Subtle cognitive disturbances include attention dysfunction, perseveration, and impairment in planning complex tasks. The "study" row includes author and year of publication (reference number). NCSE refers to nonconvulsive status epilepticus; NR, not reported.*

visual spatial skills. From a psychiatric standpoint, he displayed periodic intense affective symptoms characterized by depressive thoughts, tearfulness, rumination, and panic attacks, causing him to become withdrawn. Symptoms improved following intravenous administration of lorazepam. He was not amnestic for the neuropsychologic testing performed during the ictal period. The second patient exhibited more severe cognitive disturbances, consisting of global aphasia and marked reduction in vigilance and reactivity. During the evaluation, she continuously stared at the examiner, exhibited manual automatisms, and could perform only simple motor tasks, including the copying of simple hand movements. There was a temporary improvement in her aphasia such that she could copy single words and follow simple commands and verbal instructions, at which point she exhibited perseveration and echolalia of the instructions she had received during the neuropsychologic testing. She gradually became more reactive after intravenous treatment with 5 mg of diazepam. The third patient presented with a nonfluent aphasia but was able to retain verbal memory function. He retained a normal level of vigilance and was fully reactive despite exhibiting a defensive withdrawal tendency as he lay in bed in a fetal position and avoided any contact. His spontaneous speech improved significantly following treatment with 5 mg of diazepam administered intravenously. The fourth patient presented with cognitive impairment that fluctuated in severity throughout the neuropsychologic testing. For example, she had periods during which she could name objects and could read and carry out written body commands but with impaired comprehension of spoken language. These periods alternated with worsening of her aphasia, which was associated with apraxia, reduced reactivity, and hand automatisms. Upon improvement of her cognitive function, she reacted to the examiner by laughing inappropriately, was able to solve simple mathematical tasks, and demonstrated an improvement in her apraxia, with better performance on tests of visuoconstructive abilities. The improvement of cognitive function was associated with remission of automatisms. Following intravenous therapy with 5 mg of diazepam, her cognitive function normalized. She was able to remember the neuropsychologic testing performed during the ictal period. The fifth patient exhibited disturbances in verbal memory tasks and reported having symptoms of depression with suicidal ideation and feelings of being unable to cope with his life and appropriately carry out the responsibilities of his job. His cognitive deficits remitted following intravenous administration of 5 mg of diazepam. Finally, the sixth patient displayed global impairment of higher cognitive function, while remaining responsive to the examiner. He was able to follow commands (both written and verbal) and could copy written words. From a psychiatric standpoint, he displayed a depressed mood. All deficits remitted with treatment, and he was able to recall the neuropsychologic testing performed during the ictal period.

There are several case studies of iatrogenic CPSE in patients treated with high doses of tiagabine (19,20). These episodes are often misdiagnosed as psychiatric episodes, particularly in patients with psychiatric disorders. Lowering or discontinuing tiagabine leads to complete remission. One review of medical and EEG records of all inpatients with refractory localization-related epilepsy treated with tiagabine found that 7 patients (7.8%) had episodes of NCSE (20). Serial EEGs showed deterioration with dose increments and normalization in all patients after the drug was stopped.

## PSYCHIATRIC ICTAL SYMPTOMS AS EXPRESSIONS OF ABSENCE STATUS EPILEPTICUS

In 1945, Lennox coined the term *petit mal status* after an initial description in 1938 of a cousin whose EEG showed continuous spike-wave discharges following insulin-induced hypoglycemia (21). The patient was described as obtunded and partially responsive. Subsequently, various investigators have divided ASE into typical and atypical forms (22), the former being the expression of status epilepticus in patients with primary generalized epilepsy and the latter occurring in patients with Lennox-Gastaut syndrome. Advances in clinical neurophysiology in the last 2 decades, and the advent of magnetoencephalography, have shown that patients previously diagnosed with ASE may actually have CPSE of mesial frontal origin.

Typical ASE starts abruptly, without an aura, and is often associated with segmental myoclonic jerks (perioral, eyelids, and extremities) that vary in severity. In reviewing a series of 27 patients, Lennox emphasized the mild clouding of consciousness, but poor communication is a frequent manifestation (23). Usually, patients with ASE are alert, attentive, and cooperative. Expressive and receptive language function is relatively well preserved, but expressive language is often slow, with stereotypic and usually monosyllabic answers. Typical ASE may end with a generalized tonic-clonic seizure (22).

In a series of 84 patients with ASE, Roger et al separated the patients' clouding of consciousness into 4 categories (24): (1) slight clouding, described as "slowing of ideation and expression and psychological effects noted particularly on activities requiring sustained attention, sequential organization and spatial structuring"; (2) marked clouding, consisting of "confusion and marked disorientation and, at its most severe, immobility and mutism, simple voluntary actions performed only after repeated requests, long delays in verbal responses, [and] monosyllabic and hesitant speech"; (3) somnolence, consisting of an obtunded state with rare motor responses; and (4) lethargy, in which the patient is "motionless, reacting only to strong painful stimuli, unable to eat and incontinent."

Other authors have supported these observations with respect to the occurrence of mild clouding of consciousness. Agathonikou and colleagues detailed the following self-reports of patients with ASE: "My mind slows down ... I am able to understand but it takes me longer to formulate answers," or "I become slow but I can communicate verbally with others," or "I feel that I am like in a trance ... missing pieces of conversation" (25). Also, "I have the sensation of viewing the world through a different medium"; "a feeling of not being in the same world as everyone else;" "uncontrollable rush of thoughts"; "a feeling of fear of losing control of my mind"; "a feeling of closeness"; "a funny feeling that I can not elaborate"; "a strange feeling of not being myself"; "edgy, worried, and uncomfortable"; "my character changes completely, I become extremely snappy ... have a severe headache"; or "weird" (25,26). These authors have observed that patients often cannot recognize people other than close relatives in the midst of ASE and appear disoriented and quiet (25). Isolated behavior problems are often noticed by relatives or friends. Examples include a patient who made coffee twice or who put on trousers over his pajamas (25). The relatives of 1 patient described an unusual behavior lasting several days: "After a shower, he was unable to dress himself and roamed about his house until his wife could assist him. He went to bed with coat and boots on. After driving to work, he could not open his locker and when assisted he stated, 'I can't get my truck started.' He put two cups in an empty dishwasher and ran it without detergent. He lit a cigarette as if to smoke but stared at it for several minutes" (27). Neurologic evaluation showed orientation to person, place, year, and hospital but difficulty concentrating and limited short-term recall. He was unable to draw a clock face after several attempts. An EEG demonstrated generalized spikes and polyspikes and waves. His mental status improved within minutes of treatment with intravenously administered lorazepam. When asked again to draw a clock face, he was able to do so.

Psychiatric phenomena in typical ASE occur significantly less frequently than in CPSE. Occasionally, however, some patients become depressed, agitated, and hostile during ASE. When psychotic and behavioral disturbances are identified, they are more likely to correspond with atypical ASE. Dongier reported episodes of catatonia, paranoid delusions, and hallucinations in patients with "seemingly" typical ASE (28). Aggressive behavior and impulsivity have been reported (29). The higher frequency of psychiatric phenomena in CPSE was also demonstrated by Rohr Le-Floch and colleagues in their semiologic comparison of 32 patients with ASE and 28 with CPSE (13).

Among patients with ASE, indifference (22%), agitation, (12.5%) and an anxious and frightened attitude (11%) were the most frequently identified psychiatric symptoms.

Atypical ASE occurs in patients with Lennox-Gastaut syndrome. Its clinical manifestations may be indistinguishable from those of typical ASE, but atypical ASE is often of longer duration, does not stop with the occurrence of a generalized tonic-clonic seizure, and frequently fails to respond to intravenous administration of benzodiazepines (22).

As with CPSE, ASE can present as a catatonic state. One 78-year-old man presented with 1-week episodes of mutism, alternating with psychomotor agitation (30). On examination, he was awake but had a fixed stare. Occasionally, upon repeated questioning, he would answer with appropriate but fragmented words, in a whisper. His extremities were maintained in the same position for long periods when placed by the examiner in a bizarre posture. There were no focal neurologic signs, and he had no previous history of epilepsy or psychiatric illness. The EEG showed continuous, generalized spike-and-wave discharges (1.5-2 Hz), suggestive of atypical

ASE. A detailed interview with his wife revealed that the patient had abruptly discontinued the use of benzodiazepines. Administration of diazepam resulted in remission of the abnormal behavior and of the catatonic posture. Without EEG recordings, the ictal origin of the catatonia would have remained unrecognized.

ASE can occur in patients without prior epilepsy and may be the sole epileptic manifestation (31). Thomas and colleagues reported on 11 patients (10 women; mean age 58.6 years) with ASE. Eight were receiving high doses of psychotropic drugs, and the onset of ASE followed benzodiazepine withdrawal in 8. Other potential triggers included excessive use of other psychotropic drugs, including neuroleptic drugs, tricyclic antidepressants, and lithium, as well hypocalcemia, hyponatremia, and chronic alcoholism. Clinical and EEG presentation was similar to that of ASE in patients with prior epilepsy. No patient had a second episode of ASE, even without the subsequent use of AEDs. By reviewing the literature, the authors identified 64 patients with de novo ASE presenting in the seventh decade in whom withdrawal of benzodiazepines was also a frequent trigger. Given their comorbid psychiatric history, these patients illustrate the potential for misdiagnosis of ASE as psychiatric conditions.

ASE can also be triggered iatrogenically, as illustrated by a review of 2 patients with primary generalized epilepsy treated with carbamazepine who were misdiagnosed as having a primary psychiatric disorder (32). The first was a 14-year-old girl who had a generalized tonic-clonic seizure at age 12 years, preceded by monthly episodes of confusion, with awkward behavior since age 9 years. She had been treated with carbamazepine, and the episodes of confusion became more frequent, leading to a diagnosis of a dissociative disorder. An EEG during 1 of these episodes established the diagnosis of ASE. Substitution of valproic acid for the carbamazepine resulted in remission of the ASE. The second patient was a 23-year-old woman who presented at age 16 years with a generalized tonic-clonic seizure. Since early adolescence, she had had episodes of depressive mood, worsened school performance, and facial tics. Carbamazepine treatment caused worsening of the depressive episodes and facial tics. An EEG during a typical episode showed ASE. Once again, substitution of valproate for the carbamazepine led to seizure freedom and behavior improvement.

## ARE THE PSYCHIATRIC MANIFESTATIONS ICTAL OR POSTICTAL?

Postictal psychiatric symptoms and episodes occur characteristically within the first 12 to 96 hours following a seizure or, more frequently, after clusters of seizures, particularly secondarily generalized tonic-clonic seizures (33). They are relatively frequent in patients with pharmacoresistant partial seizure disorders. In a study of 100 consecutive patients with pharmacoresistant partial epilepsy who underwent video-EEG monitoring in our epilepsy center, 43 had postictal symptoms of depression after most of their seizures in the prior 3 months; 13 had a cluster of symptoms that mimicked a major depression (except for the shorter duration) (34). Five additional patients exhibited irritability and poor tolerance of frustration, without other dysphoric symptoms. Forty-five patients experienced postictal symptoms of anxiety; 9 had symptoms of obsessions and compulsions; 7 had psychotic symptoms; and 2 experienced hypomanic symptoms. The duration of postictal psychiatric symptoms ranged from 30 minutes to 148 hours, with a median duration of 24 hours. Of note, 14 patients had only postictal cognitive symptoms, and 8 had no postictal symptoms. Most patients with postictal psychiatric symptoms also had postictal cognitive symptoms, but the latter were of shorter duration.

Postictal psychiatric symptoms may cluster and mimic discrete psychiatric disorders. The prevalence of postictal psychiatric episodes in the general population of patients with epilepsy has yet to be established. Reported postictal psychiatric episodes have focused almost exclusively on postictal psychosis (PIP) identified in the course of video-EEG monitoring studies. In 1 study, the yearly incidence of postictal psychiatric episodes during video-EEG was 7.9% among patients with partial epilepsy (35). The majority (6.4% of the total) had PIP, which presented as a delusional psychosis in 4 patients and mimicked a mixed manic-depressive psychosis in 1, a psychotic depression disorder in 2, a hypomanic psychosis in 1, and a manic psychosis in another 1. The tenth patient presented with bizarre behavior and a thought disorder. In every case, the onset of symptoms lagged by a mean of 24 hours (range, 12 to 72 hours) after the last seizure. The mean duration of the PIP was 70 hours (range, 24 to 144 hours). The psychotic episode remitted with low doses of neuroleptic medication (2-5 mg/day of haloperidol) in 5 patients, 1 patient required high doses (40 mg/day of haloperidol), and remission occurred without pharmacotherapy in 4 patients. Six of 10 patients had PIP episodes (an average of 2.4) prior to video-EEG. In the remaining 4 patients, the PIP was the first episode ever. Other authors have reported similar findings with respect to clinical characteristics, course, and response to pharmacotherapy (35-40). These case series reported the following characteristics of PIP: (1) delay between the time of the last seizure and the onset of psychiatric symptoms, (2) relatively short duration, (3) affect-laden symptoms, (4) clustering of symptoms into delusional and affectivelike psychosis, (5) increase in the frequency of secondarily generalized tonic-clonic seizures preceding the onset of PIP, and (6) onset of PIP after having seizures for a mean of more than 10 years.

## PSYCHIATRIC AND COGNITIVE DISTURBANCES AS EXPRESSIONS OF PARAICTAL PHENOMENA IN ELECTROGRAPHIC NONCONVULSIVE STATUS EPILEPTICUS

In certain epileptic disorders, psychiatric and cognitive disturbances are the most prominent clinical expression and cause of disability. Such is the case in 2 types of epileptic encephalopathies: the acquired epileptic aphasia of childhood, also known as LKS, and the syndrome of electrical status epilepticus during sleep, also known as CSWS. These 2 syndromes have in common the presence of electrographic status epilepticus during sleep that may or may not persist during the awake state.

## LANDAU-KLEFFNER SYNDROME

LKS is an acquired epileptic aphasia or verbal auditory agnosia occurring in children who have already developed age-appropriate language function. It is thought to result from an epileptogenic lesion arising in the speech cortex during a critical period of development. It was first described in 1957 by Landau and Kleffner in a report of 6 patients (41). LKS has a clearly defined set of clinical and electrographic characteristics. These characteristics include a receptive speech disturbance or verbal auditory agnosia (42), followed soon thereafter by disturbances of expressive speech, which can evolve to a state of complete mutism. The onset of speech disturbance coincides with that of seizure activity. The symptoms of LKS appear between the ages of 2 and 8 years. The initial language disturbances include problems with verbal comprehension (verbal auditory agnosia) that often can be mistaken for acquired deafness (43). Soon after, speech output is affected, and paraphasias and phonologic errors appear. Symptoms may progress in a steady or fluctuating manner to a state of complete mutism, during which the child fails to respond to even familiar nonverbal sounds, such as the doorbell or the telephone ringing or the dog barking. Another important diagnostic criterion for LKS is the relative isolation of the behavior deficit in the linguistic and auditory perceptual spheres, ie, children show relatively normal performance on nonverbal cognitive tasks (44).

The speech disturbances are associated with behavior changes, which may include motor hyperactivity in up to 50% of children, and sleep disturbances. At the height of the auditory agnosia, some autistic-like features, such as self-stimulatory behavior, may be identified. The child with LKS, however, never loses the ability to relate to family members and to understand social cues. The onset of the language disorder is concurrent with that of seizures or electrographic evidence of epileptiform activity presenting characteristically, but not exclusively, as spike-wave discharges with a bilateral distribution, maximal in the posterior temporal regions of each hemisphere. This EEG pattern typically occupies more than 80% of slow-wave sleep, and the condition is known as CSWS. Twenty percent to 30% of children will never exhibit any evidence of clinical seizures (45). Seizures are often nocturnal. Their clinical phenomena vary widely and are often very subtle. Seizures, unlike the language disorder, respond readily to treatment with AEDs and generally subside by the age of 15 years (45). Although some children with LKS have spontaneous remission of cognitive deficits, others may require treatment with steroids or surgery to improve. Unfortunately, in children whose cognitive disturbances fail to remit spontaneously or with AEDs, abolition of epileptiform activity with steroid therapy or epilepsy surgery does not always result in remission of the disorder. In most children, the epileptic activity remits in adolescence. When language impairment persists unabated for more than a year, spontaneous language recovery is unlikely by adulthood.

Morrell suggested the following hypothesis to explain the development of LKS (46):

> *It is well known that different neural systems have critical periods in development during which the adult patterns of synaptic engagement are gradually established. At such times, there is first a superabundant outgrowth of axon terminals resulting in a temporary hyperinnervation of the synaptic target; this extravagant outgrowth appears to be entirely under genetic control. Over the remainder of the critical period, the synaptic contacts are extensively pruned. The pruning is selective; it is dependent on and controlled by synaptic use, ie, environmental input. Synaptic contacts activated by use become cemented, so to speak, whereas those not environmentally engaged wither away. Neural networks for linguistic function develop late, and their circuitry remains malleable during the first 8 to 10 years of life. We hypothesize, then, that the impact of epileptic activity originating from this anlage of speech cortex may result in chaotic and behaviorally meaningless activation of synaptic contacts that would have been "pruned" under normal circumstances. Such epileptic activity may set up permanent, inappropriate, and nonfunctional linkages.*

Data from experimental studies in animals support Morrell's hypothesis, showing that epileptogenic lesions induced during a critical period for circuit development cause the emergence and fixation of long-lasting or permanent aberrant connections (47,48). Morrell's hypothesis and other data provide an explanation for the development of language deficits associated with the temporal gap between the onset of epileptiform activity (or seizures or both) and the failure to regain language function after remission of electrographic epileptiform activity (48,49). (For further information on LKS and pediatric NCSE, see Chapters 17, 19, and 21.)

## ELECTROGRAPHIC STATUS EPILEPTICUS IN SLOW-WAVE SLEEP

LKS is not the only epileptic encephalopathy with a CSWS electrographic pattern. The electrical status epilepticus during sleep syndrome was initially described by Patry and colleagues in 1971 as "subclinical electrical status epilepticus during sleep" (49) and then retitled by Tassinari as electrical status epilepticus during sleep in a report of 6 children, aged 7 to 12 years, 5 of whom were mentally retarded, and all of whom exhibited language disturbances, epileptic seizures, and very abnormal EEG recordings consistent with a CSWS pattern (50). The epileptic seizures were of various types, including tonic, atonic, clonic, generalized tonic-clonic, and atypical absences. The severity of mental retardation was related to the age of onset. Tassinari later changed the name of this syndrome to CSWS syndrome.

The following differences between LKS and the CSWS syndrome can be identified based on data from publications by Beaumanoir (51) and Bureau (52) that include analyses of clinical and electrographic findings in 71 children with LKS and 103 children with CSWS syndrome. LKS tends to affect a slightly younger population, presenting first with language dysfunction and behavior deterioration. In CSWS, affected children tend to be slightly older, presenting with more global neuropsychologic and behavior deterioration, in addition to the language dysfunction. The severity of the seizures and EEG abnormalities are more pronounced in CSWS, and seizures are often more frequent, including atonic seizures with falls, absence and atypical absences, generalized tonic-clonic, and hemiclonic seizures. The spike-and-wave discharges are maximal in the centro-temporal or posterior-temporal regions in LKS and in the frontal head regions in CSWS. Seizures in CSWS are often difficult to control, primarily among the subgroup of patients with atypical absence seizures and drop attacks, which are resistant to treatment with AEDs. Patients with CSWS syndrome also have more frequent abnormalities on magnetic resonance imaging scans (33%) than do children with LKS (13%). Interestingly, seizure remission is comparable between the 2 groups after the CSWS pattern resolves.

## DIAGNOSIS OF NONCONVULSIVE STATUS EPILEPTICUS

NCSE is often confused with nonepileptic conditions, such as postictal states, metabolic encephalopathies, obtundation due to alcohol or drug intoxication, psychosis or delirium, or simply as emotional lability (1). Table 5.2 summarizes various conditions that are frequently considered in the differential diagnosis. Based on the data reviewed in this chapter, the diagnosis of NCSE requires, first and foremost, a high degree of clinical suspicion, even in patients without prior epilepsy. The use of EEG is essential, and an EEG should be strongly considered in a patient presenting with any of the following: (1) a prolonged (> 1 hour) postictal period after a generalized tonic-clonic seizure; (2) altered mental status with a fluctuating course, particularly if associated with blinking or myoclonic facial or appendicular jerks; (3) altered mental status of unexplained etiology; or (4) altered mental status (with or without epilepsy) after recent discontinuation of benzodiazepines.

**TABLE 15.2** DIFFERENTIAL DIAGNOSIS

1. Postictal state
2. Intoxications
3. Psychogenic or psychotic states
4. Factitious disorders
5. Mental retardation
6. Toxic or metabolic encephalopathy
7. Transient global amnesia
8. Psychotropic drug withdrawal

For practical reasons, an immediate EEG is not always available. Husain and colleagues evaluated whether clinical features can help predict which patients have a high probability of being in NCSE (53). They showed that eye-movement abnormalities (nystagmoid movements, hippus, repeated blinking, and persistent eye deviation) and remote risk factors for seizures (including previous stroke, neurosurgical intervention, brain tumor, and history of meningitis) have a very high combined sensitivity for NCSE. No clinical feature had a high sensitivity and specificity individually, but the combined sensitivity for "remote risk factors for seizures" and "eye-movement abnormalities" was 100%.

As above, SPSE may be difficult to confirm because scalp EEG can be unrevealing, especially in cases in which the ictal focus is in the amygdala. In such cases, EEG recordings with sphenoidal electrodes placed under fluoroscopic guidance can demonstrate the epileptiform activity (54), but cheek and anterior temporal skin electrodes may be sufficient. Supra-orbital electrodes and double-density electrodes, positioned in and around the midline, may also be useful in the case of suspected epileptogenic areas in mesial and orbito-frontal regions (55).

Imaging techniques can also be useful in diagnosing NCSE. Transient focal abnormalities associated with edema in the epileptogenic area may be identified on magnetic resonance imaging scans as hyperintensities on T2-weighted images. An increased signal on diffusion-weighted imaging may also reflect focal increased perfusion. These abnormalities usually resolve after cessation of status epilepticus. Ictal single-photon emission computed tomography studies can also be helpful in demonstrating an area of hyperperfusion in SPSE, particularly in demonstrating the presence of NCSE of frontal lobe origin.

Particularly challenging is the diagnosis of NCSE in patients with cognitive impairment at baseline (eg, mental retardation or dementia) or in patients with prior psychiatric disorders (see also Chapter 19). A detailed clinical history is extremely valuable in these cases. The "baseline status" of the patient should be delineated and should include examples of the patient's daily activities. Changes from baseline status, duration of the events, presence or absence of "asymptomatic" intervals, timing in relation to the sleep-wake cycle, and presence or absence of subtle motor phenomena and automatisms are important components of this diagnostic evaluation.

## CONCLUSIONS

Psychiatric phenomena are relatively frequent in NCSE, particularly in complex partial status of frontal and temporal lobe origin, and may be seen as the main or only expression of ASE. Thus, misdiagnosis with a psychiatric condition is relatively frequent. A high level of suspicion is necessary to reach the correct diagnosis. Postictal psychiatric episodes must be distinguished from NCSE, but one may follow the other, and EEG is often necessary to distinguish between them. Finally, psychiatric phenomena can be an expression of a paraictal process in syndromes with electrographic status epilepticus.

## REFERENCES

1. Kaplan PW. Behavioral manifestations of nonconvulsive status epilepticus. Epilepsy Behav 2002;3:122-139.
2. Falret J. De l'état mental des épileptiques. Arch Gen Med Fifth Ser 1860;16:661-679; 1861;17:461-469.
3. Jackson JH. Case of epilepsy with tasting movements and "dreamy state"—Very small patch of softening in the left uncinate gyrus. In: Selected Writings by John Hughlings Jackson. Vol 1. Nijmergen: The Netherlands, N.J.M. Arts; 1996:458-463.
4. Walker M, Cross H, Smith S, Young C, Aicardi J, Appleton R, Aylett S, Besag F, Cock H, DeLorenzo R, Drislane F, Duncan J, Ferrie C, Fujikawa D, Gray W, Kaplan P, Koutroumanidis M, O'Regan M, Plouin P, Sander J, Scott R, Shorvon S, Treiman D, Wasterlain C, Wieshmann U. Nonconvulsive status epilepticus: Epilepsy Research Foundation workshop reports. Epileptic Disord 2005;7:253-296.

5. Seshia SS, McLachlan RS. Aura continua. Epilepsia 2005;46:454-455.
6. McLachlan RS, Blume WT. Isolated fear in complex partial status epilepticus. Ann Neurol 1980;8:639-641.
7. Wieser HG, Hailemariam S, Regard M, Landis T. Unilateral limbic epileptic status activity: stereo EEG, behavioral, and cognitive data. Epilepsia 1985;26:19-29.
8. Zappoli R. Two cases of prolonged epileptic twilight state with almost continuous "wave-spikes." Electroencephalogr Clin Neurophysiol 1955:7:421-423.
9. Sowa MV, Pituck S. Prolonged spontaneous complex visual hallucinations and illusions as ictal phenomena. Epilepsia 1989:30:524–526.
10. Oishi M, Otsubo H, Kameyama S, Wachi M, Tanaka K, Masuda H, Tanaka R. Ictal magnetoencephalographic discharges from elementary visual hallucinations of status epilepticus. J Neurol Neurosurg Psychiatry 2003;74:525-527.
11. Sawchuk KS, Churchill S, Feldman E, Drury I. Status epilepticus amauroticus. Neurology 1997;49:1467-1469.
12. Barry E, Sussman NM, Bosley TM, Harner RN. Ictal blindness and status epilepticus amauroticus. Epilepsia 1985;26:577-584.
13. Rohr-Le Floch J, Gauthier G, Beaumanoir A. Confusional states of epileptic origin. Value of emergency EEG. Rev Neurol 1988;144:425-436.
14. Thomas P, Zifkin B, Migneco O, Lebrun C, Darcourt J, Andermann F. Nonconvulsive status epilepticus of frontal origin. Neurology 1999;52:1174-1183.
15. Lim J, Yagnik P, Schraeder P, Wheeler S. Ictal catatonia as a manifestation of nonconvulsive status epilepticus. J Neurol Neurosurg Psychiatry 1986;49:833-836.
16. Vuilleumier P, Despland PA, Regli F. Failure to recall (but not to remember): pure transient amnesia during nonconvulsive status epilepticus. Neurology 1996;46:1036-1039.
17. Lee BI, Lee BC, Hwang YM, Sohn YH, Jung JW, Park SC, Han MH. Prolonged ictal amnesia with transient focal abnormalities on magnetic resonance imaging. Epilepsia 1992;33:1042-1046.
18. Profitlich T, Hoppe C, Reuber M, Helmstaedter C, Bauer J. Ictal neuropsychological findings in focal nonconvulsive status epilepticus. Epilepsy Behav 2008;12:269-275.
19. Koepp MJ, Edwards M, Collins J, Farrel F, Smith S. Status epilepticus and tiagabine therapy revisited. Epilepsia 2005;46:1625-1632.
20. Schapel G, Chadwick D. Tiagabine and nonconvulsive status epilepticus. Seizure 1996;5:153-156.
21. Lennox WG. The treatment of epilepsy. Med Clin North Am 1945;29:1114–1128.
22. Shorvon S. Clinical forms of status epilepticus: complex partial status epilepticus. In: Status Epilepticus: its Clinical Features and Treatment in Children and Adults. Cambridge, UK: Cambridge University Press; 1994:116-129.
23. Lennox WG. Epilepsy and Related Disorders. Boston, MA: Little Brown; 1960.
24. Roger J, Lob H, Tassinari CA. Status epilepticus. In: Vinken PJ, Bruyn GW, eds. Handbook of Neurology, Vol. 15: The Epilepsies. Amsterdam: North-Holland; 1974;145-188.
25. Agathonikou A, Panayiotopoulos CP, Giannakodimos S, Koutroumanidis M. Typical absence status in adults: diagnostic and syndromic considerations. Epilepsia 1988;39:1265-1276.
26. Panayiotopoulos CP. Syndromes of idiopathic generalized epilepsies not recognized by the International League Against Epilepsy. Epilepsia. 2005;46(Suppl 9):57-66.
27. Olnes MJ, Golding A, Kaplan PW. Nonconvulsive status epilepticus resulting from benzodiazepine withdrawal. Ann Int Med 2003:139:956-958.
28. Dongier S. Statistical study of clinical and electroencephalographic manifestations of 536 psychotic episodes occurring in 516 epileptics between clinical seizures. Epilepsia 1959/1960;1:117-142.
29. Goldensohn ES, Gold AP. Prolonged behavioral disturbances as ictal phenomena. Neurology 1960;10:1-9.
30. Kanemoto K, Miyamoto T, Abe R. Ictal catatonia as a manifestation of de novo absence status epilepticus following benzodiazepine withdrawal. Seizure 1999;8:364-366.
31. Thomas, P, Beaumanoir A, Genton P, Dolisi C, Chatel M. 'De novo' absence status of late onset. Report of 11 cases. Neurology 1992;42:104-110.
32. Marini C, Parmeggiani L, Masi G, D'Arcangelo G, Guerrini R. Nonconvulsive status epilepticus precipitated by carbamazepine presenting as dissociative and affective disorders in adolescents. J Child Neurol 2005;20:693-696.

33. Kanner AM. Psychosis of epilepsy: a neurologist's perspective. Epilepsy Behav 2000:1:219-227.
34. Kanner AM, Stagno S, Kotagal P, Morris HH. The incidence of postictal psychiatric events in prolonged video-EEG monitoring studies. Arch Neurol 1996,53:258-263.
35. Kanner AM, Soto A, Gross-Kanner H. Prevalence and clinical characteristics of postictal psychiatric symptoms in partial epilepsy. Neurology 2004;62:708-713.
36. Logsdail SJ, Toone BK. Postictal psychosis. A clinical and phenomenological description. Br J Psychiatry 1988;152:246-252.
37. Savard G, Andermann F, Olivier A, Remilliard GM. Postictal psychosis after complex partial seizures: a multiple case study. Epilepsia 1991; 32:225-231.
38. Devinsky O, Abrahmson H, Alper K, FitzGerald LS, Perrine K, Calderon J, Luciano D. Postictal psychosis: a case control study of 20 patients and 150 controls. Epilepsy Res 1995;20:247-253.
39. Umbricht D, Degreef G, Barr WB, Lieberman JA, Pollack S, Schaul N. Postictal and chronic psychosis in patients with temporal lobe epilepsy. Am J Psychiatry 1995;152:224-231.
40. Kanemoto K, Kawasaki J, Kawai J. Postictal psychosis: a comparison with acute interictal and chronic psychoses. Epilespia 1996;37:551-556.
41. Landau WM, Kleffner F. Syndrome of acquired aphasia with convulsive disorder in children. Neurology 1957;7:523-530.
42. Deonna T. Acquired epileptiform aphasia in children (Landau-Kleffner syndrome). J Clin Neurophysiol 1991;8:288-298.
43. Beaumanoir A. The Landau-Kleffner syndrome. In: Roger J, Dravet C, Bureau M, Dreifuss FE, Wolf P, eds. Epileptic Syndromes in Infancy, Childhood and Adolescence. London, England: John Libbey Eurotext; 1985:181-191.
44. Deonna T, Beaumanoir A, Gaillard F, Assal G. Acquired aphasia in childhood with seizure disorder: a heterogenous syndrome. Neuropediatrics 1977;8:263-273.
45. Morrell F, Whisler WW, Smith MC, Hoeppner TJ, de Toledo-Morrell L, Pierre-Louis SJ, Kanner AM, Buelow JM, Ristanovic R, Bergen D. Landau-Kleffner syndrome: treatment with subpial intracortical transection. Brain 1995;118:1529-1546.
46. Morrell, F. Electrophysiology of CSWS in Landau-Kleffner syndrome. In: Beaumanoir A, Bureau M, Deonna T, Mira L, Tassinari CA, eds. Continuous Spikes and Waves During Slow Sleep. Electrical Status Epilepticus During Slow Sleep. Acquired Epileptic Aphasia and Related Conditions. London, England: John Libbey Eurotext;1995:77-90.
47. Baumbach HD, Chow KL. Visuocortical epileptiform discharges in rabbits: differential effects on neuronal development in the lateral geniculate nucleus and superior colliculus. Brain Res 1981;209:61-76.
48. Grigonis AM, Murphy EH. The effects of epileptic cortical activity on the development of callosal projections. Dev Brain Res 1994;77:251-255.
49. Patry G, Lyagoubi S, Tassinari CA. Subclinical "electrical status epilepticus" induced by sleep in children. Arch Neurol 1971;24:242-252.
50. Tassinari CA, Bureau M, Dravet C, Genton P, Wolf P. Epilepsy with continuous spikes and waves during slow sleep. In: Roger J, Bureau M, Dravet C, Dreifuss FE, Wolf P, eds. Epileptic Syndromes in Infancy, Childhood and Adolescence, 2nd ed. London, England: John Libbey; 1992:245-256.
51. Beaumanoir A, Bureau M, Deonna T, Mira L, Tassinari CA, eds. Continuous Spikes and Waves During Slow Sleep: Electrical Status Epilepticus During Slow Sleep. London, England: John Libbey;1995.
52. Bureau M. Outstanding cases of CSWS and LKS analysis of the data sheets provided by the participants. In: Beaumanoir A, Bureau M, Deonna T, Miram L, Tassinari CA, eds. Continuous Spikes and Waves During Slow Sleep: Electrical Status Epilepticus During Slow Sleep. London, England: John Libbey; 1995:213-216.
53. Husain AM, Horn GJ, Jacobson MP. Non-convulsive status epilepticus: usefulness of clinical features in selecting patients for urgent EEG. J Neurol Neurosurg Psychiatry 2003;74:189-191.
54. Kanner AM, Ramirez L, Jones JC. The utility of placing sphenoidal electrodes under the foramen ovale with fluoroscopic guidance. J Clinical Neurophysiol 1995;12:1:72-81.
55. Kanner AM. Psychogenic seizures and the supplementary sensory motor area. In: HO Lüders HO, ed. The Supplementary Sensory Motor Area. Advances in Neurology. Vol. 70. New York, NY: Raven Press; 1996:461-466.

PART V

# NONCONVULSIVE STATUS EPILEPTICUS IN POPULATIONS AT RISK AND BY AGE

CHAPTER 16

# NONCONVULSIVE STATUS EPILEPTICUS IN INFANTS

CHRISTIAN M. KORFF AND DOUGLAS R. NORDLI, JR.

Nonconvulsive status epilepticus (NCSE) has been defined by a group of experts as a "clear and persistent clinical change in behavior (which includes changes in cognition, memory, arousal, or motor behavior), confirmed by comparisons with previous functioning observations or by neuropsychologic examination, or both, in the presence of continuous paroxysmal electrographic activity, and in the absence of clonic, tonic or tonic-clonic seizures" (1). It is commonly divided into subcategories that differ in terms of etiology, prognosis, and management. One might identify various broad situations in which infantile NCSE is found. These include de novo presentations in previously healthy infants, conditions and epilepsies with prominent tendencies for NCSE, and infants with epileptic encephalopathies. Aspects of neonatal status epilepticus, which often manifests as nonconvulsive electrographic seizures, are also discussed.

## THE DIFFICULT RECOGNITION OF NONCONVULSIVE STATUS EPILEPTICUS IN NEONATES AND INFANTS

The diagnosis and management of neonatal seizures have been subject to much controversy among clinicians for two main reasons. First, the particular clinical characteristics of neonatal seizures and the acute circumstances in which they usually occur make their recognition more difficult than in older children (2). Second, the electroclinical correlation of seizures is limited in the neonatal period. Some clinicians require seizures to be clinical events with a clear association with concurrent electrographic discharges, whereas others consider isolated electrographic or clinical manifestations as sufficient. As a result, neonatal seizures and status epilepticus were assumed to be rare until the increased use of the electroencephalograph (EEG) in neonatal units proved this wrong. In a study on electrographically confirmed seizures in term and in preterm babies, pure electrographic seizures were more common than electroclinical seizures (3). In another series of 393 seizures recorded in 41 patients, 79% of the episodes were occult, ie, completely nonconvulsive (4). It is therefore likely that most episodes of neonatal status epilepticus are nonconvulsive as well.

Neonatal status epilepticus has been defined as "continuous electrographic seizure activity for 30 minutes or at least 50% of recording time" (5). This usually takes the form of repeated short seizures rather than a single prolonged seizure. Increasing evidence shows that status epilepticus is frequent in newborns. In one study, this was particularly true for term babies with seizures, of whom 33% had status epilepticus, compared with 9% of premature babies (5). According to Clancy, it is likely that a significant number of neonates with neurologic insults had status epilepticus for the entire acute period of their illnesses, before a progressive decrease in the seizure frequency occurred during clinical improvement (6).

Until recently, NCSE was not commonly reported in infants. Few articles were devoted to the subject before 2006. Still, recent reports of infants and children monitored in intensive care units (ICUs) show that many infants have nonconvulsive seizures and status epilepticus when systematically examined by continuous EEG (7-9).

Why has this phenomenon been underappreciated in very young patients? Recent reports give some clues: at least half of the time, infants with NCSE had previously been healthy and may have had only short isolated seizures in the acute illness immediately prior to NCSE (7,9). In a report of 19 children with NCSE (aged one month to 17 years), 26% of patients were less than one year old, and 42% could rightfully be considered infants (less than two years) (7). Four infants had a suggestion of prior cerebral hypoxia, two had metabolic disorders, one had an infection, and one had traumatic brain injury. All infants were stuporous or comatose, and 6 did not have convulsive status before the development of NCSE. Three had only isolated seizures prior to NCSE, and two had no seizures prior to NCSE. No ictal patterns were generalized. Focal ictal patterns arose from the posterior regions and involved the temporal, parietal, and occipital areas in isolation or in various combinations. Most ictal patterns were composed of repeated sharp waves, but one infant (83 days old) had rhythmic theta-delta activity. Six infants were treated with phenobarbital and combinations of other drugs; two were given phenytoin alone. Duration of the NCSE ranged from 0.5 hours in one infant to 672 hours in the most severely affected child, for an average of 130 hours. Excluding the two outliers, the average NCSE duration was 61 hours. Another report on pediatric patients in the ICU described 23 patients with nonconvulsive seizures, and 48% were younger than 12 months of age. Most infants were previously healthy, and clinical features were similar to those in the previous report (9), but NCSE was not observed in this cohort. A third study of EEG findings in 178 children admitted to the ICU in an unresponsive state found that 36% of the infants (defined as younger than one year of age) had NCSE (10). These reports show an alarmingly high incidence of NCSE in infants presenting to the ICU in a nonresponsive state. They also highlight the value of EEG in the evaluation of the unresponsive infant.

The subtlety of infantile focal seizures contributes to the difficulty of detecting NCSE (11-13). Infants offer few distinctive clues to the presence of focal seizures. Instead, they may simply pause ongoing activities and have a change in respiration. Distal limb automatisms, dystonic postures, and secondary generalization are rare. These features become more noticeable as the infant matures and are more prominent in patients 6 years of age and older (14).

On the other hand, infants may also present with paroxysmal nonepileptic movements that mimic seizures. Consequently, some true epileptic seizures may be missed, even by the most experienced observers. In addition to seizures, the differential diagnosis of paroxysmal episodes in children includes gastroesophageal reflux disease, chronic gastric volvulus, breath-holding spells, so-called "shuddering attacks," and syncope, all of which may be manifested for prolonged periods. Some present as apparent life-threatening events. According to a recent review, seizures are among the common diagnoses made in children presenting with apparent life-threatening events, accounting for 11% of all cases (15). All of these clinical symptoms are common and contribute to a great number of requests for video-EEG recording in the first year of life. Their identification is not always easy to make on the basis of history and clinical examination alone. Some recently reported observations might be helpful in that perspective. Careful examination of neonatal (16) and infantile (17) seizures have shown that the eyes are usually open at some point during seizures. Therefore, if the eyes stay closed throughout the event, seizures are unlikely. Unfortunately, such subtle clinical signs are difficult to observe in infants, particularly for parents in a frightening context.

Another factor that can make detection of NCSE in infants challenging is the complexity of the EEG background and the general lack of familiarity with ictal patterns in the immature infant. Well-organized generalized spike-wave discharges, for example, are a relatively rare ictal feature in infants, although they are seen more often in children aged three years and older (18). Detection of NCSE is particularly challenging in the setting of an encephalopathy with a disorganized chaotic EEG, such as is seen in many pediatric patients with epileptic encephalopathies. A better understanding of the nature of NCSE in infants will likely aid its detection in other babies with this serious neurologic condition.

## CLASSIFICATION OF NONCONVULSIVE STATUS EPILEPTICUS

NCSE is commonly subdivided into absence status epilepticus (ASE), simple partial status epilepticus (SPSE) or complex partial status epilepticus (CPSE), status epilepticus in patients with learning difficulties, and status epilepticus in coma. Additional entities, such as atypical ASE, tonic status epilepticus, or autonomic status epilepticus, have also been considered as categories of NCSE observed in specific epilepsy syndromes or neurologic conditions.

### ABSENCE STATUS EPILEPTICUS

ASE is characterized by a prolonged confusional state associated with generalized EEG discharges. Because patients with ASE have occasional jerks of the face and limbs, confusion with myoclonic status epilepticus is possible. Both entities are most often noted in children with idiopathic generalized epilepsies. The prognosis of ASE is very good, except for its strong tendency to recur. ASE is rare in infants.

### COMPLEX PARTIAL STATUS EPILEPTICUS

As in ASE, the primary clinical manifestation of CPSE is confusion. Symptoms may also include amnesia, aphasia, bizarre behavior, or hemiparesis. Patients with partial epilepsy frequently exhibit their typical seizure patterns, but a history of epilepsy is not always present (19). The prognosis of CPSE is controversial. Case reports and limited series data indicate that permanent cognitive sequelae might be observed after CPSE in adults (20), but this remains to be confirmed by larger trials. CPSE is seen much more often in school-aged children and adolescents than in infants.

### NONCONVULSIVE STATUS EPILEPTICUS IN PATIENTS WITH LEARNING DIFFICULTIES

This category includes several conditions that share varying degrees of developmental delay and epochs of continuous or near-continuous electrographic epileptic activity. It might be divided into atypical ASE, tonic status epilepticus, and electrical status epilepticus during sleep (ESES) (21).

Atypical ASE and tonic status epilepticus occur in 50% to 75% of patients with Lennox-Gastaut syndrome (22), which is also characterized by additional seizure types, developmental delay, and interictal slow spike-and-waves on the EEG. ESES consists of diffuse 1.5- to 3.5-Hz spike-and-wave discharges occurring in 85% to 100% of non-rapid eye movement sleep (21). It is often associated with idiopathic pediatric epilepsy syndromes such as typical or atypical benign epilepsy with centrotemporal spikes, Landau-Kleffner syndrome, or continuous spike-and-waves during sleep. The significance of electrographic abnormalities in the prognosis of these patients is uncertain (1,23). Cognitive changes occur sometimes, but not always, in parallel with EEG findings. The persistence of cognitive deficits in some patients could depend on the age at which ESES is observed (1).

### NONCONVULSIVE STATUS EPILEPTICUS IN COMA

Most neonatal NCSE episodes occur in acutely ill or comatose patients. Common etiologies include asphyxia, infections, vascular injuries, specific epilepsy syndromes, and metabolic disorders. A retrospective study of NCSE in 19 children showed that 18 were in a comatose or stuporous state at the time of diagnosis (7). Five presented with overt convulsions at the onset. The remainder had either isolated or no seizures prior to the onset of NCSE.

Current pediatric data on NCSE are insufficient to establish definite evaluation and treatment recommendations. Because clinical recognition of NCSE in young patients is notoriously difficult, however, the threshold for performing an EEG in neonates and infants who present with unexplained alteration of consciousness should be low. The prognosis of neonatal status epilepticus in coma is highly dependent on its underlying etiology, and the contribution of the electrographic seizure activity itself is unclear (2).

## AUTONOMIC STATUS EPILEPTICUS

Most cases of pediatric autonomic status epilepticus have been observed in the Panayiotopoulos syndrome, an idiopathic localization-related childhood epilepsy. Patients often present with infrequent prolonged seizures. Clinical manifestations include nausea, vomiting, pupillary abnormalities, and cardiorespiratory and thermal alterations (1). Some episodes end in convulsions, but they are considered to be autonomic NCSE because of the large predominance of vegetative features.

## ASSOCIATED CONDITIONS AND EPILEPSY SYNDROMES

### *Ring chromosome 20 syndrome*

Ring chromosome 20 syndrome is a condition that strongly predisposes infants to developing NCSE. It is a rare entity, the most important clinical characteristics of which include intractable seizures and repeated episodes of NCSE. It is hypothesized that gene loss from the terminal segment of the long arm of chromosome 20 is responsible for the epilepsy. This region includes genes that code for the nicotinic cholinergic receptor CHRNA4, which implicated in autosomal-dominant nocturnal frontal lobe epilepsy, and for the potassium-channel KCNQ2, which is associated with the syndrome of benign familial neonatal convulsions (24,25).

### *Myoclonic status epilepticus in nonprogressive encephalopathies*

Dalla Bernardina and colleagues described myoclonic status epilepticus in nonprogressive encephalopathies (MSNE) years ago (26). Recently, the International League Against Epilepsy task force on syndrome classification recommended that it be recognized as a syndrome (27).

One of the best-recognized related conditions is Angelman syndrome, a genetically determined disorder linked to chromosome 15q11-q13 and involving the *UBE3A* gene in most cases. Children have developmental delay, mild facial dysmorphism, ataxia, hypotonia, and a cheerful disposition. The interictal EEG often shows a characteristic pattern sometimes referred to as "notched" delta. This refers to the prominent rhythmic slowing with associated spikes with an inconsistent relationship to the slow waves so that the spike can appear to "ride" on the descending phase of the slow wave. The notched delta may be prominent frontally or occipitally. The pattern can occur without any clear clinical manifestation, but these infants or children often have prolonged periods of altered responsiveness, with admixed myoclonias and eye blinking associated with the rhythmic EEG activity (28).

Patients with Angelman syndrome accounted for 15 of the 29 MSNE cases reported on by Caraballo and colleagues (29). In this series, MSNE was also observed in various additional conditions, such as chromosome 4p deletion (Wolff-Hirschhorn syndrome), Rett syndrome, and perinatal anoxic encephalopathy. In 6 cases, no etiology was found. Myoclonic status appeared at the mean age of 16 months. Three subgroups were identified. The first included patients with these genetic abnormalities. They presented with episodes of brief myoclonic absences and rhythmic myoclonias followed by a clinically quiet period correlated with delta-theta waves and superimposed spikes. In many patients, these episodes could last for years despite numerous treatments. Either cortical malformations or no etiology was found in the second group. They exhibited dystonic postures, dyskinesias, and myoclonias in association with multifocal spike-and-wave discharges predominating in posterior regions. Three of these 5 patients died during status. The third group comprised 6 children who had suffered perinatal asphyxia. They presented with mild cognitive impairment and partial seizures at onset, and, later, a progressive appearance of continuous myoclonias of the face and limbs, which correlated with generalized spike-and-waves or notched delta waves. Most had cognitive deterioration in parallel with status and showed some improvement when the episode was controlled. As a consequence, the authors proposed classifying MSNE as an epileptic encephalopathy (29).

### *Dravet syndrome*

Dravet syndrome (severe myoclonic epilepsy of infancy) is an important, but probably underrecognized, form of epilepsy that invariably begins in infancy (30). Infants often have febrile convulsions, but afebrile focal seizures, atypical absence seizures, and myoclonic seizures may follow. Initial EEGs may be normal, but focal or multifocal interictal epileptiform discharges often develop later in infancy, and there is an evolution to generalized spike-wave discharges in toddlers (31). NCSE occurs in 30% to 40% of cases and usually occurs after the age of 2 years, but earlier presentations have been noted. NCSE can be admixed with erratic myoclonias and may continue for hours or days. Dravet and colleagues referred to this as *obtundation status*. In contrast with the ictal EEG of NCSE in older children or adults, the ictal EEG in Dravet syndrome shows arrhythmic slow waves with admixed spike and sharp waves, often maximal in fronto-central regions.

### *Migrating partial seizures in infancy*

Migrating partial seizures in infancy is another neglected epilepsy syndrome, although it is far less common than Dravet syndrome. It was described by Coppola and colleagues in 1995 (32). Since 2001, it has been considered a syndrome in development, but it has been reported worldwide, and the most recent work of the International League Against Epilepsy taskforce has recommended that it be recognized as a syndrome. Infants have normal development before the onset of seizures, which usually begin in the first 6 months. There are nearly continuous focal seizures that shift from one area of the brain to another so that the seizures have a migrating appearance. Clinical manifestations may be very subtle, with behavioral arrest, version, or other minor manifestations (18). Although migrating partial seizures of infancy are not often formally described as NCSE, patients with this syndrome have prolonged and nearly continuous electroclinical seizures with subtle manifestations and altered responsiveness.

## EPILEPTIC ENCEPHALOPATHIES

In addition to the NCSE described earlier, many infants have pronounced epileptic encephalopathies and share similar characteristics. Examples include early infantile epileptic encephalopathy (EIEE) described by Ohtahara, early myoclonic epilepsy (EME) described by Aicardi and colleagues, and West syndrome. These infants virtually always have some degree of apparent altered awareness and responsiveness. Although these conditions are not always labeled NCSE, the altered state of consciousness and the chaotic, disorganized, and profoundly abnormal nature of the EEGs make a case for considering them to be NCSE. Just as infants with Dravet syndrome do not show rhythmic EEG discharges during episodes of NCSE, so it may be with patients with other forms of infantile epilepsy.

### *Early infantile epileptic encephalopathy*

EIEE is a rare epileptic encephalopathy characterized by early tonic seizures and burst-suppression EEG patterns, which tend to be continuous and independent of the state of arousal. Hemiconvulsions can be observed, but myoclonias are rare. The onset of seizures is most often during the first 10 days of life but can be as late as three months. Etiologies are heterogeneous and include brain malformations, migration disorders, and mitochondrial or metabolic defects. Most cases, however, are associated with structural cerebral malformations. The prognosis of EIEE is ominous—many infants die during the first year, and the remaining children have severe developmental delay and intractable seizures (33). West syndrome and Lennox-Gastaut syndrome are often diagnosed as they evolve. Some authors question whether EIEE and EME are truly separate entities or represent a continuum (34). Indeed, both syndromes share common clinical and EEG findings. These authors hypothesize that the variability of predominant seizure types in both syndromes may reflect the severity of brainstem involvement at the time of presentation. This could explain why tonic seizures, reputedly provoked by brainstem dysfunction, are usually absent at the onset of EME but, over time, may be observed in many patients (34).

### EARLY MYOCLONIC EPILEPSY

EME is characterized by similar EEG features, but the burst-suppression pattern seems to predominate during sleep. Seizures also appear in the neonatal period but mainly consist of myoclonias. Partial seizures are almost invariably noted later in development. Metabolic diseases, such as nonketotic hyperglyicyne, have been diagnosed in some patients, and familial cases have been reported. Usually, however, no specific etiology is identified. The prognosis is grim, as in EIEE (33).

### WEST SYNDROME

West syndrome is characterized by the triad of infantile spasms, developmental delay or regression, and hypsarrhythmia on EEG. Spasms typically present around the age of 6 months. The jerks can occur in flexion or in extension and can be unilateral or bilateral, and they are usually followed by a brief tonic posture of the trunk and arms. Their electrographic correlate is a high-amplitude slow wave followed by a period of generalized attenuation (electrodecrement) with superimposed low-voltage fast activity. They appear in clusters that can be prolonged, during which alertness, although difficult to assess formally, is probably impaired (35).

## TREATMENT

Treatment of NCSE is controversial. First, the harmful potential of NCSE has not been demonstrated clearly in humans. Second, it is unclear whether treating the episodes of NCSE improves the long-term prognosis of the patients. Third, antiepileptic drugs all have potential side effects that must be taken into consideration. Current recommendations include the use of oral benzodiazepines in most situations, including for infants. An exception to this rule is NCSE in comatose patients, for whom the prognosis is often grim. In those acute situations, frequently symptomatic of a severe underlying injury, the potential risks of continuous seizure activity probably outweigh those of medications, and aggressive treatment, such as that used for convulsive status epilepticus, is recommended. In neonates, treatment with phenobarbital, phenytoin, or benzodiazepines is common practice.

## CONCLUSIONS

The use of continuous EEG recording in ICUs has contributed to a dramatic increase in the diagnosis of NCSE. Nevertheless, different expressions of NCSE produce different EEG and clinical manifestations, making their recognition challenging in infancy. NCSE is still likely underrecognized, and a high index of suspicion remains necessary to avoid a delayed or missed diagnosis. NCSE has been reported to occur in association with certain conditions, such as immediately following convulsive seizures. Of particular concern, however, it may also present in previously healthy infants with acute encephalopathies. NCSE is also common in certain epilepsy syndromes that begin in infancy, but it often does not develop until later in those syndromes.

Despite increasing recognition of NCSE, several questions remain. It is, for example, uncertain if particular EEG features represent ictal or interictal activity. Should EME, EIEE, and West syndrome be considered as NCSE? EEG abnormalities in these syndromes have been considered interictal thus far, but children with these disorders often present with concomitant cognitive impairment, possibly related to the electrographic abnormalities. What about neonates who present with prolonged electrographic abnormalities of uncertain origin, without concomitant apparent seizures? Treatment also raises questions. There is currently no consensus, but available data favor a parsimonious use of oral benzodiazepines in most situations. Aggressive treatment is probably warranted only in those situations in which the prognosis is considered poor, such as NCSE in comatose patients.

## REFERENCES

1. Walker M, Cross H, Smith S, Young C, Aicardi J, Appleton R, Aylett S, Besag F, Cock H, DeLorenzo R, Drislane F, Duncan J, Ferrie C, Fujikawa D, Gray W, Kaplan P, Koutroumanidis M, O'Regan M, Plouin P, Sander J, Scott R, Shorvon S, Treiman D, Wasterlain C, Wieshmann U. Nonconvulsive status epilepticus: Epilepsy Research Foundation workshop reports. Epileptic Disord 2005;7:253-296.
2. Wical BS. Neonatal seizures and electrographic analysis: evaluation and outcomes. Pediatr Neurol 1994;10:271-275.
3. Scher MS, Aso K, Beggarly ME, Hamid MY, Steppe DA, Painter MJ. Electrographic seizures in preterm and full-term neonates: clinical correlates, associated brain lesions, and risk for neurologic sequelae. Pediatrics 1993;91:128-134.
4. Clancy RR, Legido A, Lewis D. Occult neonatal seizures. Epilepsia 1988;29:256-261.
5. Scher MS, Hamid MY, Steppe DA, Beggarly ME, Painter MJ. Ictal and interictal electrographic seizure durations in preterm and term neonates. Epilepsia 1993;34:284-288.
6. Clancy RR. The contribution of EEG to the understanding of neonatal seizures. Epilepsia 1996;37(Suppl 1):S52-S59.
7. Tay SK, Hirsch LJ, Leary L, Jette N, Wittman J, Akman CI. Nonconvulsive status epilepticus in children: clinical and EEG characteristics. Epilepsia 2006;47:1504-1509.
8. Jette N, Claassen J, Emerson RG, Hirsch LJ. Frequency and predictors of nonconvulsive seizures during continuous electroencephalographic monitoring in critically ill children. Arch Neurol 2006;63:1750-1755.
9. Saengpattrachai M, Sharma R, Hunjan A, Shroff M, Ochi A, Otsubo H, Cortez MA, Snead OC 3rd. Nonconvulsive seizures in the pediatric intensive care unit: etiology, EEG, and brain imaging findings. Epilepsia 2006;47:1510-1518.
10. Hosain SA, Solomon GE, Kobylarz EJ. Electroencephalographic patterns in unresponsive pediatric patients. Pediatr Neurol 2005;32:162-165.
11. Acharya JN, Wyllie E, Lüders HO, Kotagal P, Lancman M, Coelho M. Seizure symptomatology in infants with localization-related epilepsy. Neurology 1997;48:189-196.
12. Nordli DR Jr, Bazil CW, Scheuer ML, Pedley TA. Recognition and classification of seizures in infants. Epilepsia 1997;38:553-560.
13. Duchowny MS. Complex partial seizures of infancy. Arch Neurol 1987;44:911-914.
14. Nordli DR Jr, Kuroda MM, Hirsch LJ. The ontogeny of partial seizures in infants and young children. Epilepsia 2001;42:986-990.
15. McGovern MC, Smith MB. Causes of apparent life threatening events in infants: a systematic review. Arch Dis Child 2004;89:1043-1048.
16. Bauder F, Wohlrab G, Schmitt B. Neonatal seizures: eyes open or closed? Epilepsia 2007;48:394-396.
17. Korff CM, Nordli DR Jr. Paroxysmal events in infants: persistent eye closure makes seizures unlikely. Pediatrics 2005;116:e485-e486.
18. Korff CM, Nordli DR Jr. The clinical-electrographic expression of infantile seizures. Epilepsy Res 2006;70(Suppl 1):S116-131.
19. Cascino GD. Nonconvulsive status epilepticus in adults and children. Epilepsia 1993;34(Suppl 1):S21-28.
20. Krumholz A, Sung GY, Fisher RS, Barry E, Bergey GK, Grattan LM. Complex partial status epilepticus accompanied by serious morbidity and mortality. Neurology 1995;45:1499-1504.
21. Walker MC. Diagnosis and treatment of nonconvulsive status epilepticus. CNS Drugs 2001;15:931-939.
22. Arzimanoglou A, Guerrini R, Aicardi J. Lennox-Gastaut syndrome. In: Arzimanoglou A, Guerrini R, Aicardi J, eds. Aicardi's Epilepsy in Children. 3rd ed. Philadelphia, PA: Lippincott Williams & Wilkins; 2004:38-50.
23. Scholtes FB, Hendriks MP, Renier WO. Cognitive deterioration and electrical status epilepti-

cus during slow sleep. Epilepsy Behav 2005;6:167-173.
24. Inoue Y, Fujiwara T, Matsuda K, Kubota H, Tanaka M, Yagi K, Yamamori K, Takahashi Y. Ring chromosome 20 and nonconvulsive status epilepticus. A new epileptic syndrome. Brain 1997;120:939-953.
25. Augustijn PB, Parra J, Wouters CH, Joosten P, Lindhout D, van Emde Boas W. Ring chromosome 20 epilepsy syndrome in children: electroclinical features. Neurology 2001;57:1108-1111.
26. Dalla Bernardina B, Fontana E, Darra F. Myoclonic status in nonprogressive encephalopathies. Adv Neurol 2005;95:59-70.
27. Engel J Jr. Report of the ILAE classification core group. Epilepsia 2006;47:1558-1568.
28. Williams CA. Neurological aspects of the Angelman syndrome. Brain Dev 2005;27:88-94.
29. Caraballo RH, Cersosimo RO, Espeche A, Arroyo HA, Fejerman N. Myoclonic status in nonprogressive encephalopathies: study of 29 cases. Epilepsia 2007;48:107-113.
30. Dravet C, Bureau M, Oguni H, Fukuyama Y, Cokar O. Severe myoclonic epilepsy in infancy: Dravet syndrome. Adv Neurol 2005;95:71-102.
31. Korff CM, Laux L, Kelley Kr, Goldstein J, Koh S, Nordli DR Jr. Dravet syndrome (severe myoclonic epilepsy in infancy): a retrospective study of 16 patients. J Child Neurol 2007;22:185-194.
32. Coppola G, Plouin P, Chiron C, Robain O, Dulac O. Migrating partial seizures in infancy: a malignant disorder with developmental arrest. Epilepsia 1995;36:1017-1024.
33. Aicardi J, Ohtahara S. Severe neonatal epilepsies with suppression-burst traces. In: Roger J, Bureau M, Dravet C, Genton P, Tassinari CA, Wolf P, eds: Epileptic Syndromes in Infancy, Childhood and Adolescence, 4th ed. London, England: John Libbey Eurotext; 2005;39-50.
34. Djukic A, Lado FA, Shinnar S, Moshé SL. Are early myoclonic encephalopathy (EME) and the Ohtahara syndrome (EIEE) independent of each other? Epilepsy Res 2006;70(Suppl 1):S68-S76.
35. Dulac O, Tuxhorn I. Infantile spasms and West syndrome. In: Roger J, Bureau M, Dravet C, Genton P, Tassinari CA, Wolf P, eds. Epileptic Syndromes in Infancy, Childhood and Adolescence, 4th ed. London, England: John Libbey Eurotext; 2005;53-72.

# CHAPTER 17

# NONCONVULSIVE STATUS EPILEPTICUS IN CHILDREN

*James J. Riviello, Jr.*

Status epilepticus is defined as an epileptic seizure or a series of seizures without a return to consciousness between seizures, lasting greater than 30 minutes (1). Status epilepticus occurs with any seizure type. Semiologically, status epilepticus may be either convulsive (CSE), with obvious convulsive activity, or nonconvulsive (NCSE), without obvious convulsive activity. A recent operational definition proposed that any convulsive seizure with a duration longer than 5 minutes should be considered to be status epilepticus and treated (2). Because patients with NCSE have altered awareness without obvious convulsive activity, electroencephalography (EEG) is crucial to confirm the diagnosis. This chapter shall primarily discuss NCSE in children and includes the special syndromes of childhood status epilepticus with sleep-activated epileptiform activity: Landau-Kleffner syndrome (LKS) and continuous spike waves of slow sleep (CSWS) (3). The entity of nonconvulsive seizures (NCSzs) is included in a discussion of NCSE because these disorders are a continuum. NCSE, NCSzs, and electrical status epilepticus of sleep (ESES) all require EEG for identification. NCSzs are referred to as subclinical seizures, silent seizures, or electrographic seizures. A more detailed discussion of neonatal and infantile NCSE is in other chapters.

These terms need definition. NCSE is electrographic status epilepticus, either generalized or focal, with associated altered awareness. Drislane lists three criteria: (1) clinical neurologic deficits, especially altered awareness; (2) an epileptiform EEG with either typical discrete seizures or continuous discharges; and (3) a clinical and EEG response to anticonvulsant drugs (4). Clinical or EEG improvement following treatment, usually with a benzodiazepine, is considered part of the diagnostic criteria by some experts. Granner and Lee reported that, in NCSE, the epileptic discharge frequency is usually less than 3 Hz, and the morphology varies (5). NCSzs are defined as electrographic patterns, lasting longer than 10 seconds, of (1) repetitive focal or generalized spikes, sharp waves, or spike-and-wave complexes with a frequency greater than 3 Hz; (2) repetitive generalized or focal spikes, spike-and-wave or sharp-and-slow complexes with a frequency less than 3 Hz; or (3) a secondary criterion, a significant improvement in clinical state or EEG after treatment (6-8). The strict definition of ESES requires epileptiform activity in more than 85% of non-rapid eye movement sleep (9,10). Few data exist from children with NCSE and NCSzs, whereas ESES is rare in adults.

Treiman and colleagues identified NCSE as the end-stage of CSE, when continuous epileptiform discharges evolve into periodic epileptiform discharges (11). Mikati and colleagues demonstrated this same sequence in the developing brain (12). NCSE may also occur after the successful termination of CSE. De Lorenzo and colleagues, in the Richmond Study, reported NCSE in 14% of patients following the treatment of CSE (13). In a study of NCSE in children, 5 of 19 patients (26%) had NCSE detected after treatment of CSE (14).

The definition of neonatal status epilepticus has evolved from an overt clinical seizure to clinical seizures combined with the abundance of epileptiform activity. Monod, Udaeta Mora, Olmos-Garcia, and colleagues included repetitive clinical or subclinical seizures associated with an abnormal interictal neurologic state (15-17). The following EEG characteristics were added: generalized high-voltage paroxysmal discharges with two or more discharges occurring every 10 seconds for at least 20 minutes (17). Scher and colleagues defined neonatal status epilepticus as continuous seizure activity for at least 30 minutes or recurrent seizures for at least 50% of a 1- to 3-hour recording (18). Wertheim and colleagues referred to continuous seizure activity in one or more EEG channels for at least 4 hours or separated for only short periods by activity with frequent sharp waves or spikes (19). Ortibus and colleagues referred to neonatal status epilepticus as a seizure duration longer than 30 minutes or seizures and periodic discharges exceeding 50% of the EEG recording (20). These variations in definitions make it difficult to compare studies (20). Neonatal NCSzs and NCSE have no convulsive movements and are referred to as electroencephalographic seizures or silent seizures (21).

Coma may be the only manifestation of NCSE. In a study of 236 comatose patients without overt seizure activity, 19 (8%) had NCSE on EEG (22). The EEG criteria consisted of discrete electrographic seizures, continuous spike-and-wave activity, or rhythmic recurrent epileptiform activity, with marked improvement after intravenous administration of a benzodiazepine. Three of these were children, with ages from 5 weeks to 18 years. The 5-week-old had a slow EEG background, with bilaterally independent periodic discharges and spike-and-wave discharges with brief intervals; the 12-year-old also had brief intervals of 1- to 2-Hz, generalized, sharp and rhythmic slow waves; and the 18-year-old had 2-Hz, continuous, generalized spike-and-wave discharges. In another study, NCSE occurred in 22 of 210 patients (10.5%) admitted to an intensive care unit with altered mental status (23). Two were children, aged 6 and 17 years, both with known epilepsy and altered awareness, but one had twitching of the hands and face.

Claassen and colleagues found seizures in 19% of adults and children undergoing continuous EEG recordings (CEEG); seizures were exclusively nonconvulsive in 92% (24). Electrographic seizures were more likely to occur in the setting of coma, in patients younger than 18 years of age or with history of epilepsy, and when convulsive seizures had occurred before CEEG monitoring. Of special importance regarding the length of monitoring needed to detect seizures, seizures occurred within 24 hours in 88% of patients and by 48 hours in 93%. In the presence of coma, seizures were first recorded after 24 hours in 20%, versus in only 5% of noncomatose patients. In an analysis of only children, Jette and colleagues reported similar findings (25). In 117 patients monitored by CEEG, seizures were recorded in 51 (44%). Seizures were completely nonconvulsive in 75%, both convulsive and nonconvulsive in 16%, and convulsive alone in 10%. Status epilepticus was recorded in 27 children, 24 of whom had only NCSE; of all monitored patients, 70% had in-hospital seizures prior to CEEG monitoring, 91% had convulsive seizures, and 22% had generalized CSE. Compared with data in adults, in children, earlier epilepsy, in-hospital seizures before CEEG, or stupor and coma only trended toward significance as risk factors for the development of seizures, whereas hypoxic injury showed a trend toward a lower incidence of NCSzs. EEG factors that independently predicted seizures included periodic lateralized epileptiform discharges and lack of normal background reactivity. Regarding the monitoring duration needed, seizures were seen immediately in 15%, within one hour in 50%, within 24 hours in 80%, and within 48 hours in 87%.

Tay and colleagues used a strict definition for NCSE in children (14), requiring both clinical findings and a response to treatment (6,7). Periodic discharges without evolution were not included unless there was a clinical correlate or improvement with treatment. Nineteen children were identified over a 3.5-year period. The mean age was 67 months, and 26% were younger than one year of age. Etiologies included hypoxic-ischemic encephalopathy in 5, exacerbation of a metabolic disorder in 4, change in anticonvulsant medications or infection in three each, and intracranial hemorrhage or refractory epilepsy in two each. Five of 19 patients had NCSE after treatment of CSE, two after initial treatment, and three following refractory status epilepticus.

Hyllienmark and colleagues reported NCSE in 4 of 24 children who had status epilepticus evaluated with CEEG (26). These four presented with altered awareness and without overt seizures and had generalized epileptiform activity on EEG. Abend and Dlugos reported on 20 children with NCSE, which often occurred in those children with prior epilepsy or congenital heart disease. Neurologic presentation included isolated seizures in 55%, CSE in 20%, and change in mental status in 25% (27).

There is a continuum from NCSzs to NCSE. Saengpattrachai and colleagues defined NCSzs as deterioration of consciousness accompanied by at least one episode of an electrographic seizure lasting longer than 10 seconds (28). They distinguished NCSzs from NCSE, diagnosing NCSE only when the EEG showed continuous or nearly continuous electrographic seizure activity. To detect NCSzs, they included children with unexplained altered awareness without overt clinical seizures, in whom an EEG was done within 24 hours of admission to the pediatric intensive care unit. Among 141 patients, 23 (16%) had NCSzs. The mean age was 40 months; 43% had no earlier neurologic illness.

In a recent study of 100 patients (mostly adults) with NCSE, the mortality was 18% and morbidity 39% (29). As with CSE, the prognosis was related to the underlying etiology, with a mortality rate of 27% in those with an acute medical insult versus only 3% in those with underlying epilepsy. Niedermeyer and Ribeiro caution that the EEG findings in what has recently been called NCSE in patients with an acute encephalopathy may actually be the expression of a very severe encephalopathy, rather than the NCSE that occurs with absence status epilepticus (ASE) or complex partial status epilepticus (CPSE) (30).

## ABSENCE STATUS EPILEPTICUS, COMPLEX PARTIAL STATUS EPILEPTICUS, AND AUTONOMIC STATUS EPILEPTICUS

NCSE also occurs in the idiopathic generalized epilepsies, such as absence epilepsy (with ASE), and juvenile myoclonic epilepsy (31). ASE is rare and occurs in children with known absence epilepsy, in whom typical absence seizures, with 3-Hz, spike-and-wave activity evolves into ASE, with near-continuous discharges. New-onset ASE, however, has been reported in an 8-year-old without prior absence seizures (32). The term spike-wave stupor has been used for ASE (33). Adults may develop "isolated" ASE, whereas, in children, ASE usually occurs in those with known epilepsy (34).

In the symptomatic generalized epilepsies and epileptic encephalopathies, such as Lennox-Gastaut syndrome, atypical absence seizures, with a slow spike-and-wave discharge, are more common and can be very prolonged. NCSE has been reported to occur in patients with ring chromosome 20 (35) and with Angelman syndrome (36).

CPSE is relatively rarely reported in children. The EEG shows focal rather than generalized electrographic status epilepticus. The reported symptoms and signs include altered awareness, a lack of recognition of familiar people, staring, decreased visual tracking, eye deviation, automatisms, crying, lip smacking, amaurosis, and hypotonia (37,38). The incidence of CPSE will increase with adoption of the 5-minute operational definition for status epilepticus.

It is increasingly recognized that antiepileptic drugs (AEDs) may exacerbate seizures. This has been well described with carbamazepine used in primary generalized epilepsy (39). Tiagabine has caused NCSE (40), and ASE and myoclonic status epilepticus have occurred following treatment with phenytoin, carbamazepine, vigabatrin, and gabapentin (41). This typically occurs in the setting of treating a primarily generalized epilepsy with an AED more suited for focal epilepsy. Status epilepticus manifesting as epileptic negative myoclonus has also been described (42).

The entity of Panayiotopoulos syndrome has been reclassified from an occipital epilepsy to an autonomic epilepsy (43). It occurs in about 6% of childhood epilepsies. Alternate diagnoses made in these children include encephalitis, syncope, migraine, sleep disorder, and gastroenteritis (44). The seizures have more of an autonomic component, with altered awareness rather than overt convulsions, with status epilepticus occurring in a large percentage of cases (45). A recently developed consensus statement has defined autonomic status epilepticus as epileptic activity manifesting as autonomic dysfunction at seizure onset, lasting longer than 30 minutes. It emphasizes that autonomic seizures also occur in childhood symptomatic epilepsies (rarely in adults) and are not limited to the Panayiotopoulos syndrome (46). One previously reported case of CPSE (a 7-year-old boy with two prolonged episodes of altered awareness, facial pallor, headache, and vomiting) most likely had autonomic status epilepticus (38).

## SPECIAL SYNDROMES OF STATUS EPILEPTICUS

Electrographic status epilepticus appears in specific epileptic syndromes with sleep-activated epileptiform activity that occurs continuously (3,47). This marked sleep activation is referred to as ESES or CSWS (9,10). Clinical seizure activity rarely occurs during the actual ESES. This is considered a special syndrome of NCSE in children (3). Although these are specific epileptic syndromes, not all affected children have overt clinical seizures. The term *epileptic encephalopathy* refers to conditions in which the epileptiform abnormalities contribute to a progressive cognitive dysfunction (47,48).

When pronounced, such as in ESES, sleep-activated epileptform activity typically presents with cognitive regression. In the two specific pediatric epilepsy syndromes with ESES, language regression predominates in LKS (47,49), and a more global neuropsychiatric regression occurs in the specific epileptic syndrome of CSWS (9,10,47). Both syndromes have the EEG pattern of ESES and marked behavior problems. Cognitive regression should raise concern for ESES, especially when underlying developmental problems are present.

It is important to distinguish the EEG finding of ESES from the epileptic syndrome of ESES (CSWS): the first describes the sleep-activated EEG, whereas the epileptic clinical syndrome includes the EEG findings plus the associated clinical characteristics (50). The EEG pattern ESES occurs in both LKS and CSWS. The clinical presentation depends on the location of the EEG abnormalities: in ESES with more focal features, especially posterior, language regression may predominate, whereas, with a more generalized pattern, neurobehavioral dysfunction predominates (51). In 17 children with ESES, 5 had LKS, and the EEG showed diffuse activity with accentuation in the centrotemporal region, whereas the others had widespread discharges (52). LKS and ESES have sometimes been considered "benign" because the EEG may improve over time. Given the devastating neuropsychologic deficits that occur in these epileptiform encephalopathies, we consider them "malignant" epileptic syndromes.

## LANDAU-KLEFFNER SYNDROME

LKS is a rare epileptic syndrome, occurring in 0.2% of pediatric epilepsies (53). LKS usually develops in a previously normal child older than four years of age (54) and may first manifest as an apparent word deafness, a "verbal auditory agnosia." Seizures and behavior disturbances, particularly hyperactivity, each occur in approximately two thirds of the children (47). Most cases are classified as idiopathic, but LKS may be caused by any pathologic process affecting auditory cortex. We have seen "symptomatic" cases, one with a left temporal lobe tumor and another with a left middle cranial fossa arachnoid cyst. Therefore, neuroimaging is needed.

The term "LKS variant" applies to children without the classic features (55). These include children with involvement of more anterior language areas and a dysfunction characterized by an expressive disorder with oral-motor apraxia, sialorrhea, seizures, and an abnormal EEG (centro-temporal spikes similar to those seen with benign focal epilepsy); children with progressive developmental delay with language regression (autism) and abnormal EEGs; and even children with congenital aphasias (also called developmental language disorders) with epileptiform EEGs. In our experience, children with progressive developmental delay comprise the largest group of the variants.

The EEG in LKS shows sleep-activated, bilateral, multifocal spikes, and spike-and-wave discharges, usually occurring posteriorly, especially in the temporal or the parietal regions. Epileptiform discharges occur in many locations, however, and may even be generalized. Some centers require ESES to diagnose LKS, but the strict ESES definition would exclude many cases. The EEG may improve over time, either spontaneously or with treatment (56,57), raising the possibility that the EEG abnormalities may be an epiphenomenon (58).

The evaluation of LKS includes a baseline history, physical examination, sleep-deprived EEG, a formal neuropsychologic evaluation, neuroimaging (magnetic resonance imaging preferred), and long-term video-EEG monitoring. Hearing tests are always performed to exclude peripheral auditory dysfunction. In certain cases, spike mapping or functional neuroimaging with either single-photon emission computed tomographic or positron emission tomographic scan and magnetoencephalography might be helpful, especially in the child with medically refractory LKS. The frequency-modulated auditory evoked response may differentiate an expressive from a receptive aphasia (59,60) and may localize to the superior temporal gyrus, but this type of study is not widely available. All children should have intensive speech therapy.

## CONTINUOUS SPIKE WAVES OF SLEEP

CSWS is rare, also occurring in only 0.2% of pediatric epilepsies (53). The strict definition of CSWS requires finding epileptiform activity in 85% of slow-wave sleep (9,10). There are symptomatic and cryptogenic cases, determined by etiology and whether normal neurologic or psychomotor development was present before the onset of the CSWS.

These children commonly have seizures, but the hallmark feature is regression in cognitive function and behavior but not primarily in language, as occurs in LKS. Tassinari reported on 29 children with CSWS (10). All but one had seizures; one had a single seizure, and one had only three seizures. Eighteen had normal and 11 had abnormal psychomotor development prior to onset. Of the 18 with normal development, all had severe loss of IQ and behavior disturbances, defined as decreased attention span, hyperactivity, aggression, and difficulties with interaction and inhibition, and two patients developed a psychotic state. In the 11 with abnormal psychomotor development, mental deterioration occurred in all, three developed marked hyperactivity, and one showed "massive regression," including in language, and a loss of interest in all activities.

## TREATMENT AND PROGNOSIS FOR LANDAU-KLEFFNER SYNDROME AND CONTINUOUS SPIKE WAVES OF SLOW SLEEP

The treatment of LKS and CSWS is similar, and the goal should be complete elimination of the epileptiform discharges, or a "normalization" of the EEG. Standard AEDs, corticosteroids (ACTH or prednisone), high-dose benzodiazepines, intravenously administered immunoglobulins, or multiple subpial transection are all used. In LKS, the conventional wisdom has been that AEDs may control seizures but not the aphasia, whereas corticosteroid treatment decreases the epileptiform activity and improves the seizures and aphasia (61-63). Early corticosteroid treatment has been considered the treatment of choice, especially for LKS (63). Because relapse may occur, LKS often requires long-term corticosteroid treatment, which increases the risk of the patients developing adverse effects (64). Despite either AED or corticosteroid treatment, many children continue to have language dysfunction. Regardless of treatment, 50% to 80% of children have long-term language or neurobehavior abnormalities (65-67).

Landau and Kleffner reported aphasia improvement with AED treatment (49). There is no good evidence to support the use of one AED over others, but we prefer AEDs with antiepileptogenic properties (spike-suppressors), compared with those with anticonvulsant properties (68). Anticonvulsant refers to suppression of seizures, whereas antiepileptogenic refers to suppression of the development of epilepsy or the underlying process that leads to epilepsy (68). Of the older AEDs, carbamazepine and valproate have been the most widely used. We prefer the spike-suppressing AEDs that are able to "normalize" the EEG, as compared with AEDs that don't control the epileptiform activity, because the complete control of epileptiform activity is the treatment goal. The better spike suppressors include valproic acid (VPA), lamotrigine, levetiracetam, and the benzodiazepines. VPA is an AED with, theoretically, both anticonvulsant and antiepileptogenic properties. Carbamazepine may worsen the generalized epilepsies and may even worsen focal spike-and-wave discharges and activate the EEG (39,69,70). Lamotrigine is also a good spike suppressor (71), and levetiracetam has been used in LKS (72) and ESES (73). Nevertheless, we have seen deterioration with every AED used. In general, if standard AEDs fail for either LKS or ESES, high-dose corticosteroids are used. Corticosteroids have anticonvulsant activity, with GABAergic effects, in addition to immune modulation (74).

We now use a high-dose diazepam treatment prior to using corticosteroids in children with LKS that has not responded to AEDs. De Negri and colleagues introduced a high-dose diazepam protocol for electrical status epilepticus (75), including a rectal dose of 1 mg/kg with EEG monitoring and a continued dose of 0.5 mg/kg orally for several weeks in patients who respond to this treatment. Those on chronic benzodiazepine treatment did not respond as well. When a clinical relapse occurred, this dosing schedule was repeated. In De Negri's group with electrical status epilepticus, only one child had LKS, and one had ESES. We modified this high-dose diazepam protocol, using 1 mg/kg, either orally or rectally, under EEG guidance, but then treated all children with a dose of 0.5 mg/kg, orally, for 3 to 4 weeks (76). If the EEG showed no improvement, we rapidly tapered the diazepam. If the EEG did show an improvement, we then tapered by 2.5 mg per day per month. In our series, every child who initially responded and then had a rapid diazepam taper had either a clinical or electrographic regression. We now continue a maintenance diazepam dose, usually at 2.5 to 5 mg per day, for two years. The best responders to high-dose diazepam have been children with idiopathic LKS.

Tassinari and colleagues recommend trials with several different drugs and report a long-lasting effect with VPA along with clobazam, lorazepam, and clonazepam (77). Smith and Hoeppner recommend initial treatment with high-dose VPA, with or without a benzodiazepine, and, in the absence of response, several months of corticosteroid therapy (78). Inutsuka and colleagues (79) reported their treatment results in 15 children, using the following protocol: (1) VPA at levels greater than 100 mg/L, (2) a combination of VPA plus ethosuximide, (3) short cycles of high-dose diazepam, or (4) intramuscular injections of ACTH. Treatment with short cycles of ACTH (a duration of 11 to 43 days) or diazepam (a duration of 6 to 7 days) did not achieve long-term remission, whereas either high-dose VPA alone (n = 7) or valproate in combination with ethosuximide (n = 3) achieved remission in 10 children (67%). We retrospectively analyzed our experience with ESES treatment in 12 children (80). Only one responded initially to VPA. We used prednisone for 6 months in 6 children, with the dose schedule outlined in Table 17.1 (81); 5 of 6 children had a positive response, but 4 of 5 relapsed and required another course of treatment. Before corticosteroids are used electively, the patient's immunizations should be up to date.

Alternate treatments, including immunoglobulins and the ketogenic diet, have been tried, with case reports documenting efficacy, but limited long-term follow-up data (82-86). Multiple subpial transection has been performed in selected children whose symptoms

**TABLE 17.1** SIX-MONTH DOSING SCHEDULE FOR ORAL PREDNISONE[a]

| |
|---|
| 2 mg kg$^{-1}$ day$^{-1}$ for 1 month (maximum dose: 60 mg/day) |
| 1.5 mg kg$^{-1}$ day-1 for 1 month |
| 1 mg kg$^{-1}$ day-1 for 1 month |
| 1 mg/kg every other day for 1 month |
| 0.75 mg/kg every other day for 1 month |
| 0.5 mg kg$^{-1}$ day$^{-1}$ every other day for 1 month |

*Reprinted from the American Academy of Child and Adolescent Psychiatry (81).*

[a] *We ensure that all immunizations are up to date, including varicella and influenza, prior to treatment.*

have not responded to medical therapy, and this treatment may provide benefit (87,88).

In general, cognitive dysfunction persists in the majority of children (78), but the outcome of epilepsy is favorable in both LKS and CSWS (89). The LKS prognosis varies. In a follow-up study of the original 9 children reported on by Landau and Kleffner, Mantovani and Landau reported full recovery in 4; one had a mild language disability, and four had moderate disability (90). In a literature review of studies that included 45 children, however, Bishop reported that outcome was related to the age of onset of symptoms and was worse if onset was before 4 years of age (54). Shinnar and colleagues reported language dysfunction in 88% of children with language regression, with most having autism or autistic features (65). Deonna and colleagues reported normal language in only one patient, and 6 patients had varying degrees of language deficits, some with a complete lack of language (91). Soprano and colleagues reported that 9 of 12 patients had a variable degree of persistent language deficit (92).

CSWS has a poor prognosis (93). In a follow-up study of 7 adult patients, only two had been in a normal school setting (94). The IQ was normal in the two patients with LKS, whereas mental retardation was present in the 5 with ESES. Scholtes and colleagues performed a long-term follow-up of 10 children with ESES, with good recovery in only one and a partial recovery in four (95). CSWS is more likely than LKS to have residual deficits because it is more likely than LKS to have a symptomatic etiology, rather than the idiopathic etiology that is more likely to exist in LKS.

## REFERENCES

1. Dodson WE, DeLorenzo RJ, Pedley TA, Shinnar S, Treiman DM, Wannamaker BB. The treatment of convulsive status epilepticus: Recommendations of the Epilepsy Foundation of America's Working Group on Status Epilepticus. JAMA 1993;270:854-859.
2. Lowenstein DH, Bleck T, Macdonald RL. It's time to revise the definition of status epilepticus. Epilepsia 1999;40:120-122.
3. Riviello JJ. Status epilepticus in children. In: Drislane FW, ed. Status Epilepticus: a Clinical Perspective. Totowa, NJ: Humana Press; 2005:313-338.
4. Drislane FW. Presentation, evaluation, and treatment of nonconvulsive status epilepticus. Epilepsy Behav 2000;1:301-314.
5. Granner MA, Lee SI. Nonconvulsive status epilepticus: EEG analysis in a large series. Epilepsia 1994;35:42-47.
6. Young GB, Jordan KG, Doig GS. An assessment of nonconvulsive seizures in the intensive care unit using continuous EEG monitoring: an investigation of variables associated with mortality. Neurology 1996;47:83-89.
7. Chong DJ, Hirsch LJ. Which EEG patterns warrant treatment in the critically ill? Reviewing the evidence for treatment of periodic epileptiform discharges and related patterns. J Clin Neurophysiol 2005;22:79-91.
8. Jirsch J, Hirsch LJ. Nonconvulsive seizures: Developing a rational approach to the diagnosis and management in the critically ill population. Clin Neurophysiol 2007;118:1660-2670.
9. Patry G, Lyagoubi S, Tassinari A. Subclinical "electrical status epilepticus" induced by sleep in children. A clinical and electroencephalographic study of six cases. Arch Neurol 1971;24:242-252.
10. Tassinari CA, Bureau M, Dravet C, Dalla Bernardina B, Roger J. Epilepsy with continuous spikes and waves during slow sleep-otherwise described as ESES (epilepsy with electrical status epilepticus during slow sleep. In: Roger J, Bureau M, Dravet C, Dreifuss FE, Perret A,

Wolf P. Epileptic Syndromes in Infancy, Childhood, and Adolescence, 2nd ed. London, England: John Libbey and Co; 1992:245-256.

11. Treiman DM, Walton NY, Kendrick C. A progressive sequence of electroencephalographic changes during generalized convulsive status epilepticus. Epilepsy Res 1990;5:49-60.
12. Mikati MA, Werner S, Shehab L, Shamseddine A, Simaan E, Liu Z, Tarif S, Stafstrom C, Holmes G. Stages of status epilepticus in the developing brain. Epilepsy Res 2003;55:9-19.
13. DeLorenzo RJ, Waterhouse EJ, Towne AR, Boggs JG, Ko D, DeLorenzo GA, Brown A, Garnett L. Persistent nonconvulsive status epilepticus after the control of generalized convulsive status epilepticus. Epilepsia 1998;39:833-840.
14. Tay SKH, Hirsch LJ, Leary L, Jette N, Wittman J, Akman CI. Nonconvulsive status epilepticus in children: clinical and EEG characteristics. Epilepsia 2006;47:1504-1509.
15. Monod N, Dreyfus-Brisac C, Sfaello Z. Detection and prognosis of neonatal seizures according to the electroclinical study of 150 cases. Arch Fr Pediatr 1969;26:1085-1102.
16. Udaeta Mora E, Olmos-Garcia de Alba G, Villaneuva Garcia D, Malagon Valdez J. Neonatal status epilepticus I: Clinical aspects. Clin Electroencephalogr 1984;15;193-196.
17. Olmos-Garcia de Alba G, Udaeta Mora E, Malagon Valdez J, Villaneuva Garcia D, Valarezo Crespo F. Neonatal status epilepticus II: Electroencephalographic aspects. Clin Electroencephalogr 1984;15:197-201.
18. Scher MS, Hamid MY, Steppe DA, Beggarly ME, Painter MJ. Ictal and interictal electrographic seizure durations in preterm and term neonates. Epilepsia 1993;34:284-288.
19. Wertheim D, Mercuri E, Faundez JC, Rutherford M, Acolet D, Dubowitz L. Prognostic value of continuous electroencephalographic recording in full term infants with hypoxic ischaemic encephalopathy. Arch Dis Child 1994;71:F97-102.
20. Ortibus EL, Sum JM, Hahn JS. Predictive value of EEG for outcome and epilepsy following neonatal seizures. Electroencephalogr clin Neurophysiol 1996; 98:175-185.
21. Clancy RR, Legido A. The exact ictal and interictal duration of electroencephalographic neonatal seizures. Epilepsia 1987:28:537-541.
22. Towne AR, Waterhouse EJ, Boggs JG, Garnett LK, Brown AJ, Smith JR Jr, DeLorenzo RJ. Prevalence of nonconvulsive status epilepticus in comatose patients. Neurology 2000;54:340-345.
23. Narayanan JT, Murthy JMK. Nonconvulsive status epilepticus in a neurological intensive care unit in a developing country. Epilepsia 2007;48:900-905.
24. Claassen J, Mayer SP, Kowalski RG, Emerson RG, Hirsch LJ. Detection of electrographic seizures with continuous EEG monitoring in critically ill patients. Neurology 2004;62:1743-1748.
25. Jette N, Claassen J, Emerson RG, Hirsch LJ. Frequency and predictors of nonconvulsive seizures during continuous electroencephalographic monitoring in critically ill children. Arch Neurol 2006;63:1750-1755.
26. Hyllienmark L, Amark P. Continuous EEG monitoring in a paediatric intensive care unit. Eur J Paediatr Neurol 2007;11:70-75.
27. Abend NS, Dlugos DJ. Nonconvulsive status epilepticus in a pediatric intensive care unit. Pediatr Neurol 2007;37:165-170.
28. Saengpattrachai M, Sharma R, Hunjan A, Shroff M, Ochi A, Otsubo H, Cortez MA, Snead, III OC. Nonconvulsive seizures in the pediatric intensive care unit: etiology, EEG, and brain imaging findings. Epilepsia 2006;47:1510-1518.
29. Shneker BF, Fountain NB. Assessment of acute morbidity and mortality in nonconvulsive status epilepticus. Neurology 2003;61:1066-1073.
30. Niedermeyer E, Ribeiro M. Considerations of nonconvulsive status epilepticus. Clin Electroencephalogr 2000;31:192-195.
31. Kimura S, Kobayashi T. Two patients with juvenile myoclonic epilepsy and nonconvulsive status epilepticus. Epilepsia 1996;37:275-279.
32. Benson PJ, Klein EJ. New-onset absence status epilepticus presenting as altered mental status in a pediatric patient. Ann Emerg Med 2001;37:402-405.
33. Niedermeyer E, Khalifeh R. Petit-mal status ("spike-wave stupor"). An electro-clinical appraisal. Epilepsia 1965;6:250-262.
34. Fujiwara T, Watanabe M, Nakamura H, Kudo T, Yagi K, Seino M. A comparative study of absence status epilepticus between children and adults. Jpn J Psychiatry Neurol 1988;42:497-508.
35. Inoue Y, Fujiwara T, Matsuda K, Kubota H, Tanaka M, Yagi K, Yamamori K, Takahashi Y. Ring chromosome 20 and nonconvulsive status epilepticus. A new syndrome. Brain 1997;120: 939-953.
36. Matsumoto A, Kumagai T, Miura K, Miyazaki S, Hayakawa C, Yamanaka T. Epilepsy in

Angelman syndrome associated with chromosome 15q deletion. Epilepsia 1992;33:1083-1090.

37. McBride MC, Dooling EC, Oppenheimer EY. Complex partial status epilepticus in young children. Ann Neurol 1981;9:526-530.
38. Wakai S, Ito N, Sueoka H, Kawamoto Y, Hayasaka H, Tsutsumi H, Chiba S. Complex partial status epilepticus in childhood. Pediatr Neurol 1995;13:137-141.
39. Snead OC 3rd, Hosey LC. Exacerbation of seizures in children by carbamazepine. N Engl J Med 1985;313:916-921.
40. Jette N, Cappell J, van Passell L, Akman CI. Tiagabine-induced nonconvulsive status epilepticus in an adolescent without epilepsy. Neurology 2006;67:1514-1515.
41. Thomas P, Valton L, Genton P. Absence and myoclonic status epilepticus precipitated by antiepileptic drugs in idiopathic generalized epilepsy. Brain 2006;129:1281-1292.
42. Gambardella A, Aguglia U, Oliveri RL, Russo C, Zappia M, Quattrone A. Negative myoclonic status due to antiepileptic drug tapering: report of three cases. Epilepsia 1997;38:819-823.
43. Panayiotopoulos syndrome: a consensus view. Dev Med Child Neurol 2006;48:236-240.
44. Covanis A. Panayiotopoulos syndrome: a benign childhood autonomic epilepsy frequently imitating encephalitis, syncope, migraine, sleep disorder, or gastroenteritis. Pediatrics 2006;118:e1237-e1243.
45. Panayiotopoulos CP. Autonomic seizures and autonomic status epilepticus peculiar to childhood:diagnosis and management. Epilepsy Behav 2004;5:286-295.
46. Ferrie CD, Caraballo R, Covanis A, Demirbilek V, Dervent A, Fejerman N, Fusco L, Grunewald RA, Kanazawa O, Koutroumanidis M, Lada C, Livingston JH, Nicotra A, Oguni H, Martinovic Z, Nordli DR Jr, Parisi P, Scott RC, Specchio N, Verrotti A, Vigevano F, Walker MC, Watanabe K, Yoshinaga H, Panayiotopoulos CP. Autonomic status epilepticus in Panayiotopoulos syndrome and other childhood and adult epilepsies: a consensus view. Epilepsia 2007;48:1165-1172.
47. Hadjiloizou S, Riviello JJ. Epileptic and Epileptiform Encephalopathies. Neurology, eMedicine from WebMD. http://www.emedicine.com/neuro/topic547.htm. Updated May 15, 2006. Accessed June 16, 2008.
48. Engel J Jr. A proposed diagnostic scheme for people with epileptic seizures and with epilepsy: Report of the ILAE task force on classification and terminology. Epilepsia 2001;42:796-803.
49. Landau W, Kleffner FR. Syndrome of acquired aphasia with convulsive disorder in children. Neurology 1957;7:523-530.
50. Veggiotti P, Beccaria F, Guerrini R, Capovilla G, Lanzi G. Continuous spike-and-wave activity during slow-wave sleep: syndrome or EEG pattern? Epilepsia 1999;40:1593-1601.
51. Guilhoto LM, Morrell F. Electrophysiological differences between Landau-Kleffner Syndrome and other conditions showing the CSWS electrical pattern. Epilepsia 1994;35(Suppl 8):126.
52. Guilhoto LM, Machado-Haertel LR, Manreza ML, Diament AJ. Continuous spike wave activity during sleep. Electroencephalographic and clinical features. Arq Neuropsiquiatr 1997;55:762-770.
53. Kramer U, Nevo Y, Neufeld MY, Fatal A, Leitner Y, Harel S. Epidemiology of epilepsy in childhood: a cohort of 440 consecutive patients. Pediatri Neurol 1998;18:46-50.
54. Bishop DVM. Age of onset and outcome in acquired aphasia with convulsive disorder (Landau-Kleffner Syndrome). Dev Med Child Neurology 1985;27:705-712.
55. Connolly AM, Chez MG, Pestronk A, Arnold ST, Mehta S, Deuel RK. Serum autoantibodies to brain in Landau-Kleffner variant, autism, and other neurologic disorders. J Pediatr 1999;134:607-613.
56. Bolanos A, Mikati M, Holmes G, Helmers S, Riviello J. Landau-Kleffner Syndrome: clinical and EEG features. [abstract] Neurology 1995;45(Suppl 4):180.
57. Bolanos A, Urion DK, Helmers SL, Lombroso CT, Mikati M, Duffy FH, Holmes GL, Riviello J. Serial electroencephalographic changes in children with Landau-Kleffner Syndrome. [abstract] Epilepsia 1997;38(Suppl 3):27.
58. Holmes GL, McKeever M, Saunders Z. Epileptiform activity in aphasia of childhood: an epiphenomenon? Epilepsia 1981;22:631-639.
59. Stefanatos GA, Foley C, Grover W. Steady-state auditory evoked responses to pulsed frequency modulations in children. Electroencephalogr Clin Neurophysiol 1997;104:31-42.
60. Duffy FH, Riviello JJ. Changes in frequency-modulated steady state auditory evoked response (FM-AER) after treatment in Landau-Kleffner Syndrome (LKS) and LKS variants (LKSV). [abstract] Epilepsia 1999;40(Suppl 7):84-85.

61. McKinney W, McGreal DA. An aphasic syndrome in children. Can Med 1974;110:637-639.
62. Marescaux C, Finck S, Maquet P, Schlumberger E, Sellal F, Metz-Lutz MN, Alembik Y, Salmon E, Franck G, Kurtz D. Landau-Kleffner Syndrome: A pharmacologic study of five cases. Epilepsia 1990;31:768-777.
63. Lerman P, Lerman-Sagie T, Kivity S. Effect of early corticosteroid therapy for Landau-Kleffner Syndrome. Dev Med Child Neurology 1991;33:257-260.
64. Verhelst H, Boon P, Buyse G, Ceulemans B, D'Hooghe M, Meirleir LD, Hasaerts D, Jansen A, Lagae L, Meurs A, Coster RV, Vonck K. Steroids in intractable childhood epilepsy: clinical experience and review of the literature. Seizure 2005;14:412-421.
65. Shinnar S, Rapin I, Arnold S, Tuchman RF, Shulman L, Ballaban-Gil K, Maw M, Deuel RK, Volkmar FR. Language regression in childhood. Pediatr Neurol 2001;24:183-189.
66. Mantovani JF. Autistic regression and Landau-Kleffner syndrome: progress or confusion? Dev Med Child Neurol 2000;42:349-353.
67. Soprano AM, Garcia EF, Caraballo R, Fejerman N. Acquired epileptic aphasia: neuropsychologic follow-up of 12 patients. Pediatr Neurol 1994;11:230-235.
68. Silver JM, Shin C, McNamara JO. Antiepileptogenic effects of conventional anticonvulsants in the kindling model of epilepsy. Ann Neurol 1991;29:356-363.
69. Kochen S, Giagante B, Oddo S. Spike-and-wave complexes and seizure exacerbation caused by carbamazepine. Eur J Neurol. 2002;9:41-47.
70. Gansaeuer M, Alsaadi TM. Carbamazepine-induced seizures: a case report and review of the literature. Clin Electroencephalogr 2002;33:174-177.
71. Akman CI, Holmes GL. The effect of lamotrigine on the EEGs of children and adolescents with epilepsy. Epilepsy Behav 2003;4:420-423.
72. Kossoff EH, Boatman D, Freeman JM. Landau-Kleffner Syndrome responsive to levetiracetam. Epilepsy Behav 2003;4:571-575.
73. Aeby A, Posnanski N, Verheulpin D, Wetzberger C, Van Bogaert P. Levetiracetam in epileptic syndromes with continuous spike and waves during slow sleep: experience in 12 cases. Epilepsia 2005;46:1937-1942.
74. Mtchedlishvili Z, Kapur J. A presynaptic action of the neurosteroid pregnenolone sulfate on GABAergic synaptic transmission. Mol Pharmacol 2003;64:857-864.
75. De Negri M, Baglietto MG, Battaglia FM. Treatment of electrical status epilepticus by short diazepam (DZP) cycles after DZP rectal bolus test. Brain Dev 1995;17:330-333.
76. Riviello JJ, Holder DL, Thiele E, Bourgeois BFD, Bergin AM, Duffy FH, Holmes GL. Treatment of continuous spikes and waves during slow wave sleep with high dose diazepam. [abstract] Epilepsia 2001;42(Suppl 7):56.
77. Tassinari CA, Rubboli G, Volpi L, Meletti S, d'Orsi G, Franca M, Sabetta AR, Riguzzi P, Gardella E, Zaniboni A, Michelucci R. Encephalopathy with electrical status epilepticus during slow sleep or ESES syndrome including the acquired aphasia. Clin Neurophysiol 2000:111(Suppl 2):S94-S102.
78. Smith MC, Hoeppner TJ. Epileptic encephalopathy of late childhood: Landau-Kleffner Syndrome and the syndrome of continuous spikes and waves during slow sleep. J Clin Neurophysiol 2003;20:462-472.
79. Inutsuka M, Kobayashi K, Oka M, Hattori J, Ohtsuka Y. Treatment of epilepsy with electrical status epilepticus of sleep and its related disorders. Epilepsy Behav 2006;28:281-286.
80. Albaradie RS, Bourgeois BFD, Thiele E, Duffy FH, Holmes GL, Riviello JJ. Treatment of continuous spike and wave during slow wave sleep. [abstract] Epilepsia 2001;42(Suppl 7):46-47.
81. Stefanatos GA, Grover W, Geller E. Case study: Corticosteroid treatment of language regression in pervasive developmental disorder. J Am Acad Child Adolesc Psychiatry 1995;34:1107-1111.
82. Fayad MN, Choueiri R, Mikati M. Landau-Kleffner Syndrome: consistent response to repeated intravenous gamma-globulin doses: a case report. Epilepsia 1997;38:489-494.
83. Mikati MA, Saab R. Successful use of intravenous immunoglobulin as initial monotherapy in Landau-Kleffner syndrome. Epilepsia 2000;41:880-886.
84. Mikati MA, Saab R, Fayad MN, Choueiri RN. Efficacy of intravenous immunoglobulin in Landau-Kleffner syndrome. Pediatr Neurol 2002;26:298-300.
85. Lagae LG, Silberstein J, Gillis PL, Casaer PJ. Successful use of intravenous immunoglobulins in Landau-Kleffner syndrome. Pediatr Neurol 1998;18:165-168.
86. Prasad AN, Stafstrom CF, Holmes GL. Alternative epilepsy therapies: the ketogenic diet,

immunoglobulins, and steroids. Epilepsia 1996;37(Suppl 1):81-95.

87. Morrell F, Whisler WW, Smith MC, Hoeppner TJ, de Toledo-Morrell L, Pierre-Louis SJ, Kanner AM, Buelow JM, Ristanovic R, Bergen D, et al. Landau-Kleffner syndrome. Treatment with subpial intracortical transection. Brain 1995;118:1529-1546.
88. Irwin K, Birch V, Lees J, Polkey C, Alarcon G, Binnie C, Smedley M, Baird G, Robinson RO. Multiple subpial transection in Landau-Kleffner syndrome. Dev Med Child Neurol 2001;43:248-252.
89. Bureau M. Outstanding cases of CSWS and LKS: analysis of the data sheets provided by the participants. In: Beaumanoir A, Bureau M, Deonna T, Mira L, Tassinari, eds. Continuous Spikes and Slow Waves During Slow Sleep Electrical Status Epilepticus During Slow Sleep: Acquired Epileptic Aphasia and Related Conditions. London, England: John Libbey; 1995:213-216.
90. Mantovani JF, Landau WM. Acquired aphasia with convulsive disorder: course and prognosis. Neurology 1980;30:524-529.
91. Deonna T, Davidoff V, Maeder-Ingvar M, Zesiger P, Marcoz JP. The spectrum of acquired cognitive disturbances in children with partial epilepsy and continuous spike-waves during sleep. A 4-year follow-up case study with prolonged reversible learning arrest and dysfluency. Eur J Paediatr Neurol 1997;1:19-29.
92. Soprano AM, Garcia EF, Caraballo R, Fejerman N. Acquired epileptic aphasia: Neuropsychologic follow-up of 12 patients. Pediatr Neurol 1994;11:230-235.
93. Morikawa T, Seino M, Watanabe M. Long-term outcome of CSWS syndrome. In: Beaumanoir A, Bureau M, Deonna T, Mira L, Tassinari, eds. Continuous Spikes and Slow Waves During Slow Sleep Electrical Status Epilepticus During Slow Sleep: Acquired Epileptic Aphasia and Related Conditions. London, England: John Libbey; 1995:27-36.
94. Praline J, Hommet C, Barthez M-A, Brault F, Perrier D, Du Passage G, Lucas B, Bonnard J, Billard C, De Toffel B, Autret A. Outcome at adulthood of continuous spike waves of slow sleep and Landau-Kleffner Syndrome. Epilepsia 2003;44:1434-1400.
95. Scholtes FB, Hendriks MP, Renier WO. Cognitive deterioration and electrical status epilepticus during slow sleep. Brain Dev 2005;6:167-173.

CHAPTER 18

# NONCONVULSIVE STATUS EPILEPTICUS IN THE ELDERLY

FRANK W. DRISLANE

## EPIDEMIOLOGY

After childhood, the incidence and prevalence of epilepsy increases monotonically with age, such that its prevalence in the elderly is about twice that in the general population. The annual incidence of new seizures is 127 per 100,000 persons older than 60 years of age, increasing with each decade (1). Most are acute symptomatic seizures due to strokes, head injury, and metabolic abnormalities. The prevalence of epilepsy is 0.9% at age 55 years and older and 1.2% at age 85 to 94 years (2). In nursing home residents, it can exceed 5% (3). Most studies use 60 years or older as defining the elderly and that will be assumed in this review, except where noted otherwise.

The increased seizure risk arises from the many illnesses of older age. Cerebrovascular disease accounts for up to 40% of new epilepsy in the elderly (4,5). In a population-based study, 6% of patients without earlier seizures had seizures within the first week after stroke; 5% had a first seizure later, and 3% developed epilepsy, a risk 17 times that in the general population (6). Systemic illnesses, head injury, tumors, and dementing illnesses such as Alzheimer disease are also frequent causes of seizures and epilepsy.

Acute symptomatic seizures are three times more common in subjects aged 75 and older, as compared with the general population (7). The most common causes are stroke, trauma, medication withdrawal, and central nervous system infections. Many are caused or precipitated by medications or changes in medications, especially with multidrug therapy, high doses, and in the presence of other illnesses (8). Discontinuation of sedating medications is one cause, particularly with barbiturates and benzodiazepines (9). Other medications, particularly at higher doses, or when used at "typical" doses in more vulnerable elderly patients, may precipitate seizures. These include meperidine, isoniazid, bupropion, phenothiazines, theophylline, tricyclic antidepressants, and some antibiotics (8,10).

In one study of 80 hospitalized patients older than 60 years of age with new seizures, about half had generalized convulsions (11). Almost all of the seizures were symptomatic of underlying illnesses, with 41% of patients having acute symptomatic seizures, 40% remote symptomatic seizures, and another 11% progressive encephalopathies; 6% had convulsive status epilepticus. Cerebral infarction or hemorrhage caused 54% of all seizures.

## DIFFERENT CLINICAL MANIFESTATIONS OF SEIZURES AND EPILEPSY IN THE ELDERLY

Clinical manifestations of seizures change with age and are often quite different in the elderly, as compared with presentation in younger adults (4,5). Older patients often have no earlier history of epilepsy, and epilepsy is more likely to be misdiagnosed in the elderly than in younger patients and in those with earlier seizures (12). Many patients' histories are unreliable, sometimes because the patients have cognitive impairment or dementia. When elderly people live alone, there may be no witnesses to describe seizure manifestations. The elderly are more likely to have more than one illness at a time.

Psychiatric illnesses, such as depression, increase with age and may complicate the diagnosis. A Veterans Affairs study demonstrated a mean delay of 1.7 years from the first medical contact until the correct diagnosis of epilepsy (13). Generalized convulsions were easier to diagnose, but only 20% of complex partial seizures were diagnosed correctly initially.

Most newly diagnosed epilepsy in the elderly has evidence of focal onset (4), sometimes progressing to generalized convulsions (14). Frequently, the focal onset is difficult to discern. Idiopathic (primary) generalized epilepsy is rarely diagnosed for the first time in the elderly.

In large Veterans Affairs studies, complex partial seizures were the primary seizure type in patients older than 65 years, but were a minority in patients younger than 40 years of age (15,16). In these studies, younger adults with focal-onset seizures more often had mesial temporal sclerosis and presented with more typical symptoms of temporal lobe epilepsy; half had seizure onsets characterized by staring or altered consciousness. In the elderly, strokes were more common and led to a wider variety of cortical injuries, such that simple motor and sensory symptoms were more common than "psychic" symptoms. There are more extratemporal seizure foci in the elderly, particularly in frontal and parietal areas (4). Clinical manifestations and motor components of partial seizures, such as automatisms, may become less prominent in the elderly (17). A video-electroencephalogram (EEG) study showed that elderly patients with seizures exhibited fewer motor phenomena than did younger patients (18). Generalized convulsions occur less frequently than in younger adults, also making the diagnosis more difficult (4).

Simple partial and complex partial seizures may last longer in the elderly, and postictal confusion can last for hours or even weeks, compared with briefer episodes in younger adults. If there are frequent or prolonged seizures and prolonged postictal states, patients can appear to have chronic degenerative illnesses or dementia adversely affecting cognitive function. Frequent complex partial seizures may lead to longer-lasting memory deficits (19). The different clinical manifestations and more extensive differential diagnosis probably yield an underestimate of epilepsy incidence in the elderly (4).

## DIFFERENTIAL DIAGNOSIS OF SEIZURES AND EPILEPSY IN THE ELDERLY

Cardiovascular disease is the most common alternate diagnosis — both accurately and inaccurately. Cardiac arrhythmias, orthostatic hypotension, vasovagal episodes, and marked fluctuations in blood glucose are frequent causes of episodic events mistaken for seizures, and vice versa (20). Syncope is more common in older individuals, but recovery is usually faster than with seizures. Transient ischemia usually has focal neurologic features. Both ischemia and epilepsy can lead to prolonged dysfunction in the elderly. Transient global amnesia is usually distinctive and should not be mistaken for epilepsy unless it is repeated often. Migraine, medication effects, and sleep disorders should be considered.

It is common for encephalopathies, dementias, and seizures to be confused in older patients. Some patients are thought to have dementing illnesses when they have frequent and prolonged complex partial seizures, and some patients have both. Having Alzheimer disease and other dementias is associated with a 6-fold increased risk of having unprovoked seizures (21).

Nocturnal paroxysmal spells may be epileptic, but there are many other causes, and polysomnography or video-EEG monitoring may be necessary to make the proper diagnosis. Such spells include periodic leg movements in sleep and rapid eye movement sleep behavior disorder. A monitoring study of nonepileptic physiologic attacks mistaken for epilepsy found cataplexy, hypotension, nocturnal confusion, episodic vomiting, nonepileptic myoclonic jerks, transient ischemia, and behavior abnormalities (22).

The detailed history should include questions about earlier similar episodes; any confusion spells, remote head injury, or cerebral infection; and a complete list of medications. With any new diagnosis of seizures or epilepsy in the elderly, magnetic resonance imaging is appropriate to look for a causative lesion. A single seizure in an elderly person does not necessarily warrant treatment with antiepileptic drugs (AEDs), and side effects are more likely to occur in the elderly, but, among elderly people with new seizures, 80% of seizures recur within 6 months (23).

## ELECTROENCEPHALOGRAPHY IN THE ELDERLY

EEG can be harder to interpret in the elderly than in younger patients. Focal slowing on an EEG is of interest in younger patients because it indicates an area of physiologic disturbance that might be related to seizures. By contrast, focal slowing is so common in older patients (often due to vascular disease and other injuries) that it is less useful in diagnosing paroxysmal episodes.

Elderly patients who have epilepsy are less likely than younger patients to have interictal epileptiform activity (24). In patients older than 60 years of age who have new seizures, most EEGs are abnormal, but few include epileptiform abnormalities (23), and interictal epileptiform discharges are less specific. Most epileptiform discharges in the elderly are focal (24), but focal discharges in patients with seizures after stroke are not a good predictor of subsequent epilepsy (23). In one study, 76% of patients diagnosed with epilepsy had epileptiform discharges on the EEGs, but 26% with nonepileptic events did so as well (22). Many patients with nonepileptic physiologic and psychogenic events that are misdiagnosed as epilepsy are put on AEDs (22). A study of more than 10,000 nursing home residents found that 11% of the residents were taking AEDs, many without a clear diagnosis of epilepsy (3).

Overinterpretation of EEGs and misdiagnosis of epilepsy can be a significant disservice to patients. Interictal EEG, whether positive or negative, is clearly insufficient for diagnosis (22). Especially when events are frequent, EEG monitoring with video recording is often the best way to make an accurate diagnosis and direct the patient to appropriate therapy or to avoid inappropriate therapy with adverse effects (25). In a group of 67 patients older than 60 years of age who had episodes of an uncertain nature, about half had nonepileptic physiologic disturbances, and about 20% had psychogenic nonepileptic seizures (often thought to be relatively rare in older people) (22). Several patients had both epileptic and nonepileptic attacks.

## STATUS EPILEPTICUS IN THE ELDERLY

### EPIDEMIOLOGY AND TYPES OF SEIZURES

Up to 40% of all status epilepticus occurs in the elderly (26). Among subjects older than 60 years of age, the incidence increases with each decade and reaches nearly one per 1000 per year, at least double that of younger people (27,28). Up to one third of new seizures in the elderly begin with an episode of status epilepticus, a much greater risk of status epilepticus than in the general population (29). Status epilepticus is significantly underdiagnosed in the elderly (26).

Acute symptomatic causes of status epilepticus predominate in the elderly. Cerebrovascular disease is by far the most common. Acute strokes or remote symptomatic seizures from earlier strokes cause two thirds of all status epilepticus in the elderly (26). About 7% of acute strokes provoke at least one epileptic seizure. Five percent of patients have early (first-week) seizures after stroke, and 20% to 25% of these have status epilepticus, ie, 1% of all strokes lead to status epilepticus (30); subsequent epilepsy causes more status epilepticus. Patients with larger ischemic strokes, hemorrhagic strokes, and subdural hematomas are an even greater risk of having seizures. Reduced levels of AEDs and remote symptomatic causes are also common. Many of the remainder are multifactorial, with contributions from acute metabolic or infectious precipitants (or medications or medication changes) superimposed upon an already impaired brain affected by vascular or "degenerative" diseases (31,32).

Compared to the case with younger adults, focal-onset status epilepticus is significantly more common than generalized status epilepticus in older patients (28). In one study, focal-onset seizures with secondary generalization were shown to be the seizure type in 45% of elderly patients with status epilepticus (26); 29% had focal seizures, and 26% had generalized seizures with no clear focal onset. Thus, status epilepticus with focal onset constituted 75% of status epilepticus in this group of elderly patients. In general, etiology influences the type of status. Metabolic derangements often lead to generalized status epilepticus, whereas vascular disease and other focal lesions cause partial seizures and status epilepticus (33).

## OUTCOME AND MORTALITY

Mortality from status epilepticus in the elderly is high (34). In a comprehensive epidemiologic study, status epilepticus mortality was 25% in adults overall, increasing to 45% at age 60 years or older, and 54% at age 80 years and older (27). In a study of elderly patients with status epilepticus, generalized seizures had a 49% mortality; partial seizures, 30%; and partial seizures with a secondary generalization, 36% (26). Myoclonic status epilepticus in the elderly (often symptomatic of severe underlying illness) has a mortality approaching 100%.

In a study of 41 patients with new status epilepticus arising during hospitalization (median age, 65 years), mortality was 61% (35). Half had earlier epilepsy but were usually on inadequate AEDs when the status epilepticus developed. Two thirds had focal brain lesions, usually strokes. Major metabolic derangements were also common.

The underlying etiology for status epilepticus is the most important determinant of mortality (26,34). Many cases of status epilepticus result from acute symptomatic causes, some of which are life threatening. Patients without earlier seizures have a much higher mortality than do those with old seizures (48% vs 25%, respectively), ie, exacerbations of earlier seizures are a better prognostic sign (26). Anoxic status epilepticus in the elderly has a mortality of at least 90%. Also exceeding a 30% mortality rate are metabolic disorders, systemic or central nervous system infections, cerebral hemorrhages, tumors, hypoxia, strokes, and trauma. Decreased AED levels, alcohol withdrawal, and idiopathic seizure disorders have mortality rates less than 6%.

# NONCONVULSIVE STATUS EPILEPTICUS IN THE ELDERLY

## EPIDEMIOLOGY

There have been many studies of the epidemiology of seizures, epilepsy, and even status epilepticus in the elderly, but data are not so readily available for NCSE in the elderly. NCSE may constitute one fourth of all status epilepticus (36). A population-based estimate of the incidence of status epilepticus is 80 per 100,000 persons per year (but this has been suggested to be an underestimate) (27), whereas NCSE is estimated at 45 cases per 100,000 per year (37). Status epilepticus incidence increases with age, and status epilepticus in the elderly constitutes about 40% of all status epilepticus (26). It is reasonable to conclude that NCSE in the elderly constitutes about 20% to 30% of status epilepticus in the elderly and possibly 10% of all status epilepticus in the larger population. It is not a rarity.

Most NCSE in the elderly is "symptomatic" of an underlying illness, especially vascular disease. Tumors, trauma, and metabolic disturbances may cause 10% each (14). Many older patients have combinations of etiologies, such as acute metabolic disorders and infection, or medications (or medication changes) superimposed on remote symptomatic lesions (such as strokes) or a chronic degenerative illness, such as Alzheimer disease (31,32). Relatively few cases of NCSE, perhaps 10%, are exacerbations of earlier epilepsy. In one study, 14 of

18 NCSE patients older than 75 years of age had acute medical causes of their NCSE; only two cases were attributed to epilepsy, although 35% of patients had had earlier epilepsy (38).

## DIAGNOSTIC DIFFICULTY IN THE ELDERLY

NCSE in the elderly can present very subtly and may be mistaken for other causes of prolonged or fluctuating confusion, with failure of diagnosis for several days (39). Many older people have other illnesses that cause hypotension, delirium, or "confusional episodes." Clinical manifestations of NCSE may be diagnosed incorrectly as being due to metabolic abnormalities, medication toxicity, transient global amnesia, psychiatric conditions, or other causes (40). This produces not only difficulties in epidemiologic ascertainment, but also clinical problems for individual patients.

Diagnosis requires a high level of clinical suspicion. Often, the diagnosis can be made readily with an EEG, but one cannot treat NCSE appropriately if the diagnosis is not considered. Of 23 patients seen in an emergency room with NCSE and the wrong or delayed diagnosis, 10 were elderly (40). They were labeled as having postictal, psychiatric, or confusional states. Even once the diagnosis was made, patients often required more than 24 hours for their conditions to respond successfully to AEDs.

When a patient has cognitive impairment at baseline, it can be difficult to tell if his or her condition is worse, and, hence, the diagnosis may be delayed. With prolonged amnestic spells during the seizures, and with prolonged postictal periods, seizures can cause a protracted memory loss, sometimes mimicking a dementia. Tatum and colleagues described 5 elderly patients with substantial memory impairment and confusion, presumed to have dementias, but later diagnosed with complex partial seizures as the cause of altered mental status (41). The seizures in all but one patient improved with the use of AEDs.

EEG and prolonged video-EEG monitoring can help to overcome the difficulty of diagnosing NCSE in the elderly. Video-EEG should be considered in elderly patients with prolonged and otherwise unexplained episodes of confusion. McBride and colleagues reviewed such monitoring for 94 elderly patients (average age, 70 years) with known or suspected seizures (22). Three quarters of the patients had their usual events of interest recorded, and about half had epileptic seizures. NCSE was infrequent, but this study did not include patients in the intensive care unit.

## THE ELECTROENCEPHALOGRAM OF NONCONVULSIVE STATUS EPILEPTICUS

Granner and Lee provided the most informative description of EEGs in NCSE, covering 85 episodes in 78 patients, diagnosed by both EEG and a good clinical response to AEDs (42). Waveform morphologies were remarkably variable and were seldom simply a typical spike-and-slow-wave pattern. Discharge frequencies were generally from 1.0 to 3.5 Hz (mean 2.2 Hz). Most discharges were generalized, but they often became focal once AEDs were initiated. Most focal discharges were frontal. Older patients were more likely to have focal discharges, again indicating that NCSE in the elderly tends to be "symptomatic" or arise from a focal lesion. The mean age in the series was 51 years, but those with focal discharges had a mean age of 69 years.

Periodic lateralized epileptiform discharges (PLEDs) are generally not considered to represent seizures or status epilepticus themselves, but PLEDs may be seen during seizures or status epilepticus, with their clinical significance differing in individual cases. One report of 7 elderly patients described recurrent confusional episodes associated with PLEDs (43). Patients had no structural lesions, and EEG discharge intervals were as long as four seconds. Clinical deficits resolved with a slowing of the EEG discharges, whether spontaneous or in response to intravenously administered diazepam. Carbamazepine appeared to prevent recurrences, and patients' conditions relapsed when the drug dose was decreased. The authors considered

PLEDs to be an "unusual status epilepticus of the elderly." Clinicians should keep an open mind about the significance of PLEDs.

## TYPES OF NONCONVULSIVE STATUS EPILEPTICUS

NCSE in the elderly takes many forms, including idiopathic (primary) generalized epilepsy (such as absence status epilepticus [ASE]); complex partial status epilepticus (CPSE), secondarily generalized NCSE, and "subtle" or electrographic generalized status epilepticus, which is often seen in comatose patients.

### *Idiopathic generalized nonconvulsive status epilepticus*

Primary generalized idiopathic epilepsy leads to nonconvulsive generalized status epilepticus (such as typical ASE) relatively seldom in the elderly (26). Almost always, there has been an earlier diagnosis of absence seizures or idiopathic generalized epilepsy. Some patients may have had the genetic trait without earlier clinical expression. Others may have had episodes of NCSE that went unrecognized (44). *De novo* ASE of "late onset" (mean age, 59 years) is frequently attributed to benzodiazepine or other medication withdrawal (9).

### *Complex partial status epilepticus*

Most NCSE in the elderly is not primarily generalized but, instead, has a focal onset and, thus, usually constitutes CPSE (14,26,42). CPSE may include an "epileptic twilight state" with a lack of responsiveness or confusion and bizarre, and particularly fluctuating, behavior (45-49). At times, there are automatisms. It can represent a prolonged complex partial seizure or a series of seizures. It has been estimated that about 1.5% of patients with complex partial seizures have an episode of status in a given year (37). In one series, the rate of CPSE accounted for only 2% of status epilepticus in the elderly (26). In another series of 10 elderly patients with NCSE, all had CPSE, some with generalization (50).

In one study of NCSE, the mean age was 70 years, and almost all patients had CPSE without any motor abnormalities (39). Altered mood and neglect were noted, and two thirds of patients had had earlier similar episodes. All had protracted confusion. Some had fluctuation in the level of consciousness. Attention and concentration were impaired, and speech was reduced to simple phrases. Younger patients were somewhat more aggressive, and older patients appeared depressed. Patients were often misdiagnosed (with dementia, transient ischemia, or metabolic disorders) for days, even in those with previous similar episodes. Three patients were thought to have definite psychiatric depression. Imaging studies were of minimal value, but EEG and video-EEG studies were diagnostic in all. Most were treated successfully with AEDs.

### *Secondarily generalized nonconvulsive status epilepticus*

Most generalized NCSE in the elderly is not "typical" ASE but, rather, "atypical" NCSE or secondarily generalized status epilepticus with a focal onset (see also Chapters 2 and 12). It could be labeled CPSE, but some cases appear generalized at the beginning of the EEG, and no focal onset is evident. There is some alteration of consciousness, but it is often not a complete loss of consciousness and, thus, is harder to detect. The manifestations of frontal NCSE can be very similar to those of ASE, possibly with generalization of discharges from a frontal focus (51). In a large series of patients with a frontal NCSE, indifference, loss of initiative, and irritability were common (52).

NCSE of frontal origin typically has an underlying lesion, although the lesion may be small. Some presentations include very subtle cognitive and behavior changes, without marked alteration of consciousness. Thomas and colleagues described 10 patients with frontal NCSE, all with presumed focal onset and 6 without earlier seizures; half were 60 years of age or older (53). Presentations were uncharacteristic enough that there was a mean delay to diagnosis of 48 hours. Seven patients had mood changes with behavior disinhibition or near abulia, but without obvious confusion. The EEGs had normal backgrounds, with unilateral frontal epileptiform discharges. Patients were able to carry out routine activities such as walking or eating and even gave correct addresses and telephone numbers and followed simple commands, but more complex tasks were disturbed by impaired attention. Several were disinhibited or hypomanic, and some had fluctuation of symptoms. Perseveration was prominent.

A second group of three patients had impaired consciousness with bilateral (but asymmetric) frontal epileptiform activity and abnormal EEG backgrounds. Confusion was more prominent, and behavior could be very disruptive. Attention and cooperation were diminished to the point of catatonia or stupor with progression of the NCSE.

### *Electrographic status epilepticus in the elderly*

Finally, ongoing, rapid, rhythmic epileptiform discharges strongly indicative of status epilepticus are relatively common in the elderly, particularly among very sick patients in the intensive care unit who have several illnesses. Most patients with electrographic seizure activity have secondarily generalized NCSE, often following earlier convulsions or generalized convulsive status (GCSE), usually with minimal or no convulsive motor activity at the time. Many are comatose, in the setting of major illness such as anoxia, sepsis, serious cerebrovascular disease, or severe toxic and metabolic encephalopathies (54,55). They have been labeled with several different diagnoses. Those with minimal movement after GCSE have been said to be in "subtle" status epilepticus (56); others are labeled as having electrographic status epilepticus (ESE) (54). Some clinicians refer to this as "status epilepticus in coma," although not all patients with ongoing epileptiform discharges are comatose. Some clinicians refer to these patients with severe medical illness as having "epileptic encephalopathies," indicating that the underlying disease causing the encephalopathy is the key diagnosis and that the epileptic component is not primary and may not respond to AEDs. This term, however, is probably best reserved for childhood conditions such as Landau-Kleffner syndrome and ESE in sleep.

ESE is usually nonconvulsive, but it is an ominous finding, with or without clinical seizures. It is often fatal, essentially always due to the underlying severe medical or neurologic illnesses (54). Nevertheless, some patients improve on AEDs (57). ESE is not simply an encephalopathy with spikes. Given the EEG pattern suggesting status epilepticus; the frequent clinical seizures before, during, and after the EEG; and the occasional positive response to AEDs, ESE is part of the spectrum of status epilepticus. See also Chapter 13.

ESE is not rare. Of 164 patients who had EEGs after apparent control of clinical status epilepticus in one large series, 48% had continued seizure discharges, and 14% were considered to be in NCSE (58). In a Veterans Affairs study of GCSE treatment, 20% of patients whose clinical status epilepticus appeared to stop had subsequent evidence of ongoing status epilepticus on the EEG (56). Similarly, 8% of patients with a number of different causes of coma and similar monitoring were found to have NCSE, without clinical signs of seizures (59). Among 112 patients with ESE seen in our medical center, two thirds were older than 60 years of age (median age, 69 years) (54). In 75% of patients, the diagnosis was unsuspected for days before the EEG was obtained.

## OUTCOME OF NONCONVULSIVE STATUS EPILEPTICUS IN THE ELDERLY

Among all patients with status epilepticus, mortality is about 22% (28). NCSE in the elderly is generally no more benign, but the risk varies a great deal with the type of NCSE, and it is determined primarily by the underlying cause (31). See also Chapter 22.

Patients with typical ASE do not appear to incur any significant mortality, long-term morbidity, or neurologic residua (60,61). Patients with CPSE and underlying vascular and other diseases are harder to treat and may not respond to AEDs until after a significant delay. In a group of 10 patients with frontal NCSE, treatment was difficult, but none appeared to suffer long-term cognitive sequelae (53). In one study, CPSE in the elderly had a mortality of about 30% (26).

In a report of 15 patients with NCSE and a mean age of 90 years (!), none had an earlier history of epilepsy (62). There were no convulsive seizures, and all had acute and severe medical illnesses. Six could not attain control of seizures and died, and most others died within 6 months, often from aspiration pneumonia. It was unclear in this study that the NCSE affected mortality, given the advanced age and severe underlying illnesses.

Generally, worsened outcome of NCSE in the elderly correlates with more serious etiologies and with worsened level of consciousness (31,38). In a series of 24 patients aged 65 years or older (mean age 77) with critical medical and neurologic illnesses and NCSE (most with generalized discharges) mortality was 54% and correlated with the severity of medical illness (32). All but one had acute insults or traumatic brain injuries. Very few had earlier epilepsy. Increasing doses and numbers of AEDs did not appear helpful, and 6 of 16 patients treated with intravenously administered benzodiazepines had immediate respiratory depression requiring intervention. The authors concluded that patients died from the underlying medical illnesses, and NCSE may not have been a significant contributor to mortality. This was not a randomized study, and it is unclear whether some particularly ill patients were selected for treatment with benzodiazepines. Patients who died were more severely ill.

In all of these reports, most patients with generalized NCSE had features that were probably similar to those described elsewhere as "subtle" status epilepticus or ESE (54,56). Comatose patients in the intensive care unit who are in NCSE usually do very poorly, with a mortality exceeding 50% in many series (35,54,63). Whatever their age, patients with earlier epilepsy (usually younger) have a better prognosis than do those with anoxia (often older). Generalized NCSE can have a mortality of 90% in the elderly (26). For ESE in one study, survival was 40% for patients younger than 70 years of age and 30% for those older than 70 (64). In that series, if patients with anoxia (usually older) were excluded, survival was nearly identical at all ages, again suggesting that etiology is more important than age.

Many elderly patients with generalized NCSE have ischemic and hemorrhagic strokes, tumors, anoxia, infections, and other severe medical and neurologic illnesses and prolonged status epilepticus. The severe illness determines the outcome, and it is unclear that age confers an independent risk for mortality. The markedly elevated mortality among elderly patients with NCSE is almost always attributable to the etiology (34). Given this major influence of etiology of status epilepticus, and the frequent comorbidities, it appears unlikely that there will be studies powerful enough to dissect out an independent risk for age alone.

## TREATMENT OF NONCONVULSIVE STATUS EPILEPTICUS

Treatment of NCSE is strikingly easy in some cases (if the underlying cause is relatively benign) but can be complicated and difficult in others, given the life-threatening etiologies and concomitant medical illnesses often accompanying NCSE in the elderly. Given the lack of evidence for neuronal damage from NCSE in most patients and because AEDs can have harmful effects (32), many clinicians recommend a relatively cautious approach to the treatment of NCSE, especially in the elderly (65). Most NCSE in the elderly may not need particularly aggressive treatment, but some refractory cases might.

Many patients with NCSE respond well to typical AED treatment (42,61,66). Patients with primary generalized ASE usually recover with modest doses of benzodiazepines. Valproate is often helpful. *De novo* ASE of late onset is usually very easy to treat with benzodiazepines, sometimes even orally (9). Once the precipitating cause of the NCSE has resolved, many patients do not require long-term AEDs (9,61). See also Chapter 20 on treatment.

Focal-onset and secondary generalized NCSE are often more difficult to treat. In one of the largest series, only 60% of focal-onset NCSE responded successfully to intravenously administered benzodiazepines (vs 90% with generalized EEGs) (42). Also, the response to AEDs is frequently delayed, sometimes for several days. CPSE is typically due to some underlying lesion and often requires long-term medication.

In a study of 22 elderly patients (median age, 70 years) with protracted confusion as a manifestation of NCSE, 18 were treated successfully with phenytoin, with 8 of these patients also receiving lorazepam (39). Two patients with primary generalized seizures were treated successfully with intravenously administered valproate. Two others required pentobarbital-induced coma for 2 to 7 days to control the NCSE. All recovered eventually. The authors recommended aggressive early treatment of ambulatory patients with prolonged confusion and NCSE, in an attempt to break the status epilepticus while patients were still healthy otherwise. The ambulatory population in this study was relatively free of severe medical illnesses, possibly explaining the excellent outcome.

In another study of patients with frontal NCSE that proved difficult to treat, only 2 of 10 patients responded well to initial intravenously administered benzodiazepines (53). Six others eventually responded to phenytoin, but two required more aggressive treatment, including pentobarbital in 1.

Comatose patients in the intensive care unit who have severe underlying illnesses have a high mortality rate, whatever the treatment. Hypotension, respiratory complications, and infection make medication use more complex. Patients in ESE and coma should probably have more aggressive treatment, but with the understanding that treatment may be ineffective and frustrating in many cases. Often, the ongoing rhythmic electrical activity of ESE indicates an illness so severe that treatment will not be sufficient to save the patient. Nevertheless, some patients do improve on AEDs (57).

Treatment must cover concomitant medical illnesses such as cardiac and respiratory failure, as well as metabolic abnormalities and infections—which all contribute to the increased incidence of confusion and adverse effects from medication use, such as hypotension, as well as troublesome drug interactions. Adverse effects of AEDs and other medications can increase in the setting of organ failure, and older brains are more vulnerable to such adverse effects (32). Most elderly patients with NCSE can be treated successfully if the underlying illness is relatively benign, but there is a need for good clinical judgment balancing the severity of the seizures with the complications of treatment.

### *Individual antiepileptic drugs in the elderly*

For primary generalized (e.g., absence or *de novo* absence) NCSE, benzodiazepines and valproate have been effective frequently, as noted earlier. CPSE and other focal-onset NCSE are often treated with the same AEDs used in GCSE, but usually less aggressively. Phenytoin and carbamazepine are avoided if the NCSE might be primarily generalized because these drugs may worsen the status epilepticus (67).

In the largest study of AEDs for GCSE, 44% of patients were at least 65 years of age (average, 73 years), and 70% had remote symptomatic neurologic injuries as the cause of status epilepticus (68). Lorazepam was superior to phenytoin as an initial treatment for the study overall, but phenobarbital was the most successful medication in the elderly, stopping overt convulsive status epilepticus in 71% of cases, with lorazepam following at 63%, diazepam plus phenytoin 53%, and phenytoin alone 42%. For patients with "subtle" status epilepticus, phenobarbital was successful in 31% of cases, lorazepam 14%, phenytoin 12%, and the diazepam-phenytoin combination 8%. Treiman estimated that 30% of all GCSE had a subtle presentation, with clinical manifestations including subtle motor phenomena such as nystagmus or twitching in the face or in the limbs or torso (56). That study suggested that phenobarbital was particularly helpful in the treatment of electrographic or subtle status epilepticus in the elderly, but this was a secondary finding and not the primary aim of the study, and these results did not reach statistical significance. The authors still argued for the use of lorazepam as an initial treatment. It is administered over a shorter period, allowing time for the use of other AEDs if necessary.

Once status epilepticus has been controlled, most patients need longer-term treatment to prevent recurrence, but the use of AEDs and other medications is fraught with difficulty in the elderly. Diminished metabolism in the liver may cause drug levels to rise, especially with most older AEDs plus tiagabine and oxcarbazepine, but not with gabapentin and levetiracetam, and only slightly with topiramate. Reduction in glomerular filtration and creatinine clearance in patients in their later years may also increase drug levels and lead to toxicity, although less so for medications metabolized in the liver, such as carbamazepine and phenobarbital (33). Changes in absorption in the intestinal tract and loss of stomach acidity do not appear to have much effect on AED levels.

In long-term treatment, many elderly patients require much lower doses and levels of AEDs to avoid toxicity. For AEDs with strong protein binding (e.g., phenytoin and valproate), changes in the serum albumin concentration, and in the bound fraction of medications, can cause changes in free levels that are difficult to predict (69). Levetiracetam and gabapentin do not have significant effects on enzyme induction, and lamotrigine appears to have relatively little. Older maintenance AEDs (e.g., carbamazepine, phenobarbital, phenytoin, and valproic acid) can be very effective, but enzyme induction or inhibition and drug interactions can be problematic. Newer AEDs (e.g., gabapentin, lamotrigine, levetiracetam, oxcarbazepine, topiramate, and zonisamide) often have simpler pharmacologic properties and ease of use, and many are better tolerated, but they have their own adverse effects and a higher drug cost (70).

In considering longer-term treatment following NCSE, the prominence of depression in the elderly must be kept in mind, and medications such as phenobarbital, benzodiazepines, and tiagabine might exacerbate this. Some AEDs may have antidepressant effects. Long-term treatment with AEDs increases the risk of falls in elderly people. Adverse effects must be weighed and balanced against the benefits of epilepsy treatment.

Drug interactions are particularly worrisome with the many medications used in the elderly. For example, a selective serotonin reuptake inhibitor such as fluoxetine can inhibit metabolizing enzymes and lead to marked increases in levels of carbamazepine, phenytoin, and valproate, with potential toxicity. Several other antidepressants have less potential for drug interactions with AEDs. Phenytoin, carbamazepine, and phenobarbital have significant interactions with warfarin, used for anticoagulation in patients with cardiac disease and stroke. Such cardiovascular disease is increasingly prevalent among the elderly.

There are very few studies comparing the benefits and adverse effects of AEDs in the elderly. One Veterans Affairs study of 593 patients aged 60 years or older with new-onset epilepsy demonstrated reasonably good seizure control with relatively low daily doses of gabapentin (1500 mg), lamotrigine (150 mg), or carbamazepine (600 mg) (5). The primary outcome in the study was retention in the trial for a year, which largely reflected medication tolerability. Of the patients taking lamotrigine, 56% were retained for a year, compared with 49% for gabapentin and 35% for carbamazepine. Seizure control was similar across the groups. In another study, lamotrigine, 100 mg daily, was tolerated better than carbamazepine, 400 mg daily (71).

## CONCLUSION

NCSE is relatively common in elderly people. Most is "acute symptomatic," due to the illnesses that are increasingly prevalent in the elderly; there is relatively little idiopathic (primary) generalized epilepsy. Manifestations of seizures and status are different in the elderly, and, often, status epilepticus is harder to diagnose, and older patients are particularly sensitive to medication effects and drug interactions. As with younger patients, the prognosis of NCSE is heavily dependent on the etiology. Although NCSE may be harder to diagnose in the elderly, treatment can still be very beneficial, especially if the precipitating illness is not devastating, but the diagnosis of NCSE must be considered first to facilitate successful treatment.

## REFERENCES


1. Loiseau L, Loiseau P, Duché B, Guyot M, Dartigues JF, Aublet B. A survey of epileptic disorders in southwest France: seizures in elderly patients. Ann Neurol 1990;27:232-237.
2. de la Court A, Breteler MB, Meinardi H, Hauser WA, Hofman A. Prevalence of epilepsy in the elderly: the Rotterdam study. Epilepsia 1996;37:141-147.
3. Schachter SC, Cramer GW, Thompson GD, Chaponis RJ, Mendelson MA, Lawhorne L. An evaluation of antiepileptic drug therapy in nursing facilities. J Am Geriatr Soc 1998;46:1137-1141.
4. Ramsay RE, Rowan AJ, Pryor FM. Special considerations in treating the elderly patient with epilepsy. Neurology 2004;62(Suppl 2):S24-S29.
5. Rowan AJ, Ramsay RE, Collins JF, Pryor F, Boardman KD, Uthman BM, Spitz M, Frederick T, Towne A, Carter GS, Marks W, Felicetta J, Tomyanovich ML. and the VA Cooperative Study 428 group. New onset geriatric epilepsy. A randomized study of gabapentin, lamotrigine, and carbamazepine. Neurology 2005;64:1868-1873.
6. So EL, Annegers JF, Hauser WA, O'Brien PC, Whisnant JP. Population-based study of seizure disorders after cerebral infarction. Neurology 1996;46:350-355.
7. Annegers JF, Hauser WA, Lee J, Rocca WA. Incidence of acute symptomatic seizures in Rochester, Minnesota, 1935-1984. Epilepsia 1995;36:327-333.
8. Messing RO, Closson RG, Simon RP. Drug-induced seizures: a 10-year experience. Neurology 1984;34:1582-1586.
9. Thomas P, Beaumanoir A, Genton P, Dolisi C, Chatel M. "De novo" absence status of late onset: report of 11 cases. Neurology 1992;42:104-110.
10. Franson KL, Hay DP, Neppe V, Dahdal WY, Mirza WU, Grossberg GT, Chatel DM, Szwabo PA, Kotegal S. Drug-induced seizures in the elderly. Causative agents and optimal management. Drugs Aging 1995;7:38-49
11. Ettinger AB, Shinnar S. New-onset seizures in an elderly hospitalized population. Neurology 1993;43:489-492.
12. Cloyd J, Hauser W, Towne A, Ramsay R, Mattson R, Gilliam F, Walczak T. Epidemiological and medical aspects of epilepsy in the elderly. Epilepsy Res 2006;68S:S39-S48.
13. Spitz MC, Bainbridge JL. Observations on the delay and diagnosis of seizures in the elderly: update 3. Epilepsia 2003;44 (Suppl 9):18.
14. Sung CY, Chu NS. Status epilepticus in the elderly: etiology, seizure type and outcome. Acta Neurol Scand 1989; 80:51-56.
15. Mattson RH, Cramer JA, Collins JF, Smith DB, Delgado-Escueta AV, Browne TR, Williamson PD, Treiman DM, McNamara JO, McCutchen CB, et al. Comparison of carbamazepine, phenobarbital, phenytoin, and primidone in partial seizures and secondarily generalized tonic-clonic seizures. N Engl J Med 1985;313:145-115.
16. Mattson RH, Cramer JA, Collins JF. A comparison of valproate with carbamazepine for the treatment of complex partial seizures and secondarily generalized tonic-clonic seizures in adults. The Department of Veterans Affairs Epilepsy Cooperative Study No. 264 group. N Engl J Med 1992;327:765-771.
17. Tinuper P. The altered presentation of seizures in the elderly. In: Rowan AJ, Ramsay RE. eds. Seizures and Epilepsy in the Elderly. Boston, MA: Butterworth-Heinemann; 1997:123-130.
18. Kellinghaus C, Loddenkemper T, Dinner DS, Lachwani D, Lüders HO. Seizure semiology in the elderly: a video analysis. Epilepsia 2004;45:263-267.
19. Palmini AL, Gloor P, Jones-Gotman M. Pure amnestic seizures in temporal lobe epilepsy: definition, clinical symptoms, etiology, and functional anatomic considerations. Brain 1992;115:749-769.
20. Stephen L, Brodie M. Epilepsy in elderly people. Lancet 2000;355:1441-1446.
21. Hesdorffer DC, Hauser WA, Annegers JF, Kokmen E, Rocca WA. Dementia and adult-onset unprovoked seizures. Neurology 1996;46:727-730.
22. McBride A, Shih T, Hirsch L. Video-EEG monitoring in the elderly: a review of 94 patients. Epilepsia 2002;43:165-169.
23. Lühdorf K, Jensen LK, Plesner AM. Etiology of seizures in the elderly. Epilepsia 1986;27:458-463.

24. Drury I, Beydoun A. Interictal epileptiform activity in elderly patients with epilepsy. Electroencephalogr Clin Neurophysiol 1998;106:369-373.
25. Abubakr A, Wambacq I. Seizures in the elderly: Video/EEG monitoring analysis. Epilepsy Behav 2005;7:447-450.
26. DeLorenzo RJ. Clinical and epidemiologic study of status epilepticus in the elderly. In: Rowan AJ, Ramsay RE, eds. Seizures and Epilepsy in the Elderly. Boston MA: Butterworth-Heinemann; 1997:191-205.
27. DeLorenzo RJ, Towne AR, Pellock JM, Ko D. Status epilepticus in children, adults and the elderly. Epilepsia 1992;33(Suppl 4):S15-25.
28. DeLorenzo RJ, Hauser WA, Towne AR, Boggs JG, Pellock JM, Penberthy L, Garnett L, Fortner CA, Ko D. A prospective, population-based epidemiologic study of status epilepticus in Richmond, Virginia. Neurology 1996;46:1029-1035.
29. Hauser WA. Epidemiology of seizures and epilepsy in the elderly. In: Rowan AJ, Ramsay RE, eds. Seizures and Epilepsy in the Elderly. Boston, MA: Butterworth-Heinemann;1997:7-18.
30. Rumbach L, Sablot D, Berger E, Tatu L, Vuillier F, Moulin T. Status epilepticus in stroke. Report on a hospital-based stroke cohort. Neurology 2000;54:350-354.
31. Shneker BF, Fountain NB. Assessment of acute morbidity and mortality in nonconvulsive status epilepticus. Neurology 2003;61:1066-1073.
32. Litt B, Wityk RJ, Hertz SH, Mullen PD, Weiss H, Ryan DD, Henry TR. Nonconvulsive status epilepticus in the critically ill elderly. Epilepsia 1998;39:1194-1202.
33. Krämer G. Epilepsy in the elderly: some clinical and pharmacotherapeutic aspects. Epilepsia 2001;45(Suppl 3):55-59.
34. Towne AR, Pellock JM, Ko D, DeLorenzo, RJ. Determinants of mortality in status epilepticus. Epilepsia 1994; 35:27-34.
35. Delanty N, French JA, Labar DR, Pedley TA, Rowan AJ. Status epilepticus arising de novo in hospitalized patients: an analysis of 41 patients. Seizure 2001;10:116-119.
36. Celesia GG. Modern concepts of status epilepticus. JAMA 1976;235:1571-1574.
37. Shorvon S. Definition, classification, and frequency of status epilepticus. In: Shorvon S, ed. Status Epilepticus: Its Clinical Features and Treatment in Children and Adults. Cambridge, England: Cambridge University Press; 1994: 21-33.
38. Bottaro FJ, Martinez OA, Fernandez Pardal MM, Bruetman JE, Reisin RC. Nonconvulsive status epilepticus in the elderly: a case-control study. Epilepsia 2007;48:966-972.
39. Sheth R, Drazhowski JF, Sirven JI, Gidal BE, Hermann BP. Protracted ictal confusion in elderly patients. Arch Neurol 2006;63:529-532.
40. Kaplan PW. Nonconvulsive status epilepticus in the emergency room. Epilepsia 1996;37:643-650.
41. Tatum WO, Ross J, Cole AJ. Epileptic pseudodementia. Neurology 1998;50:1472-1475.
42. Granner MA, Lee SI. Nonconvulsive status epilepticus: EEG analysis in a large series. Epilepsia 1994;35:42-47.
43. Terzano MG, Parrino L, Mazzucchi A, Moretti G. Confusional states with periodic lateralized epileptiform discharges (PLEDs): a peculiar epileptic syndrome in the elderly. Epilepsia 1986;27:446-457.
44. Agathonikou A, Panayiotopoulos CP, Giannakodimos S, Koutroumanidis M. Typical absence status in adults: diagnostic and syndromic considerations. Epilepsia 1998;39:1265-1276.
45. Belafsky MA, Carwille S, Miller P, Waddell G, Boxley-Johnson J, Delgado-Escueta AV. Prolonged epileptic twilight states: continuous recordings with nasopharyngeal electrodes and videotape analysis. Neurology 1978;28:239-245.
46. Engel J, Ludwig, BI, Fetell M. Prolonged partial complex status epilepticus: EEG and behavioral observations. Neurology 1978;28:863-869.
47. Ballenger CE, King DW, Gallagher BB. Partial complex status epilepticus. Neurology 1983;33:1545-1552.
48. Treiman DM, Delgado-Escueta AV. Complex partial status epilepticus. In: Delgado-Escueta AV, Wasterlain CG, Treiman DM, Porter RJ, eds. Advances in Neurology, Vol. 34. Status Epilepticus. New York, NY: Raven Press;1983:69-81.
49. Cockerell OC, Walker MC, Sander JWAS, Shorvon SD. Complex partial status epilepticus: a recurrent problem. J Neurol Neurosurg Psychiatry 1994;57:835-837.
50. Labar D, Barrera J, Solomon G, Harden C. Nonconvulsive status epilepticus in the elderly: a case series and review of the literature—causes, treatment, and outcome in 65 patients. J Epilepsy 1998;11:74-78.

51. Shorvon S, Walker M. Status epilepticus in idiopathic generalized epilepsy. Epilepsia 2005;46:73-79.
52. Rohr-Le Floch J, Gauthier G, Beaumanoir A. État confusionnels d'origine épileptique: intérêt de l'EEG fait en urgence. Rev Neurol (Paris) 1988;144:425-436.
53. Thomas P, Zifkin B, Migneco O, Lebrun C, Darcourt J, Andermann F. Nonconvulsive status epilepticus of frontal origin. Neurology 1999;52:1174-1183.
54. Drislane FW, Schomer DL. Clinical implications of generalized electrographic status epilepticus. Epilepsy Res 1994;19:111-121.
55. Privitera M, Hoffman M, Moore JL, Jester D. EEG detection of nontonic-clonic status epilepticus in patients with altered consciousness. Epilepsy Res 1994;18:155-166.
56. Treiman DM, Meyers PD, Walton NY, Collins JF, Colling C, Rowan AJ, Handforth A, Faught E, Calabrese VP, Uthman BM, Ramsay RE, Mamdani MB. A comparison of four treatments for generalized convulsive status epilepticus. N Engl J Med 1998;339:792-798.
57. So EL, Ruggles KH, Ahmann PA, Trudeau SK, Weatherford KJ, Trenerry MR. Clinical significance and outcome of subclinical status epilepticus in adults. J Epilepsy 1995;8:11-15.
58. DeLorenzo RJ, Waterhouse EJ, Towne AR, Boggs JG, Ko D, DeLorenzo GA, Brown A, Garnett L. Persistent nonconvulsive status epilepticus after the control of convulsive status epilepticus. Epilepsia 1998;39:833-840.
59. Towne AR, Waterhouse EJ, Boggs JG, Garnett LK, Brown AJ, Smith JR, DeLorenzo RJ, Smith JR Jr. Prevalence of nonconvulsive status epilepticus in comatose patients. Neurology 2000;54:340-345.
60. Andermann F, Robb JP. Absence status: a reappraisal following review of thirty-eight patients. Epilepsia 1972;13:177-187.
61. Walker MC. Diagnosis and treatement of nonconvulsive status epilepticus. CNS Drugs 2001;15:931-939.
62. Martin Y, Artaz M-A, Bornand-Rousselot A. Nonconvulsive status epilepticus in the elderly. J Am Geriatr Soc 2004;52:476-477.
63. Barry E, Hauser WA. Status epilepticus: the interaction of epilepsy and acute brain disease. Neurology 1993;43:1473-1478.
64. Drislane FW, Blum AS, Lopez MR, Schomer DL. Outcome in refractory status epilepticus; age is not a significant risk factor when controlled for aetiology. [abstract] J Neurol 2005;252(Suppl 2):80.
65. Kaplan PW. Assessing the outcomes in patients with nonconvulsive status epilepticus: nonconvulsive status epilepticus is underdiagnosed, potentially overtreated, and confounded by comorbidity. J Clin Neurophysiol 1999;16:341-352.
66. Ellis JM, Lee SI. Acute prolonged confusion in later life as an ictal state. Epilepsia 1978;19:119-128.
67. Osorio I, Reed RC, Peltzer JN. Refractory idiopathic absence status epilepticus: a probable paradoxical effect of phenytoin and carbamazepine. Epilepsia 41;2000:887-894.
68. Treiman D, Walker MC. Treatment of seizure emergencies: convulsive and non-convulsive status epilepticus. Epilepsy Res 2006;68S:S77-82.
69. Perucca E, Berlowitz D, Birnbaum A, Cloyd JC, Garrard J, Hanlon JT, Levy RH, Pugh MJ. Pharmacological and clinical aspects of antiepileptic drug use in the elderly. Epilepsy Res 2006;68S:S49-63.
70. Waterhouse EJ, Towne AR. Seizures in the elderly: Nuances in presentation and treatment. Cleve Clin J Med 2005;72(Suppl 3):S26-37.
71. Brodie MJ, Overstall PW, Giorgi L. Multicentre, double-blind, randomized comparison between lamotrigine and cabamazepine in elderly patients with newly diagnosed epilepsy. The UK Lamotrigine Elderly Study Group. Epilepsy Res 1999;37:81-87.

CHAPTER 19

# NONCONVULSIVE STATUS EPILEPTICUS: SPECIAL CONSIDERATIONS IN THE MENTALLY RETARDED

RANDA Y. MAKHOUL AND MOHAMAD A. MIKATI

Nonconvulsive status epilepticus (NCSE) is a term used to denote a range of conditions in which electrographic seizure activity is prolonged and results in nonconvulsive clinical symptoms. This definition was suggested by an interest group that met in Oxford in April 2004, sponsored by the Epilepsy Research Foundation, to discuss the definition, diagnosis, and treatment of NCSE (1). Kaplan has stated that NCSE is also characterized by behavior or cognitive changes from baseline for at least 30 minutes with electroencephalogram (EEG) evidence of seizures (2). These cognitive changes are often incorrectly ascribed to a postictal state, intoxication, mental retardation, psychogenic symptoms, or psychiatric states.

In patients with mental retardation, NCSE can be particularly difficult to recognize because these patients have baseline abnormal cognition and often have associated psychologic or psychiatric conditions. Walker has stated that, in patients with a previous diagnosis of epilepsy, any prolonged change in personality, prolonged postictal confusion (greater than 30 minutes), or recent onset of psychosis should be investigated with EEG, as these can all be presentations of NCSE (3). NCSE can result from, and follow, convulsive status epilepticus and is an important treatable cause of persistent coma or abnormal mental state following convulsive status epilepticus.

Although EEG interpretation is usually straightforward when there are regular, continuous, and repetitive discharges, sometimes occurring in a cyclic fashion, difficulties can occur in differentiating NCSE from an encephalopathy of other causes. Thus, diagnostic EEG features should include unequivocal electrographic seizure activity consisting of periodic epileptiform or rhythmic discharges, with either clinical or electrographic response to treatment (3).

## CLASSIFICATION OF NONCONVULSIVE STATUS EPILEPTICUS IN THE MENTALLY RETARDED

A categorization of NCSE in the mentally retarded has been proposed by Brodtkorb and colleagues based on current classification of epileptic seizures (4). A differentiation between NCSE that is generalized from the onset from forms with a focal origin is essential in achieving an adequate therapeutic strategy. Generalized NCSE is also subdivided into typical absence status epilepticus (ASE) (with rhythmic 3-Hz spike and waves on the EEG) and atypical ASE (with more irregular and slower, generalized, spike-and-wave EEG patterns). The most common partial form, complex partial status epilepticus, may occur in a continuous pattern or as frequent and recurrent seizures. Because NCSE with a focal onset may have a generalized ictal EEG pattern, a classification of NCSE solely based on the seizure classification may be difficult, for example, with secondary generalized NCSE. Often, it is impossible to distinguish between continuous complex partial seizures and atypical ASE, either clinically or on the basis of EEG recordings (4).

## PRESENTATION

### COGNITIVE DYSFUNCTION AND DEMENTIA

The electrographic seizure activity of NCSE is responsible for diverse clinical symptoms, including impairment of mental function, sometimes manifested as dementia. One example is that of a 50-year-old man with mental retardation and right hemiparesis who seemed to be cured from his epilepsy and then developed physical and mental deterioration simulating dementia (5). The EEG showed marked epileptic activity characterized by spikes appearing every 10 seconds over the left temporal lobe. This activity disappeared with the introduction of carbamazepine, resulting in rapid and long-term improvement of symptoms. Thus, the "dementia syndrome" was a transient cognitive impairment caused by the "subclinical" electrical seizure activity of NCSE.

Another example with cognitive impairment is that of a 29-year-old mentally retarded woman who had had epilepsy since the age of 1 year (6). She had been treated with almost all available anticonvulsant drugs but had generalized tonic-clonic seizures and absence-like seizures regularly since the age of 12 years. She had recurrent episodes of confusion and disorientation, each lasting for one to three days, 6 times per month, over a year. The ictal EEG pattern was a monomorphic alpha activity with a generalized distribution. NCSE started and ended abruptly clinically as well as electroencephalographically, and the most characteristic clinical findings during NCSE were disorientation and delay in response even to simple questions (with some incorrect answers). Verbal memory, which was impaired interictally, was even worse during NCSE.

### CATATONIA

NCSE and catatonia share many clinical features. Distinguishing between them on the basis of the physical examination may be difficult and, at times, even impossible. This presentation of NCSE has been reported, to our knowledge, in the mentally normal (7) and only in a single case report in the mentally retarded—a 12-year-old boy with familial bilateral perisylvian polymicrogyria, mental retardation, and refractory partial seizures (8). After one week of a maintenance dose of tiagabine, 1mg/kg per day, added to sodium valproate, he developed hypoactivity and affective detachment. An EEG showed almost continuous sharp-wave discharges with irregular runs of atypical spike-wave complexes over the anterior regions of both hemispheres, consistent with a diagnosis of frontal NCSE (8). Conversely, catatonia can potentially mimic NCSE (9).

### PSYCHOSIS

One mentally retarded 26-year-old patient with complex partial seizures had NCSE, including psychotic agitation and hallucinations (12). We evaluated a 15-year-old girl with mental retardation due to perinatal hypoxia, who presented with episodes of psychotic agitation alternating with catatonia. She had intermittent uncontrolled rage attacks, hyperactivity, and agitation followed by complete mutism and unresponsiveness. She responded clinically and electroencephalographically to therapy with carbamazepine. Somatic, visual, and auditory hallucinations have also been described in many nonretarded patients with NCSE (10,11).

### ATYPICAL ABSENCE STATUS EPILEPTICUS

Atypical ASE is a common presentation of NCSE in the mentally retarded (13,14). One example involves a 9-year-old boy with congenital bilateral perisylvian syndrome and pseudobulbar palsy, mental retardation, and intractable epilepsy (13). He was born as a full-term baby to healthy parents with an uneventful perinatal course. At 8 years of age, he developed recurrent episodes of excessive drooling, fluctuating level of consciousness, frequent head drops, and subtle myoclonus of the face and limbs. Each episode lasted several days. The EEG demonstrated continuous diffuse slow spikes and waves. Intravenously administered diazepam resulted in improvement of clinical and EEG findings (13).

Occasionally, NCSE is difficult to distinguish from electrical status epilepticus in sleep, a distinct entity in which the cognitive impairment is due to the indirect effect of continuous EEG discharges in sleep on cognitive development and function. In NCSE, cognition is impaired due to the direct effect of EEG discharges during wakefulness. One report has described an 18-month-old boy who presented with global developmental delay and decreased alertness (15). He was not interested in his surroundings, was unable to walk or speak any words, and did not follow simple commands. The Denver II test showed a 9-month delay in fine and gross motor, social, and language development. The results of metabolic investigations and cranial magnetic resonance imaging were normal. The EEG obtained during sleep demonstrated continuous generalized epileptiform discharges, mainly consisting of slow-wave discharges and some spikes in between the slow-wave discharges; a waking EEG could not be recorded. The diagnosis of electrical status epilepticus in sleep was made, and intravenously administered valproic acid (15 mg/kg per day—one in four doses) was initiated. A follow-up EEG performed after 24 hours demonstrated disappearance of epileptiform activity, with some slowing. He was maintained on oral valproic acid (30 mg/kg per day) and, three months later, was able to stand up independently and verbalize a few words. He was more interested in his surroundings and able to follow simple commands. An EEG obtained during sleep was normal.

## FACTORS PREDISPOSING TO NONCONVULSIVE STATUS EPILEPTICUS

## SYNDROMES COMPLICATED BY NONCONVULSIVE STATUS EPILEPTICUS

### *Chromosomal and genetic abnormalities*

NCSE may be associated with chromosomal and genetic abnormalities resulting in syndromes such as ring chromosome 20 syndrome, Wolf-Hirschhorn syndrome (4p deletion), and congenital bilateral perisylvian polymicrogyria. Ring chromosome 20 syndrome is characterized by mild to moderate learning disability, behavior disorders, intractable epileptic seizures, and dysmorphic features including microcephaly, strabismus, micrognathia, downslanting eyelids, and ear abnormalities. Although still considered rare, this syndrome is increasingly diagnosed. One report has characterized 6 cases with epilepsy (16). All had frequent episodes of NCSE resistant to antiepileptic drug (AED) therapy. The episodes consisted of a prolonged confusional state, with or without additional motor seizures. Only one patient was mentally retarded. This 28-year-old woman with an IQ of 47 (verbal IQ: 54; performance: 56) developed seizures at the age of 7 years. She had two types of seizures, each occurring daily. One, usually lasting one to two minutes, consisted of complex motor automatisms with increased tone, downward retraction of the mouth, eye opening, and an appearance of fearfulness. The other seizures were episodes of fluctuating consciousness lasting 20 to 30 minutes, occurring two to three times daily. The ictal EEG showed bursts of diffuse high-voltage slow waves or spike-and-wave complexes. The interictal EEG showed bilateral diffuse high-voltage slow waves or spike-and-wave complexes and bilateral frontal spikes. There was no abnormal finding on the brain magnetic resonance imaging scans, but single-photon emission computed tomography showed decreased perfusion of the right frontotemporal region interictally. Seizures were extremely difficult to control with AEDs. See also Chapter 17.

An 8-year-old girl with Wolf-Hirschhorn syndrome, born at term by normal delivery, had peculiar facial features and a poor suck since birth (14). At 24 months, she presented with growth and developmental delay (weight and height below the third percentile), dysmorphic features including microcephaly, "Greek helmet" facies, and cleft lip and palate, suggesting Wolf-Hirschhorn syndrome that was confirmed by fluorescent in situ hybridization. Epilepsy started during infancy, with myoclonic seizures that progressed gradually to NCSE by 2.5 years of age. NCSE manifested as atypical absences consisting of brief episodes of impairment of consciousness and repetitive head nodding. Congenital bilateral perisylvian polymicrogyria syndrome has also been associated with NCSE, presenting as catatonia or as ASE (8,13).

*Lennox-Gastaut syndrome*

One retrospective study attempted to delineate risk factors associated with outcome in Lennox-Gastaut syndrome (LGS) (17). It reviewed the natural course of the disease over a period of 16 years, EEG changes, and intellectual function in 101 patients. Overall, the intellectual and neurologic outcome was poor. At last follow-up, 38% of the patients could not speak, 21% were unable to walk, and only 4% were free of seizures. Four independent risk factors for severe mental retardation were identified by multivariate analysis (in decreasing order of importance): NCSE (odds ratio [OR] 25.2), a previous diagnosis of West syndrome (OR 11.6), symptomatic etiology (OR 9.5), and an early age at onset of the epilepsy (OR 4.7). These results highlighted the association between NCSE and the severity of mental retardation in patients with LGS. In another report of four patients with LGS and NCSE, benzodiazepine administration resulted in complete recovery in two but was ineffective in the other two (4).

## DRUG-INDUCED NONCONVULSIVE STATUS EPILEPTICUS

Drug-induced NCSE may occur in patients with known epilepsy and in those without previous epilepsy. It is of particular interest in the mentally retarded because they are more likely to receive many of the drugs that may cause NCSE, exhibit behavioral drug-related side effects that can be confused with NCSE, and have abnormal baseline behavior abnormalities that could render recognition of NCSE more difficult.

*Diazepam*

Among 11 mentally retarded patients with NCSE, one report described precipitation of NCSE in three patients (2 with LGS) by intermittent diazepam overadministration (4). Episodes of NCSE recurred periodically several days after large doses of diazepam (30 to 50 mg rectally in 2).

*Tiagabine*

This drug has been strongly associated with NCSE in mentally retarded and normal individuals (8,17). One 30-year-old mildly retarded woman suffered from frequent complex partial seizures since late infancy, despite many AED trials (18). Tiagabine was introduced gradually, and one week after a dose of 1 mg/kg per day was reached, the patient appeared intermittently confused. On examination, she stared, reacted slowly, and answered simple questions with a delay. Ictal EEG showed a diffuse slowing of the background rhythm, with frequent spike-wave discharges. After intravenous administration of 4 mg of lorazepam, the patient's mental status rapidly returned to normal, and the EEG background improved.

*Cephalosporins*

NCSE is an occasional complication of cephalosporin therapy, especially in patients with renal failure (19). One study reported 10 such patients who developed alteration of consciousness without convulsions associated with continuous epileptiform EEG activity while receiving intravenously administered ceftriaxone, ceftazidime, or cefepime (19). They had progressive disorientation or agitation, sometimes associated with mild facial or limb myoclonus, that began 1 to 10 days after starting cephalosporins. Intravenously administered clonazepam suppressed the epileptiform activity completely in 5 patients and partially in the other 5.

*Neuroleptics*

The relationship between neuroleptics and NCSE is difficult to prove, but some case reports suggest that it exists. One 26-year-old patient who developed measles-associated encephalitis at the age of 17 years had a generalized tonic-clonic seizure at the time (12). This patient had mental retardation and complex partial seizure activity with apparent hallucinations, presumably due to NCSE. When the hallucinations were treated with chlorpromazine, the NCSE worsened. Neuroleptic therapy has also been documented to induce myoclonic status epilepticus in a patient with probable Alzheimer disease (20).

## DIAGNOSIS AND ELECTROENCEPHALOGRAPHIC FINDINGS

NCSE is an underrecognized but treatable condition with considerable associated morbidity. The diagnosis may be particularly difficult to make in mentally retarded or previously encephalopathic patients due to their baseline abnormal cognitive and behavior status. A high level of suspicion is essential to establish an early diagnosis with urgent EEG. Intravenous administration of benzodiazepines is very helpful diagnostically but, as reported previously in this book, some patients may not respond to the first treatment, and other AEDs may be needed.

Based on a group of 11 mentally retarded patients (aged 19 to 65 years), Brodtkorb et al proposed a classification of NCSE, based on ictal EEG patterns and epilepsy syndrome diagnoses (Table 19.1) (4). See also Chapter 2. Another EEG feature reported in the mentally retarded (described also in the dementia and cognitive dysfunction section) consists of ictal monomorphic alpha activity with a generalized distribution (6).

## TREATMENT

### BENZODIAZEPINES

Several randomized controlled trials show that benzodiazepines should be the initial therapy in patients with convulsive status epilepticus, but there are no controlled studies on the use of benzodiazepines in NCSE, whether in mentally retarded or mentally normal patients. Treatment has evolved as new medications have become available. At present, with few exceptions, it is generally agreed that the first drug to

**TABLE 19.1** CLASSIFICATION OF NCSE, BASED ON ICTAL EEG PATTERNS AND EPILEPSY SYNDROME DIAGNOSES

1. Nonconvulsive status epilepticus in generalized epilepsy syndromes—These patients had generalized seizure types, generalized ictal and interictal EEG changes, and no clinical evidence of a localized brain lesion. They were all diagnosed with the cryptogenic form of the LGS persisting into adulthood.
2. Nonconvulsive status epilepticus localization-related epilepsy
   a. With localized electroencephalographic features—These patients had focal epileptiform abnormalities on EEG. The clinical picture was dominated by sudden change in mental status with disorientation and mutism.
   b. With generalized EEG features—These patients had nearly continuous, bilaterally synchronous, epileptiform activity on EEG, without laterality. Complex automatisms dominated the clinical picture. In most cases, the onset of the epilepsy dated to an encephalitis.
   c. With transitional EEG features—In these patients, NCSE seemed to represent a transition between groups 2a and 2b. The EEG pattern during status alternated between focal and generalized epileptiform discharges. Clinical manifestations were consistent with cycling between the two seizure phases.
3. Undetermined NCSE—In these patients, the level of consciousness was continuously reduced without automatisms. Ictal EEG recordings showed bilaterally synchronous seizure activity with frontal predominance. NCSE in these patients was unclassifiable by EEG and other investigations, and the epilepsy syndromes could not be determined.

*Based on the study of Brodtkorb E, Sand T, Kristiansen A, and Torbergsen T (4). **Abbreviations:** NCSE, nonconvulsive status epilepticus; EEG, electroencephalogram; LGS, Lenox-Gastaut syndrome.*

be used for NCSE in the mentally retarded is an intravenously administered benzodiazepine, usually lorazepam or diazepam. Intravenously administered fosphenytoin, phenytoin, or valproate may follow next. If NCSE is resistant to first- and second-line treatments, then newer AEDs, or combinations of anesthetics and intravenously or enterally administered AEDs may be needed (22). It is not clear if patients with NCSE and mental retardation respond any differently, as compared with patients without mental retardation. Selecting a specific AED for the treatment of seizures in those with mental retardation requires a balance of the drug's likely efficacy for both seizures and comorbid disorders versus adverse events.

### VALPROATE AND VALPROATE-LAMOTRIGINE COMBINATION

For almost 40 years, valproate has been available for the treatment of generalized and partial seizures, convulsive or nonconvulsive. It is used in the treatment of epilepsy in the multiply handicapped and mentally retarded (14,23). Importantly, however, before clinicians initiate the use of valproate in the mentally retarded, they must rule out metabolic disorders that increase the risk of hepatotoxicity in patients who take valproate. At times, the combination of valproate and lamotrigine may be particularly effective. Bauer and colleagues described two patients, aged 29 and 55 years, who had suffered from epilepsy since the age of 1 and 40 years, respectively (6). The first patient was mentally retarded, whereas the second had normal psychomotor development. NCSE started and ended abruptly, clinically as well as electroencephalographically. In both patients, lamotrigine added to valproate showed significant efficacy in NCSE.

### CARBAMAZEPINE

One 50-year-old man with mental retardation and right hemiparesis developed mental and physical deterioration mimicking dementia (5). The EEG showed marked epileptic activity, but introduction of carbamazepine resulted in rapid and long-term improvement. Carbamazepine has been used as monotherapy in NCSE, but it may also precipitate or exacerbate NCSE, particularly ASE, and should generally be avoided in that condition.

### LEVETIRACETAM

Adjunctive levetiracetam therapy has been used for patients with convulsive status epilepticus and, less frequently, NCSE. In two cases of NCSE following infusion of ifosfamide chemotherapy, both patients developed confusion, lethargy, and speech deterioration on the third day of treatment, responded to intravenously administered diazepam (10 mg), and received levetiracetam as maintenance therapy (24). Another 6 patients with status epilepticus of various types (convulsive, focal, and nonconvulsive) that was refractory to treatment with at least two AEDs had complete cessation of seizures following oral administration of levetiracetam (25). Seizure control was achieved within 12 to 96 hours, and no significant adverse events were noted.

### SULTHIAME

A single case report suggests that sulthiame (10 mg/kg per day) may be effective in the treatment of "idiopathic" continuous spike-wave in slow-wave sleep syndrome (26).

### KETAMINE

In one study, ketamine, an NMDA-receptor antagonist, was orally administered to 5 children with severe epilepsy (LGS, myoclonic-astatic epilepsy, progressive myoclonic epilepsy, and pseudo-Lennox syndrome) during episodes of NCSE (27). Clinical and EEG resolution of NCSE was documented, without any significant adverse effects, in all cases within 24 to 48 hours of starting ketamine.

## OUTCOME AND LONG-TERM PROGNOSIS

The prognosis of patients with NCSE usually depends on the underlying etiology of the seizure activity. In humans with mental retardation, long-term effects of NCSE are largely undetermined, and their significance remains a subject of debate. The neurologic function of most reported cases has returned to baseline, but several well-described patients have had prolonged memory deficits. The significance of other deficits is difficult to interpret in light of the usual concomitant and underlying diseases causing neurologic dysfunction. Most morbidity appears to be attributable to the underlying illnesses rather than to the NCSE itself (3). There are data to suggest that surviving a first episode of NCSE could lower the mortality and morbidity rates associated with subsequent episodes, indicating again that underlying etiology, rather than NCSE per se, is the major determinant of outcome (3). Still, there are many other important prognostic factors. These include the initial episode of status epilepticus, the number of acute life-threatening medical problems on presentation, and a generalized EEG pattern (28). See also Chapters 20 to 22.

Litt and colleagues prospectively identified 25 episodes of altered mentation and NCSE associated with generalized, focal, or bihemispheric epileptiform EEG patterns in critically ill elderly patients (28). Thirteen resulted in death, and 12 patients survived to discharge. Death was associated with a number of acute, life-threatening medical problems on presentation and with a generalized EEG pattern. Treatment with intravenously administered benzodiazepines was associated with an increased risk of death. Higher doses or a greater number of AEDs did not improve outcome.

## REFERENCES

1. Walker M, Cross H, Smith S, Young C, Aicardi J, Appleton R, Aylett S, Besag F, Cock H, DeLorenzo R, Drislane F, Duncan J, Ferrie C, Fujikawa D, Gray W, Kaplan P, Koutroumanidis M, O'Regan M, Plouin P, Sander J, Scott R, Shorvon S, Treiman D, Wasterlain C, Wieshmann U. Nonconvulsive status epilepticus: Epilepsy Research Foundation workshop reports. Epileptic Disord 2005;7:253-296.
2. Kaplan PW. Assessing the outcomes in patients with nonconvulsive status epilepticus: nonconvulsive status epilepticus is underdiagnosed, potentially overtreated, and confounded by comorbidity. J Clin Neurophysiol 1999;16:341-352; discussion 353.
3. Walker MC. Diagnosis and treatment of nonconvulsive status epilepticus. CNS Drugs 2001;15:931-939.
4. Brodtkorb E, Sand T, Kristiansen A, Torbergsen T. Non-convulsive status epilepticus in the adult mentally retarded. Classification and role of benzodiazepines. Seizure 1993;2:115-123.
5. Tomka-Hoffmeister M, Huber B, Seidel M. Atypical epilepsy symptomatology as cause of a dementia like state in a mentally and physically retarded patient. Fortschr Neurol Psychiatr 2004;72:160-163.
6. Bauer J, Neumann M, Kolmel HW, Elger CE. Ictal generalized rhythmic alpha activity during non-convulsive status epilepticus. Eur J Neurol 2000;7:735-734.
7. Lim J, Yagnik P, Schraeder P, Wheeler S. Ictal catatonia as a manifestation of nonconvulsive status epilepticus. J Neurol Neurosurg Psychiatry 1986;49:833-836.
8. Piccinelli P, Borgatti R, Perucca E, Tofani A, Donati G, Balottin U. Frontal nonconvulsive status epilepticus associated with high-dose tiagabine therapy in a child with familial bilateral perisylvian polymicrogyria. Epilepsia 2000;41:1485-1488.
9. Louis ED and Pflaster NL. Catatonia mimicking nonconvulsive status epilepticus. Epilepsia 1995;36:943-945.
10. Takaya S, Matsumoto R, Namiki C, Kiyosu H, Isono O, Hashikawa K, Ikeda A, Fukuyama H. Frontal nonconvulsive status epilepticus manifesting somatic hallucinations. J Neurol Sci 2005;15:234(1-2):25-29.
11. Mikati MA, Lee WL, DeLong GR. Protracted epileptiform encephalopathy: an unusual form of partial complex status epilepticus. Epilepsia 1985;26:563-571.
12. Brodtkorb E, Sand T, Strandjord RE. Neuroleptic and antiepileptic treatment in the mentally retarded. Seizure 1993;2:205-211.
13. Tagawa T, Itagaki Y, Kobayashi M, Sano T, Sumi K. Nonconvulsive status epilepticus in a child with congenital bilateral perisylvian syndrome. Pediatr Neurol 1999;21:579-582.
14. Valente KD, Freitas A, Fiore LA, Kim CA. A study of EEG and epilepsy profile in Wolf-Hirschhorn syndrome and considerations

regarding its correlation with other chromosomal disorders. Brain Dev 2003;25:283-287.
15. Dirik E, Yis U, Hudaoglu O, Kurul S. Nonconvulsive status epilepticus and neurodevelopmental delay. Pediatr Neurol 2006;35:209-212.
16. Inoue Y, Fujiwara T, Matsuda K, Kubota H, Tanaka M, Yagi K, Yamamori K, Takahashi Y. Ring chromosome 20 and nonconvulsive status epilepticus. A new epileptic syndrome. Brain 1997;120(Pt 6):939-953.
17. Hoffmann-Riem M, Diener W, Benninger C, Rating D, Unnebrink K, Stephani U, Ernst HP, Korinthenberg R. Nonconvulsive status epilepticus, a possible cause of mental retardation in patients with Lennox-Gastaut syndrome. Neuropediatrics 2000;31:169-174.
18. Imperiale D, Pignatta P, Cerrato P, Montalenti E, Ravetti C, Benna P. Nonconvulsive status epilepticus due to a de novo contralateral focus during tiagabine adjunctive therapy. Seizure 2003;12:319-222.
19. Martinez-Rodriguez JE, Barriga FJ, Santamaria J, Iranzo A, Pareja JA, Revilla M, dela Rosa CR. Nonconvulsive status epilepticus associated with cephalosporins in patients with renal failure. Am J Med 2001;11:115-119.
20. Camacho A, Garcia-Navarro M, Martinez B, Villarejo A, Pomares E. Olanzapine-induced myoclonic status. Clin Neuropharmacol 2005;28:145-147.
21. Delpont E, Thomas P, Gugenheim J, Chichmanian RM, Mahagne MH, Suisse G, Dolisi C. Prolonged confusion syndrome in the course of cyclosporine treatment: a state of confusion? Neurophysiol Clin 1990;20:207-215.
22. Ruegg SJ, Dichter MA. Diagnosis and treatment of nonconvulsive status epilepticus in an intensive care unit setting. Curr Treat Options Neurol 2003;5:93-110.
23. Pellock JM. Treatment considerations: traditional antiepileptic drugs. Epilepsy Behav 2002;3:18-23.
24. Kilickap S, Cakar M, Onal IK, Tufan A, Akoglu H, Aksoy S, Erman M, Tekuzman G. Nonconvulsive status epilepticus due to ifosfamide. Ann Pharmacother 2006;40:332-335.
25. Patel NC, Landan IR, Levin J, Szaflarski J, Wilner AN. The use of levetiracetam in refractory status epilepticus. Seizure 2006;15:137-141.
26. Wirrell E, Ho AW, Hamiwka L. Sulthiame therapy for continuous spike and wave in slow-wave sleep. Pediatr Neurol 2006;35:204-208.
27. Mewasingh LD, Sekhara T, Aeby A, Christiaens FJ, Dan B. Oral ketamine in paediatric non-convulsive status epilepticus. Seizure 2003;2:483-489.
28. Litt B, Wityk RJ, Hertz SH, Mullen PD, Weiss H, Ryan DD, Henry TR. Nonconvulsive status epilepticus in the critically ill elderly. Epilepsia 1998;39:1194-1202.

PART VI

# MANAGEMENT AND PROGNOSIS OF NONCONVULSIVE STATUS EPILEPTICUS

CHAPTER 20

# PRINCIPLES OF TREATMENT OF NONCONVULSIVE STATUS EPILEPTICUS

MATHEW C. WALKER

Nonconvulsive status epilepticus (NCSE) encompasses a range of conditions with different pathophysiologies and varying prognoses (1). It is therefore difficult to make general recommendations. Further, the area is complicated by a surfeit of opinion and a lack of evidence (2). The main debate lies in how aggressively we should treat these conditions; this undoubtedly depends upon the type of NCSE and its circumstance (as will be discussed later in this chapter). In most instances, the delay to achieving adequate serum concentrations of antiepileptic drugs (AEDs) comes not from the route of administration (oral vs intravenous), but from the delay in making the diagnosis. Thus, if there is one overwhelming principle of treatment, it is to make the diagnosis as rapidly as possible.

The approach to treatment is largely determined by the morbidity and mortality associated with the status epilepticus balanced against the potential mortality and morbidity of treatment. Three key observations shape our treatment regimens:

1. Continuous seizure activity is associated with neuronal damage.
2. The longer the seizures continue, the more difficult they are to treat.
3. The drugs we use have different pharmacokinetic profiles when given acutely, compared with chronic administration, and are often cardiorespiratory depressants.

I will discuss each of these issues before describing treatments in specific forms of NCSE.

## NEURONAL DAMAGE IN STATUS EPILEPTICUS

Considerable animal evidence indicates that continuous electrographic seizure activity, even without convulsions or physiologic compromise, leads to neuronal damage (3,4) and that this damage is more severe the longer that seizures continue (5). Because animal models of NCSE have been proposed to replicate the human condition, it has been assumed that NCSE inevitably results in neuronal damage in humans. This is frequently used as an argument for aggressive treatment of status epilepticus. We should, however, be careful in defining both the type of NCSE and the setting in which it occurs. There is no evidence of pathologic damage or long-term behavior effects in an animal model of absence status epilepticus (ASE) (6), and this is largely supported by human data, which demonstrate no morbidity or mortality with ASE de novo (7). ASE is therefore likely to be relatively benign.

What about complex partial status epilepticus (CPSE)? This undoubtedly causes significant and severe neuronal damage in a variety of animal models (8). The methods of seizure generation in animals, however, do not easily translate to the human condition. Status epilepticus is induced in animals with either powerful chemoconvulsants or prolonged high-frequency repetitive stimulation. This is very different from the human condition. Furthermore, human CPSE is often characterized by lower-frequency discharges (9); reproducing this in animal models produces substantially less neuronal damage than do high-frequency discharges (10). CPSE in humans often occurs in the setting of prior epilepsy and prior treatment with AEDs; if such conditions (prior epilepsy or prior treatment with AEDs) are reproduced in animal models, then CPSE results in far less neuronal damage (11-13). Thus, prior AED use and a history of epilepsy may confer significant neuroprotection. Finally, CPSE in humans often results from an acute precipitant, such as stroke or encephalitis, and, in many cases, the etiology will likely cause much more damage than the seizure activity.

Reports from human data of CPSE causing neuronal damage are confounded by limited follow-up, etiology, concomitant illness, and treatment. Importantly, large case series of prolonged CPSE with no neurologic sequelae have been published (14). Even in the absence of an acute neurologic insult, CPSE results in significant rises in serum neuron-specific enolase, a marker for acute neuronal injury (15,16). However, the rises in serum neuron-specific enolase could partially be the result of a breakdown in the blood-brain barrier rather than an increase in neuronal death; thus, cerebrospinal fluid levels of neuron-specific enolase would be a more accurate indicator of neuronal damage (17). The degree to which serum levels of neuron-specific enolase correlate with neurologic and cognitive disability in CPSE is unknown, and it is unknown whether the results of these studies hold for the majority of patients. Neuroimaging has also been inconclusive; reversible changes do occur, and, in some selected patients, mild atrophy can be associated with CPSE (18).

## PROGRESSIVE DIFFICULTY IN TREATMENT

As status epilepticus progresses, it becomes increasingly more difficult to treat (19-21). This loss of drug efficacy is especially evident with benzodiazepines, the ED50 which increases 10-fold from 10 to 40 minutes of seizure activity (19). This appears to be due to an internalization of benzodiazepine-sensitive GABAA receptors with prolonged seizure activity (22,23). A further contributor to the progressive drug resistance of NCSE may also be the seizure-induced upregulation of multidrug transporters (24,25), which prevent drugs from reaching adequate levels at their target.

## ACUTE NEUROPHARMACOKINETICS

With parenteral administration, a drug directly enters the central (blood) compartment from where it is distributed to peripheral compartments, in particular, fat and muscle. Since most drugs given for status epilepticus are highly lipid soluble, they are rapidly redistributed into the peripheral compartment from the central compartment. This leads to an initial drop in plasma concentrations, which can be quantified as a distribution half-life. Drugs in the central compartment are also either excreted unchanged or metabolized, and this can be quantified as the elimination half-life. Many of the AEDs used in status epilepticus have a much shorter distribution half-life than elimination half-life; this can result in a very rapid initial fall in plasma levels and, consequently, brain levels following acute administration. This has led to the practice of repeat boluses and infusions to maintain adequate plasma levels. With repetitive administration, however, drugs accumulate within the peripheral compartment, and this results in two important effects (26): (1) a fall in the volume of distribution that results in higher peak levels with subsequent boluses or with continued infusions and (2) the clearance from the central compartment becomes dependent on elimination, resulting in a significant increase in apparent half-life.

These two effects are potentially very dangerous, and some of the mortality and morbidity of status epilepticus is due to injudicious use of repeated boluses or continuous infusions of lipid-soluble drugs. It has also influenced our choice of drugs that are used in status epilepticus. Diazepam has a very short distribution half-life (less than 30 minutes) but a long elimination half-life (30 hours), and, therefore, with acute administration, there is a high chance of seizure recurrence (50% within two hours)

(27,28), but, with repetitive boluses, there is a high chance of accumulation, prolonged action, higher peak levels, and cardiorespiratory arrest. Lorazepam may be preferable, as it has a long distribution half-life (3-10 hours) and, therefore, less chance of seizure recurrence (27,29).

When it comes to anesthesia in status epilepticus, different pharmacokinetic properties are needed. Barbiturates have a great propensity to accumulate with prolonged infusion, leading to long recovery times after infusions. Propofol is advantageous in that its volume of distribution is so large that accumulation is not such a problem, but, consequently, stopping propofol can result in rapid decreases in serum concentrations and rebound seizures (propofol infusions therefore have to be tapered slowly) (30,31).

## TYPICAL ABSENCE STATUS EPILEPTICUS

Typical ASE needs to be distinguished from CPSE and atypical absences seen in other syndromes. This term should perhaps be reserved for prolonged absence seizures with continuous or discontinuous 3-Hz spike and waves occurring in patients with primary generalized epilepsy (32). There is, however, late-onset ASE developing de novo, usually following drug or alcohol withdrawal (7). There is also some overlap with myoclonic status epilepticus in juvenile myoclonic epilepsy in which there is often a combination of absences and myoclonus. Some have referred to this as atypical ASE, but this term should probably be reserved for atypical absences in specific epilepsy syndromes with learning difficulties—see later in this chapter and in Chapter 19.

There is no evidence that ASE induces neuronal damage, and, thus, aggressive treatment is rarely warranted (32). Treatment can be administered either intravenously or orally. ASE responds rapidly to intravenously administered benzodiazepines, and, in my experience, lorazepam, 1 mg, administered intravenously during the EEG recording is usually sufficient, but, occasionally, higher doses (up to 4 mg) need to be used. The effect may be only transient, and a longer-acting AED may need to be given. If intravenous treatment is required, but benzodiazepines are either ineffective or contraindicated, then intravenously administered valproate (20-40 mg/kg) can be given; this is well tolerated in the elderly (33,34). Inappropriate prescription of AEDs (especially carbamazepine) in idiopathic generalized epilepsies can precipitate ASE (35). Withdrawal of these drugs is necessary; otherwise, the status epilepticus may appear to be refractory to treatment (35). Also, if the ASE has been precipitated by AED withdrawal, then the withdrawn drug should usually be reintroduced. In most cases, orally administered medication suffices. If a precipitating factor can be identified in late-onset de novo cases, then long-term therapy is not usually indicated (7). Patients with idiopathic generalized epilepsy often have repeated episodes of ASE despite optimization of treatment. This seems to be especially true with certain syndromes, including absences with eyelid myoclonus, idiopathic generalized epilepsy with phantom absences, and juvenile myoclonic epilepsy (32). In such cases, the patient should have access to orally administered benzodiazepines at home (diazepam 5-10 mg, clobazam 10 mg, or clonazepam 0.5 mg) or rectally, buccally, or nasally administered benzodiazepines, if it is not possible for the patient to take the benzodiazepines orally.

## COMPLEX PARTIAL STATUS EPILEPTICUS

The treatment of CPSE is hotly debated. First, it has to be correctly diagnosed, and even this is not straightforward. Criteria for diagnosis are unclear. CPSE has to be differentiated not only from other forms of NCSE, but also from postictal states and other neurologic and psychiatric conditions. The use of electroencephalography (EEG) may be helpful, but the scalp EEG changes may often be nonspecific, and the diagnosis is very much clinical in nature (see Chapters 4 and 5). NCSE with a generalized EEG pattern can occasionally be due to an initial focus that may become apparent only after treatment, and confusion about diagnosis and treatment has arisen in the literature from muddling idiopathic generalized status epilepticus (e.g., ASE) with focal status epilepticus with generalized EEG abnormalities—which, from the treatment viewpoint, should be considered as a form of CPSE. Further, there is difficulty in differentiating CPSE from electrographic status epilepticus in coma, which can have both focal and generalized EEG features. From the treatment perspective, I have considered this separately as NCSE in coma, partly because of its very poor prognosis (36).

The main factors in deciding how CPSE needs to be treated are the prognosis of the condition and whether any specific treatment improves this prognosis. Unfortunately, both of these considerations are inadequately studied. As in all epilepsies, the prognosis relates partly to the prognosis of the underlying etiology and any concomitant medical conditions. The question of the associated morbidity of the epilepsy itself remains at present unresolved.

Undoubtedly, the setting in which the CPSE occurs is paramount. Those patients with a prior diagnosis of epilepsy have a much lower mortality and morbidity than do those with CPSE in the setting of an acute medical illness (37). Therefore, acutely precipitated CPSE and CPSE in the setting of a person with epilepsy should be considered separately. CPSE in patients with epilepsy is usually a benign condition; patients commonly have repeated episodes with little evidence of permanent cognitive or neurologic deficits (38). These episodes respond to orally administered benzodiazepines, such as clobazam (39). A notable observation is that there is often a delayed clinical response despite EEG resolution, probably because the patient enters a postictal state. In the hospital setting, EEG is therefore helpful to monitor response to treatment.

Intravenously administered benzodiazepines, such as lorazepam, can be used if more rapid resolution of the status epilepticus is required, and response can be easily monitored with EEG. Because many patients have recurrent episodes of CPSE (38), a specific treatment plan with oral administration of benzodiazepines over a period of 2 to 3 days (even administered at home) can usually abort the status epilepticus.

In patients with acute precipitated CPSE, early recognition is a critical goal because the delay in adequate treatment usually results from failure to diagnose the condition rather than choice of therapeutic strategy (intravenous versus oral drug loading). The usual management for such patients has been similar to that of patients with convulsive status epilepticus, with intravenously administered benzodiazepine followed by intravenous phenytoin loading (40).

The medications commonly used to treat status epilepticus are not without adverse effects and can result in hypotension, respiratory depression, and, on occasion, cardiorespiratory depression. These effects are more pronounced with intravenous administration, due to rapid high serum levels. In an uncontrolled, nonrandomized study, intravenously administered benzodiazepines worsened the prognosis in a group of critically ill elderly patients, and aggressive treatment in the intensive care unit prolonged hospitalization (41). Intravenously administered valproate has been shown to be well tolerated with few cardiorespiratory adverse effects and, thus, may offer an advantage over intravenously administered benzodiazepines (34). The use of general anesthesia to treat CPSE remains a matter for speculation, and, in conscious patients, it should probably be avoided. Other possible treatments that can be considered are loading with topiramate (42) or levetiracetam (43), which is now available as a parenteral formulation, or both. Foremost, however, is treatment of the underlying condition (e.g., encephalitis, vasculitis, autoimmune syndrome, or metabolic derangement), as this often leads to resolution of the status epilepticus. Indeed, these particular etiologies need to be considered, and suitable investigations instigated. If no etiology is identified, a trial of high-dose steroids may be worth trying in refractory cases. Another etiologic factor that must be taken into account is the use of recreational (44) and prescribed drugs. The use of a wide range of medications is associated with CPSE, ranging from lithium (45) to certain antibiotics (46), and stopping of these can aid in resolving the status epilepticus.

## NONCONVULSIVE STATUS EPILEPTICUS IN LEARNING DIFFICULTIES

The most common form of NCSE in patients with learning difficulties is CPSE, but there are specific forms of status epilepticus that are associated with epilepsy syndromes in which learning difficulties form a part, e.g., Lennox-Gastaut syndrome (LGS). These can be usefully divided into status epilepticus occurring during slow-wave sleep, atypical ASE, and tonic status epilepticus. In the epileptic encephalopathies, it is appealing to speculate that the diffuse and ongoing electrographic seizure activity in these syndromes is in some way responsible for the concomitant mental deterioration via excitotoxic mechanisms, but there is no direct evidence for this.

## ELECTRICAL STATUS EPILEPTICUS DURING SLEEP

Electrical status epilepticus during sleep (ESES) is characterized by spike-and-wave discharges in 85% to 100 % of non-rapid eye movement sleep (47,48). This phenomenon is associated with certain epilepsy syndromes, including Landau-Kleffner syndrome and LGS, continuous spikes and waves during sleep, and even "benign" epilepsy with centrotemporal spikes. The clinical spectrum, response to treatment, and definition of these syndromes are still debated. ESES can also occur in the setting of an autistic syndrome alone without overt clinical seizures. There is a spectrum of developmental delay and deterioration associated with ESES, from none to severe, and patients with benign epilepsy with centrotemporal spikes with ESES can have marked associated neuropsychologic problems (belying the term 'benign') that resolve with AED treatment. ESES has a poor response to treatment with phenytoin, phenobarbital, and carbamazepine, which can precipitate or worsen this condition. This is especially important because these drugs are often used as first-line therapies in the treatment of partial epilepsy. Low-dose orally administered clobazam or clonazepam has been reported to result in a marked improvement in ESES, associated with neuropsychologic improvement (47,48). If benzodiazepines fail to resolve the symptoms, then treatment with steroids or, in refractory cases, subpial transection should be considered (49). Again, recognition of the condition is paramount, and an overnight sleep EEG should be performed in all children with epilepsy who show regression of language, unexplained behavior changes, or neuropsychologic regression.

## ATYPICAL ABSENCE STATUS EPILEPTICUS

Atypical ASE is associated with the epileptic encephalopathies such as LGS. This condition is usually poorly responsive to intravenously administered benzodiazepines, which should, in any case, be given cautiously because they can induce tonic status epilepticus in these patients (50). Orally rather than intravenously administered treatment is usually more appropriate, and the drugs of choice are valproate, lamotrigine, topiramate, clonazepam, and clobazam. Sedating medications, carbamazepine, and vigabatrin have been reported to worsen atypical absences.

## TONIC STATUS EPILEPTICUS

Tonic status epilepticusis not uncommon in patients with syndromes such as LGS. The tonic seizures may not necessarily be clinically apparent. The EEG, however, demonstrates bursts of paroxysmal, generalized fast discharges. Tonic status epilepticus is poorly responsive to conventional treatment. It can be worsened with benzodiazepines, which should be used with care. Sedating medication can worsen all seizure types in LGS and, thus, should be avoided. Orally administered lamotrigine can be effective in terminating tonic status epilepticus. In LGS, both ACTH and corticosteroids are helpful in the emergency treatment of status epilepticusof all types.

## NONCONVULSIVE STATUS EPILEPTICUS IN COMA

Electrographic status epilepticus in coma is not uncommon. NCSE in coma occurs in three groups of patients: those who had convulsive status epilepticus, those who have subtle clinical signs of seizure activity, and those with no clinical signs of seizure activity (51). Convulsive status epilepticus has, as part of its evolution, subtle status epilepticus in which there is minimal or no motor activity but on-going electrical activity (52). This condition should be treated aggressively with deep anesthesia and concomitant AEDs. The association of electrographic status epilepticus with subtle motor activity often follows hypoxic brain activity and has a poor prognosis, but aggressive therapy, as mentioned earlier in this chapter, is possibly justified because the little available evidence indicates that such treatment improves prognosis. Electrographic status epilepticus with no overt clinical signs is difficult to interpret—does it represent status epilepticus or widespread cortical damage? Since these patients have a poor prognosis, aggressive treatment is recommended in the hope that it may improve outcome. Lastly, there is a group of patients in whom there are clinical signs of repetitive movements but no electrographic seizure activity, and, in these patients, treatment with AEDs and aggressive sedation is not recommended.

## CONCLUSION

The most important principle underlying the treatment of NCSE is prompt diagnosis. Too often, patients languish, sometimes for days, before the diagnosis is even considered. In my experience, this delay is significantly greater than the hour or so delay introduced by administering oral rather than intravenous therapy. Delay in diagnosis may contribute to drug resistance, neuronal damage, and morbidity.

Resolution of NCSE often results once the underlying cause is treated, and failure to treat the underlying cause can lead to apparent drug resistance. Further, the underlying cause can often be the injudicious use of certain AEDs (e.g., carbamazepine in idiopathic generalized epilepsy). The question about how aggressively to treat once the diagnosis is made remains unresolved. It is critical to realize, however, that the treatments we give are not benign and that, on occasion, may be worse than the disease. This is especially so if anesthesia is used in the more benign forms of NCSE. Thus, the treatment approach that I recommend is more conservative than that of some other commentators, but, until we have more concrete evidence for aggressive treatment, I feel it is best to err on the side of caution.

## REFERENCES


1. Walker MC. Diagnosis and treatment of nonconvulsive status epilepticus. CNS Drugs 2001;15:931-939.
2. Kaplan PW. Assessing the outcomes in patients with nonconvulsive status epilepticus: nonconvulsive status epilepticus is underdiagnosed, potentially overtreated, and confounded by comorbidity. J Clin Neurophysiol 1999;16:341-352; discussion 353.
3. Meldrum BS. Excitotoxicity and selective neuronal loss in epilepsy. Brain Pathol 1993;3:405-412.
4. Olney JW, Collins RC, Sloviter RS. Excitotoxic mechanisms of epileptic brain damage. Adv Neurol 1986;44:857-877.
5. Fujikawa DG. The temporal evolution of neuronal damage from pilocarpine-induced status epilepticus. Brain Res 1996;725:11.
6. Wong M, Wozniak DF, Yamada KA. An animal model of generalized nonconvulsive status epilepticus: immediate characteristics and long-term effects. Exp Neurol 2003;183:87-99.
7. Thomas P, Beaumanoir A, Genton P, Dolisi C, Chatel M. 'De novo' absence status of late onset: report of 11 cases. Neurology 1992;42:104-110.
8. Walker MC, White HS, Sander JW. Disease modification in partial epilepsy. Brain 2002;125:1937-1950.

9. Granner MA, Lee SI. Nonconvulsive status epilepticus: EEG analysis in a large series. Epilepsia 1994;35:42-47.
10. Krsek P, Mikulecka A, Druga R, Hlinak Z, Kubova H, Mares P. An animal model of nonconvulsive status epilepticus: a contribution to clinical controversies. Epilepsia 2001;42:171-180.
11. Kelly ME, McIntyre DC. Hippocampal kindling protects several structures from the neuronal damage resulting from kainic acid-induced status epilepticus. Brain Res 1994;634:245-256.
12. Pitkanen A, Nissinen J, Jolkkonen E, Tuunanen J, Halonen T. Effects of vigabatrin treatment on status epilepticus-induced neuronal damage and mossy fiber sprouting in the rat hippocampus. Epilepsy Res 1999;33:67-85.
13. Najm IM, Hadam J, Ckakraverty D, Mikuni N, Penrod C, Sopa C, Markarian G, Luders HO, Babb T, Baudry M. A short episode of seizure activity protects from status epilepticus-induced neuronal damage in rat brain. Brain Res 1998;810:72-75.
14. Williamson PD, Spencer DD, Spencer SS, Novelly RA, Mattson RH. Complex partial status epilepticus: a depth-electrode study. Ann Neurol 1985;18:647-654.
15. DeGiorgio CM, Gott PS, Rabinowicz AL, Heck CN, Smith TD, Correale JD. Neuron-specific enolase, a marker of acute neuronal injury, is increased in complex partial status epilepticus. Epilepsia 1996;37:606-609.
16. DeGiorgio CM, Heck CN, Rabinowicz AL, Gott PS, Smith T, Correale J. Serum neuron-specific enolase in the major subtypes of status epilepticus. Neurology 1999;52:746-749.
17. Correale J, Rabinowicz AL, Heck CN, Smith TD, Loskota WJ, DeGiorgio CM. Status epilepticus increases CSF levels of neuron-specific enolase and alters the blood-brain barrier. Neurology 1998;50:1388-1391.
18. Lansberg MG, O'Brien MW, Norbash AM, Moseley ME, Morrell M, Albers GW. MRI abnormalities associated with partial status epilepticus. Neurology 1999;52:1021-1027.
19. Kapur J, Macdonald RL. Rapid seizure-induced reduction of benzodiazepine and Zn2+ sensitivity of hippocampal dentate granule cell GABAA receptors. J Neurosci 1997;17:7532-7540.
20. Mazarati AM, Baldwin RA, Sankar R, Wasterlain CG. Time-dependent decrease in the effectiveness of antiepileptic drugs during the course of self-sustaining status epilepticus. Brain Res 1998;814(1-2):179-185.
21. Walton NY, Treiman DM. Response of status epilepticus induced by lithium and pilocarpine to treatment with diazepam. Exp Neurol 1988;101:267-275.
22. Naylor DE, Liu H, Wasterlain CG. Trafficking of GABA(A) receptors, loss of inhibition, and a mechanism for pharmacoresistance in status epilepticus. J Neurosci 2005;25:7724-7733.
23. Goodkin HP, Yeh JL, Kapur J. Status epilepticus increases the intracellular accumulation of $GABA_A$ receptors. J Neurosci 2005;25:5511-5520.
24. Zhang L, Ong WY, Lee T. Induction of P-glycoprotein expression in astrocytes following intracerebroventricular kainate injections. Exp Brain Res 1999;126:509-516.
25. Sisodiya SM, Thom M. Widespread upregulation of drug-resistance proteins in fatal human status epilepticus. Epilepsia 2003;44:261-264.
26. Walker MC, Tong X, Brown S, Shorvon SD, Patsalos PN. Comparison of single- and repeated-dose pharmacokinetics of diazepam. Epilepsia 1998;39:283-289.
27. Walker MC, Sander JW. Benzodiazepines in status epilepticus. In: Trimble MR, Hindmarch I, eds. Benzodiazepines. Petersfield, UK: Wrightson Biomedical, 2000:73-85.
28. Prensky AL, Raff MC, Moore MJ, Schwab RS. Intravenous diazepam in the treatment of prolonged seizure activity. N Engl J Med 1967;276:779-784.
29. Cock HR, Schapira AH. A comparison of lorazepam and diazepam as initial therapy in convulsive status epilepticus. Q J Med 2002;95:225-231.
30. Walker MC. Status epilepticus on the intensive care unit. J Neurol 2003;250:401-406.
31. Walker MC, Smith SJ, Shorvon SD. The intensive care treatment of convulsive status epilepticus in the UK. Results of a national survey and recommendations. Anaesthesia 1995;50:130-135.
32. Shorvon S, Walker M. Status epilepticus in idiopathic generalized epilepsy. Epilepsia 2005;46(Suppl 9):73-79.
33. Berkovic SF, Bladin PF. Absence status in adults. Clin Exp Neurol 1983;19:198-207.
34. Sinha S, Naritoku DK. Intravenous valproate is well tolerated in unstable patients with status epilepticus. Neurology 2000;55:722-724.
35. Thomas P, Valton L, Genton P. Absence and myoclonic status epilepticus precipitated by antiepileptic drugs in idiopathic generalized epilepsy. Brain 2006;129:1281-1292.

36. Towne AR, Waterhouse EJ, Boggs JG, Garnett LK, Brown AJ, Smith JR Jr, DeLorenzo RJ. Prevalence of nonconvulsive status epilepticus in comatose patients. Neurology 2000;54:340-345.
37. Shneker BF, Fountain NB. Assessment of acute morbidity and mortality in nonconvulsive status epilepticus. Neurology 2003;61:1066-1073.
38. Cockerell OC, Walker MC, Sander JW, Shorvon SD. Complex partial status epilepticus: a recurrent problem. J Neurol Neurosurg Psychiatry 1994;57:835-837.
39. Corman C, Guberman A, Benavente O. Clobazam in partial status epilepticus. Seizure 1998;7:243-247.
40. Meierkord H, Boon P, Engelsen B, Göcke K, Shorvon S, Tinuper P, Holtkamp M. EFNS guideline on the management of status epilepticus. Eur J Neurol 2006;13:445-450.
41. Litt B, Wityk RJ, Hertz SH, Mullen PD, Weiss H, Ryan DD, Henry TR. Nonconvulsive status epilepticus in the critically ill elderly. Epilepsia 1998;39:1194-1202.
42. Reuber M, Evans J, Bamford JM. Topiramate in drug-resistant complex partial status epilepticus. Eur J Neurol 2002;9:111-112.
43. Schulze-Bonhage A, Hefft S, Oehl B. Termination of complex partial status epilepticus by intravenous levetiracetam—a case report. J Neurol Neurosurg Psychiatry 2007 (online).
44. Ogunyemi AO, Locke GE, Kramer LD, Nelson L. Complex partial status epilepticus provoked by "crack" cocaine. Ann Neurol 1989;26:785-786.
45. Kaplan PW, Birbeck G. Lithium-induced confusional states: nonconvulsive status epilepticus or triphasic encephalopathy? Epilepsia 2006;47:2071-2074.
46. Primavera A, Cocito L, Audenino D. Nonconvulsive status epilepticus during cephalosporin therapy. Neuropsychobiology 2004;49:218-222.
47. Yan Liu X, Wong V. Spectrum of epileptic syndromes with electrical status epilepticus during sleep in children. Pediatr Neurol 2000;22:371-379.
48. Tassinari CA, Rubboli G, Volpi L, Meletti S, d'Orsi G, Franca M, Sabetta AR, Riguzzi P, Gardella E, Zaniboni A, Michelucci R. Encephalopathy with electrical status epilepticus during slow sleep or ESES syndrome including the acquired aphasia. Clin Neurophysiol 2000;111(Suppl 2):94-102.
49. Irwin K, Birch V, Lees J, Polkey C, Alarcon G, Binnie C, Smedley M, Baird G, Robinson RO. Multiple subpial transection in Landau-Kleffner syndrome. Dev Med Child Neurol 2001;43:248-252.
50. Tassinari CA, Dravet C, Roger J, Cano JP, Gastaut H. Tonic status epilepticus precipitated by intravenous benzodiazepine in five patients with Lennox-Gastaut syndrome. Epilepsia 1972;13:421-435.
51. Lowenstein DH, Aminoff MJ. Clinical and EEG features of status epilepticus in comatose patients. Neurology 1992;42:100-104.
52. Treiman DM. Generalized convulsive status epilepticus in the adult. Epilepsia 1993;34 (Suppl 1):2-11.

CHAPTER 21

# PROGNOSIS AND OUTCOME OF INFANTS AND CHILDREN WITH NONCONVULSIVE STATUS EPILEPTICUS

ALEXIS ARZIMANOGLOU AND EDOUARD HIRSCH

Better delineation of several epilepsy syndromes, particularly in the last decade, and an easier access to video-electroencephalographic (EEG) monitoring (including short-duration laboratory studies for outpatients or in the emergency unit) have facilitated an increased recognition of nonconvulsive status epilepticus (NCSE) in childhood. Particularly in children, however, this condition is highly heterogeneous, in terms of both electroclinical presentation and comorbidities. Consequently, prospective or even retrospective studies on prognosis and outcome are few. Available data are usually from hospital-based series, which also include adult patients or concern specific entities (e.g., Angelman syndrome); this ascertainment bias adversely affects our ability to evaluate the effects of the NCSE itself and to differentiate the effects of NCSE from those of the underlying pathology causing NCSE. This chapter reviews the scant available data and underscores the methodologic problems in studying the outcome and prognosis of NCSE in childhood.

## METHODOLOGIC ISSUES

NCSE in children almost always occurs in those with known epilepsy (1). Such a statement should be interpreted with caution because NCSE is easily mistaken for drowsiness, inattention, or abnormal psychogenic behavior, particularly when the impairment of consciousness is mild. An occasional child may appear normal when first seen, but the parents notice a difference from the child's usual behavior. Prospective, population-based studies are nonexistent, and it is not clear if prolonged monitoring or frequently repeated routine EEGs of children with isolated seizures will increase the yield of detection of NCSE (2). In a recent retrospective review of children who underwent long-term EEG monitoring in a pediatric intensive care unit (3), NCSE occurred mostly in children with prior epilepsy (35%) or with congenital heart disease (25%). Prior to NCSE, most had had isolated seizures (55%) or convulsive status epilepticus (20%), but some had only preceding mental-status change (25%).

Making a clear-cut differentiation between generalized and partial NCSE on clinical or even electroclinical grounds is difficult and often arbitrary, further complicating a proper evaluation of prognosis and outcome. The definition depends on the criteria applied (type of seizures or epilepsy, characteristics of EEG abnormalities, and etiology). The situation is further complicated by several nosology and terminology issues (see also Chapter 12).

In old and current literature, generalized NCSE has been variably termed a*bsence status epilepticus (ASE)* (4), *petit mal status* (5), *spike-wave stupor* (6), *epilepsia minoris continua*, or an *epileptic twilight state*. None of these terms is entirely satisfactory. *ASE* may be inaccurate in cases in which only mild blunting of consciousness or slurred speech is present. *Petit mal status* implies a relationship with childhood absence epilepsy or idiopathic generalized epilepsy (IGE) that does not exist in many cases, and terms like *minor epileptic status* or *twilight state* are nonspecific (1). Some authors distinguish between cases in which the loss of awareness is sufficiently abrupt and marked to resemble typical absences (even though they admit that the degree of unawareness is rarely as profound as in brief typical absences) and those in which the disturbance of consciousness is less marked, or in which it is associated with other manifestations, such as myoclonic jerks or atonic attacks. These authors tend to relate typical ASE to the primary generalized epilepsies with typical absences and atypical ASE to Lennox Gastaut syndrome (LGS) or secondary generalized epilepsies (7). For some, the terms *absence* or *petit mal status* imply a clear change (both clinically and on EEG) at the time of the ictal event (4,5). Others include less distinct states that are marked only by subtle behavior alterations that may last for weeks or months and that may not be reversible (8,9).

Another nosologic issue is raised by the occurrence of episodes of status in children with epilepsies of a clearly partial character that are identical to those observed in primary or secondary generalized epilepsies (1). In such cases, the paroxysmal EEG activity during status is bilateral, although at times asymmetric, and deciding whether the activity should be classified as partial or generalized NCSE is difficult.

The methodologic and nosologic issues noted previously suggest that the prognosis and outcome of NCSE can only be discussed for each individual epilepsy syndrome or, by default, for a spectrum of epileptic disorders with similar predominant characteristics, e.g., for NCSE in children whose seizures at onset suggest LGS or for another form of epilepsy with predominantly myoclonic-astatic seizures or drop attacks.

Distinction must also be made regarding outcome of an ongoing episode of NCSE; risks for recurrence of status epilepticus, epilepsy, or both; and short and long-term consequences for cognition and behavior. Cohort studies including children with the same epilepsy syndrome are also needed to better evaluate if a causative link exists between an eventual cognitive deterioration and the severity of NCSE episodes, or if the characteristics of NCSE episodes reflect the gravity and progression of the underlying disorder.

## TYPICAL ABSENCE STATUS EPILEPTICUS IN CHILDREN

Typical ASE occurs almost exclusively in children with IGE. The essential symptoms are isolated clouding of consciousness of variable degree (the child remaining calm, with little or no spontaneous language or motor activity) and some eyelid jerking. The EEG of repetitive absence seizures shows largely symmetric and bilaterally synchronous spike-waves or polyspike waves faster than 2.5 to 3 Hz. This pattern may become discontinuous during the ongoing event.

If not treated, typical ASE usually lasts for an average of 3 to 4 hours, occasionally as short as 30 minutes, often exceeding 6 to 10 hours, and occasionally for 2 to 10 days. Frequency also varies from once in a lifetime to an average of 10 to 20 episodes per year (10). In children with IGE, inappropriate treatment with antiepileptic drugs (AEDs), such as vigabatrin, carbamazepine, gabapentin, or phenytoin, as well as discontinuation of appropriate anti-absence medications, are the commonest precipitants of typical ASE (10,11). According to Panayiotopoulos, it is rare for typical ASE in IGE to start during the first decade of life (10).

In one third of patients, typical ASE ends with a generalized tonic-clonic seizure. In most cases, spontaneous cessation of typical ASE is sudden, with a striking improvement of consciousness and behavior. It is exceptional for tonic-clonic seizures to precede or be interspersed with ASE (10). Administration of a benzodiazepine (e.g., buccal or intranasal midazolam, rectal diazepam, oral clonazepam) by the patient (or by caretakers when necessary) as soon as the first symptoms appear may stop ASE and prevent a convulsion (12,13). For self-administration in case of recurrence, we usually recommend the early oral administration of clobazam or clonazepam. Panayiotopoulos also suggests the oral administration of a bolus of valproate (usually twice the daily prophylactic dose) at the onset of symptoms (10).

When the diagnosis of NCSE is made in the emergency department, intravenous administration of any benzodiazepine stops ASE in most cases. Relatively low doses are usually sufficient (e.g., diazepam 0.5 mg/kg; clonazepam 1 mg/kg). Whenever possible, the benzodiazepine should be intravenously administered during an EEG recording—a key investigation to confirm the epileptic nature of the episode. The injection should be given slowly, in successive boluses over 30 to 60 seconds each, and should produce rapid disappearance of the paroxysmal activity and normalization of the EEG. Spike-wave and polyspike-wave discharges are typically replaced by low-amplitude diffuse beta activity (14).

Although controlled studies are lacking, the occurrence of typical ASE in patients with IGE appears to have no appreciable effect on subsequent seizure frequency, epilepsy severity, cognitive development (15), or natural history of the epilepsy. In a follow-up study of 194 patients with typical absence epilepsy (72 followed beyond 18 years of age), 31 cases of ASE (16%, 11 males, 20 females) were observed (16). These patients had a favorable outcome, provided the standard therapy was instituted early. In 24 patients, ASE was followed by a generalized tonic-clonic seizure later in the course. Wirrell and colleagues have suggested that ASE may be a factor predicting that childhood absence epilepsy will not remit (17).

Despite the absence of long-term neurologic damage from typical ASE, recognition of the condition and treatment with a benzodiazepine should occur as early as possible because of the risks of physical injury or a generalized convulsion.

## NONCONVULSIVE STATUS EPILEPTICUS IN CHILDREN WITH AN EPILEPTIC ENCEPHALOPATHY OR LEARNING DIFFICULTIES AND EPILEPSY

Because of the difficulty of collecting solid evidence of the precise role of NCSE in each form of epileptic encephalopathy, this section discusses children with severe forms of epilepsy such as LGS or Dravet syndrome, those with predominantly myoclonic-astatic seizures at onset, and children with learning difficulties and epilepsy not necessarily fitting into a given syndrome.

The term *atypical ASE* (or inadvertently, but sometimes with practical consequences, simply *absence status*) is often used to designate episodes of NCSE in children with LGS or in other generalized epilepsies with predominantly myoclonic-astatic seizures.

Between 50% and 75% of patients with LGS have episodes of NCSE. The most typical form consists of discontinuous atypical absences with variable degrees of altered consciousness, periodically interrupted by recurring brief tonic seizures. On the EEG, absences are marked by the occurrence of slow spike-wave complexes, whereas tonic attacks are associated with a rapid rhythm of about 10 Hz (18,19). Another common type of status is characterized by a variable degree of mental slowing, ranging from mild obtundation to coma, associated with erratic myoclonus involving the perioral and distal limb muscles, with no tonic component (1).

Such episodes may last hours or even days. In up to one half of the patients studied by Dravet and colleagues, the duration exceeded one week (20). In fact, the exact duration may be difficult to determine because one distinctive feature of most cases of LGS is the continuous fluctuation of response latencies. This is particularly true when these children go through "bad periods," characterized by an increase in seizure frequency and EEG abnormalities and apparent further deterioration of mental performance.

A similar clinical picture is observed in children with Dravet syndrome in the form of series of atypical absences, with decreased awareness, head nods, and erratic myoclonus (1,20). These episodes of NCSE last hours or even days and are often associated with unsteadiness or frank ataxia that may wrongly suggest a degenerative disease.

Episodes of NCSE are also observed in children with myoclonic-astatic seizures. They are marked by a variable blurring of consciousness (somnolence, stupor, apathy, or milder obtundation with drooling) that is often associated with erratic perioral and distal muscle twitching and by brief head nods that are due to the repeated lapses of axial muscle tone or jerking of the neck muscles (1). Sometimes muscle tone increases, with the child having a fixed rigid posture like a statue, and he or she may display mild vibratory (or subtle, tremorlike) movements (21). These episodes can begin insidiously and develop progressively and may last from minutes to hours or even weeks, often with fluctuation. The EEG correlate is often long runs of slow waves and spike-wave complexes, sometimes associated with sequences of slow spike-waves. More often, the EEG shows irregular polymorphous paroxysmal abnormalities that may be so severely disorganized that they simulate a hypsarrhythmic pattern. During such episodes, neurologic symptoms and signs may appear, especially ataxia and pseudocerebellar signs, that can suggest a degenerative condition; they may fluctuate and eventually disappear (22,23).

The outcome of episodes of atypical ASE is probably related more to the type and cause of the underlying epilepsy than to the duration of the episodes. AEDs, including benzodiazepines, sodium valproate, and ethosuximide, have been recommended, but there are no rigorous trials supporting these recommendations (Scott, in Walker and colleagues [24]). Steroids or initiation of a ketogenic diet are helpful in some cases. To our knowledge, it has never been demonstrated that efficacy of a given drug in controlling an episode of NCSE (within the setting of the syndromes discussed) constitutes proof that this drug will also be efficacious as everyday treatment of the epileptic encephalopathy and related seizures. Controlled studies are needed to avoid the natural tendency of physicians to keep these drugs "on board," usually in addition to the previously prescribed AEDs. This tendency often leads to an unacceptable overtreatment, drug-induced drowsiness, and drug interactions, with unpredictable consequences.

The effect of repeated episodes of NCSE on long-term prognosis is also largely unknown. Doose and Volzke argued that atypical ASE is strongly correlated with the development of dementia in children with myoclonic astatic epilepsy, implying a causal relationship (25). Doose included hypsarrhythmia and the "bad periods" observed in LGS in their definition of ASE (8). This is at odds with the experience of others, who have been unable to demonstrate a correlation between NCSE and cognitive outcome in children with LGS (26,27). In children with myoclonic astatic epilepsy, the repetition of severe, frequent, and long-lasting episodes of NCSE has been considered a predictor of poor cognitive outcome (28). Nevertheless, myoclonic astatic epilepsy is a rather heterogeneous category, and this study was not designed to prove that the severity and frequency of NCSE episodes worsens overall prognosis or suggests a progressive character of the disorder.

In fact, for the majority of the so-called epileptic encephalopathies, it is almost impossible to separate the impact of a profoundly abnormal baseline function from that of episodes of NCSE on cognition and behavior. Treatment plans are based on the hypothesis that epileptic discharges cause the encephalopathy, so treatment of discharges may improve outcome. There is no doubt that there is a clear change in alertness and responsiveness following control of an episode of NCSE—independent of the underlying epilepsy syndrome. In that sense, early diagnosis and appropriate treatment of NCSE are important, even if the hypothesis that control of these episodes influences overall neuropsychological outcome cannot be confirmed now. This is particularly pertinent for children with less severe forms of epilepsy and learning disabilities because NCSE may go unrecognized in these patients.

## RING CHROMOSOME 20 SYNDROME

Ring chromosome 20 syndrome is a recently described chromosomal disorder associated with a particular pattern of epilepsy (29-31). Different seizure types include focal seizures with fear, visual symptoms or hallucinations, generalized tonic-clonic or clonic seizures, and nocturnal arousals with frontal semiology. Episodes of NCSE consist of a prolonged confusional state, with long-lasting high-voltage slow waves and occasional spikes on the EEG in all cases. Duration is from 2 to 3 minutes to several hours. Cognitive evaluation during NCSE may show no or only minor deficits. Behavior disturbances are common and take the form of attention deficit disorder, obsessive behavior, or aggressive outbursts. Epilepsy may start at any time after birth (31), throughout childhood and adolescence (Plouin and O'Regan, in Walker and colleagues [24]). Onset in the neonatal period lacks specific epilepsy features, but the phenotype includes more severe mental delay. The seizures are drug resistant in almost all cases.

Progression of the disorder is probably not directly related to the frequency and severity of NCSE episodes. Locharernkul and colleagues reported on two cases, both of whom were Thai women with normal intellectual function (32). AEDs allowed a relatively easy control of seizures but had no effect on episodes of NCSE. The authors attributed the relatively benign course of the disorder in these patients to the low percentage (20%) of ring chromosome 20 mosaicism. Biraben and colleagues proposed that the long duration of seizures could result from an abnormality of endogenous seizure-terminating mechanisms (33).

## NONCONVULSIVE STATUS EPILEPTICUS IN IDIOPATHIC FOCAL EPILEPSIES

Episodes of NCSE are not a characteristic feature of Rolandic epilepsy or of late-onset occipital epilepsy of childhood (Gastaut type). In Rolandic epilepsy, episodes of status, when they occur, usually present as hemiconvulsive seizures. Still, episodes of NCSE occur in atypical forms of Rolandic epilepsy, particularly in atypical benign partial epilepsy (34) (also termed pseudo-Lennox syndrome) (35), along with atonic seizures or atypical absences. A relationship with continuous spike-waves during slow sleep can usually be established, and these atypical forms are now considered part of the spectrum of syndromes with continuous spike-waves during slow sleep (1,36). The clinical picture is characterized by infrequent, focal, and often nocturnal seizures and by periods (usually of a few weeks' duration), in which intense clinical and EEG epileptic activity are evident. During these periods, EEG abnormalities include brief discharges of spike-waves associated with falls and "continuous spike-waves of slow sleep." The active periods are separated by intervals of up to several months. Usually, only 2 to 5 episodes occur before complete recovery. The cognitive and behavior outcome of this syndrome may be favorable, but no detailed neuropsychologic follow-up study is available. Deterioration may occur, especially after multiple and long bouts of seizures. Atypical partial benign epilepsy probably represents an intermittent form of the syndrome of continuous spike-waves of sleep, and the poor cognitive outcome of some patients may be related to the duration of the paroxysmal activity, as is discussed in Chapter 17.

Nonconvulsive autonomic status is a core feature of Panayiotopoulos syndrome (PS) (37). Indeed, PS is one of the commonest epilepsies of childhood, probably accounting for 6% to 8% of children aged 1 to 13 years with seizures. Autonomic status epilepticus occurs in slightly more than half of all children with the syndrome. It is one of the commonest causes of NCSE overall and may be the commonest cause in children without other neurologic impairment (Ferrie, in Walker and colleagues [24]). Seizure manifestations are dominated by autonomic, mainly emetic (nausea, retching, and vomiting) symptoms, often with unilateral eye deviation. Other autonomic features include color changes, pupil abnormalities, cardiorespiratory and thermoregulatory alterations, and incontinence (38). Seizures are characteristically long. In a study of 86 seizures in 47 children, the median duration of the seizures was 15 minutes (range 1 minute to 7 hours). More than two-thirds lasted longer than 10 minutes, and 44% lasted longer than 30 minutes, constituting NCSE. The median duration of status epilepticus episodes was two hours (range 30 minutes to 7 hours) (38). Like the shorter seizures, episodes of status epilepticus are dominated by autonomic symptoms, but many end in hemi- or generalized tonic-clonic seizures. Prolonged seizures occur during both wakefulness and sleep.

Many features of autonomic NCSE in PS are not obviously recognizable as being epileptic in nature. Consequently, NCSE in these children is frequently misdiagnosed. Not infrequently, the children are admitted to intensive care units with suspected encephalitis or strokes. By the next day, they are usually fully recovered, to everyone's surprise (Ferrie, in Walker and colleagues [24]). If NCSE in PS is recognized, administration of a benzodiazepine (oral midazolam, rectal diazepam, or intravenous lorazepam or diazepam) will probably terminate the event (24). Regular AED treatment is not recommended in cases of typical PS. There seems to be no reason to modify this policy in children who have had an episode of NCSE, but rescue medication may be given to the family for acute seizure treatment. PS has an excellent prognosis—independent of whether episodes of NCSE occur.

## PARTIAL NONCONVULSIVE STATUS EPILEPTICUS

Partial NCSE is rarely reported in children. It occurs in the course of temporal lobe or other lesional epilepsies. The outcome of partial status epilepticus with alteration of consciousness is imperfectly known because of the small number of reported cases, the underrecognition of episodes with spontaneous resolution, the incorrect diagnoses based on a misinterpretation of EEG abnormalities, and definition problems (39). Profound memory deficit has occasionally been reported in adults (40); for a fuller discussion, see Chapter 10. Transient neuroimaging abnormalities reported following partial status include localized areas of hypodensity with enhancement on computed tomographic scanning and increased T2-weighted signal on magnetic resonance imaging, suggestive of focal edema (41-43). Such abnormalities may persist for several days. They must be distinguished from a lesion causing the NCSE.

How aggressive the management of partial NCSE should be remains a controversial issue. AED treatment of NCSE usually does not differ fundamentally from that for convulsive status. Because the degree of emergency may be less, some authors prefer to not use intravenously administered benzodiazepines and begin treatment with intravenously administered phenytoin or phenobarbital (44). Nevertheless, benzodiazepines yield good results in 62% to 73% of cases of temporal lobe or psychomotor status (44,45). See Chapter 20 for principles of treatment of NCSE.

Whether or not medical treatment is successful in controlling an episode of NCSE, most well-documented reports describe a favorable neurologic outcome—even in very prolonged episodes lasting months (46). Severe focal neurologic deficits and localized cerebral edema can occur and may be long lasting but completely reversible (43). In our case of a 6-year-old boy with drug-resistant focal (probably symptomatic) epilepsy, NCSE lasted 6 days, followed by cortical blindness that persisted nearly a week. Acutely ill patients in critical care settings often have a poor outcome, related to the underlying etiology in most cases.

The long-term prognosis for patients presenting with episodes of NCSE is also usually related to the cause. In the setting of chronic epilepsy, recurrences of NCSE are very likely, but deficits are usually reversible and usually do not influence long-term outcome.

## CONCLUSIONS

Prospective or retrospective controlled studies on the prognosis and outcome of NCSE in children are not available. Some data are provided in studies of both children and adults, but definite conclusions are difficult to reach because of the heterogeneity of the epilepsy syndromes and neurologic pathologies included, the lack of a uniform classification of NCSE types, and the confusing terminology used.

Typical ASE occurs as part of an IGE most often characterized by typical absences. Immediate prognosis is usually excellent after administration of a benzodiazepine, and NCSE in this setting does not seem to affect the natural evolution of the illness or overall long-term prognosis.

In patients with prior neurologic abnormalities or an epileptic encephalopathy, episodes of NCSE are frequent. They may prove to be difficult to control and may last several days, characterized by a continuous fluctuation of response latencies. Undoubtedly, NCSE episodes in this setting indicate exacerbation of the global clinical problem in these children and should be treated promptly. Still, no strong data exist to suggest a causative link between the severity of NCSE events and eventual deterioration of the neurodevelopmental status of a patient. Episodes of NCSE may simply reflect a progressive disorder.

The long-term prognosis of focal NCSE is also related to the cause. Isolated events are usually easy to control, and sequelae, when present, are almost always reversible. Further prospective studies are needed, especially for groups of children with similar diseases and types of NCSE, in order to better define long-term outcome and prognosis of NCSE in children.

## REFERENCES


1. Arzimanoglou A, Guerrini R, Aicardi J. Aicardi's Epilepsy in Children, 3rd ed. Philadelphia, PA: Lippincott, Williams & Wilkins; 2004.
2. Tay SK, Hirsch LJ, Leary L, Jette N, Wittman J, Akman CI. Nonconvulsive status epilepticus in children: clinical and EEG characteristics. Epilepsia 2006;47:1504-1509.
3. Abend NS, Dlugos DJ. Nonconvulsive status epilepticus in a pediatric intensive care unit. Pediatr Neurol 2007;37:165-170.
4. Gastaut H. Classification of status epilepticus. In: Delgado-Escueta AV, Wasterlain CG, Treiman DM, Porter RJ. Status Epilepticus. Advances in Neurology. Vol 34. New York, NY: Raven Press; 1983:75-81.
5. Porter RJ, Penry JK. 1983. Petit mal status. In: Wasterlain CG, Treiman DM, Porter RJ, eds. Status Epilepticus: Mechanisms of Brain Damage and Treatment. Advances in Neurology. Vol 34. New York, NY: Raven Press; 1983:61-67.
6. Niedermeyer E, Khalifeh R. Petit mal status ("spike-wave stupor"). An electro-clinical appraisal. Epilepsia 1965;6:250-262.
7. Ohtahara S, Oka E, Yamatogi Y, Ohtsuka Y, Ichiba N, Ishida S, Miyake S. Non-convulsive status epilepticus in childhood. Folia Psychiatr Neurol Jpn 1979;33:345-351.
8. Doose H. Nonconvulsive status epilepticus in childhood: clinical aspects and classification. in: Delgado-Escueta AV, Wasterlain CG, Treiman DM, Porter RJ, eds. Status epilepticus: mechanisms of brain damage and treatment. Advances in Neurology. Vol 34. New York, NY: Raven Press; 1983:83-92.
9. Hess R, Scollo-Lavizzari G, Wyss FE. Borderline cases of petit mal status. Eur Neurol 1971;5:137-154.
10. Panayiotopoulos CP. The Epilepsies: Seizures, Syndromes and Management. Oxford, UK: Bladon Medical Publishing; 2005.
11. Thomas P, Valton L, Genton P. Absence and myoclonic status epilepticus precipitated by antiepileptic drugs in idiopathic generalized epilepsy. Brain 2006;129:1281-1292.
12. Scott RC, Besag FM, Neville BG. Buccal midazolam and rectal diazepam for treatment of prolonged seizures in childhood and adolescence: a randomised trial. Lancet 1999;20;353:623-626.
13. Kutlu NO, Dogrul M, Yakinci C, Soylu H. Buccal midazolam for treatment of prolonged seizures in children. Brain Dev 2003;25:275-278.
14. Thomas P. Typical and atypical absence status epilepticus in children. In: Panayiotopoulos CP, ed. A Practical Guide to Childhood Epilepsies. Oxford, UK: Medicinae; 2006:67-71.
15. Drislane FW. Evidence against permanent neurologic damage from nonconvulsive status epilepticus. J Clin Neurophysiol 1999;16:323-331.
16. Dieterich E, Baier WK, Doose H, Tuxhorn I, Fichsel H. Longterm follow-up of childhood epilepsy with absences. I. Epilepsy with absences at onset. Neuropediatrics 1985;16:149-154.
17. Wirrell EC, Camfield CS, Camfield PR, Gordon KE, Dooley JM. Long-term prognosis of typical childhood absence epilepsy: remission or progression to juvenile myoclonic epilepsy. Neurology 1996;47:912-918.

18. Beaumanoir A, Foletti G, Magistris M, Volanschi D. Status epilepticus in the Lennox-Gastaut syndrome. In: Niedermeyer E, Degen R, eds. The Lennox-Gastaut syndrome. New York, NY: Alan R. Liss; 1988:283-299.
19. Dravet C, Natale O, Magaudda A, Larrieu JL, Bureau M, Roger J, Tassinari CA. Les états de mal dans le syndrome de Lennox-Gastaut. Rev Electroencephalogr Neurophysiol Clin 1985;15:361-368.
20. Dravet C, Bureau M, Oguni H, Fukuyama Y, Cokar O. Severe myoclonic epilepsy in infancy (Dravet syndrome). In: Roger J, Bureau M, Dravet C, Bureau M, Dreifuss FE, Wolf P, eds. Epileptic Syndromes in Infancy, Childhood and Adolescence, 4th ed. Montrouge, France: John Libbey Eurotext; 2005:89-114.
21. Guerrini R, Dravet C, Gobbi G, Ricci S, Dulac O. Idiopathic generalized epilepsies with myoclonus in infancy and childhood. In: Malafosse A, Genton P, Hirsch E, Marescaux C, Broglin D, Bernasconi R, eds. Idiopathic Generalized Epilepsies: Clinical, Experimental, and Genetic Aspects. London, UK: John Libbey; 1994:267-280.
22. Bennett HS, Selman JE, Rapin I, Rose A. Nonconvulsive epileptiform activity appearing as ataxia. Am J Dis Child 1982;136:30-32.
23. Aicardi J, Chevrie JJ. Myoclonic epilepsies of childhood. Neuropédiatrie 1971;3:177-190.
24. Walker M, Cross H, Smith S, Young C, Aicardi J, Appleton R, Aylett S, Besag F, Cock H, DeLorenzo R, Drislane F, Duncan J, Ferrie C, Fujikawa D, Gray W, Kaplan P, Koutroumanidis M, O'Regan M, Plouin P, Sander J, Scott R, Shorvon S, Treiman D, Wasterlain C, Wieshmann U. Nonconvulsive status epilepticus: Epilepsy Research Foundation workshop reports. Epileptic Disord 2005;7:253-296.
25. Doose H, Völzke E. Petit mal status in early childhood and dementia. Neuropadiatrie 1979;10:10-14.
26. Aicardi J, Gomes AL. The Lennox-Gastaut syndrome: clinical and electroencephalographic features. In: Niedermeyer E, Degen D, eds. The Lennox-Gastaut Syndrome. New York, NY: Alan R. Liss; 1988:25-46.
27. Beaumanoir A, Dravet C. The Lennox-Gastaut syndrome. In: Roger J, Bureau M, Dravet C, Bureau M, Dreifuss FE, Wolf P, eds. Epileptic Syndromes in Infancy, Childhood and Adolescence. London, UK: John Libbey;1992:115-132.
28. Kaminska A, Ickowicz A, Plouin P, Bru MF, Dellatolas G, Dulac O. Delineation of cryptogenic Lennox-Gastaut syndrome and myoclonic astatic epilepsy using multiple correspondence analysis. Epilepsy Res 1999;36:15-29.
29. Inoue Y, Fujiwara T, Matsuda K, Kubota H, Tanaka M, Yagi K, Yamamori K, Takahashi Y. Ring chromosome 20 and nonconvulsive status epilepticus. A new epileptic syndrome. Brain 1997;120:939-953.
30. Petit J, Roubertie A, Inoue Y, Genton P. Nonconvulsive status in the ring chromosome 20 syndrome: a video illustration of three cases. Epileptic Disord 1999;1:237-241.
31. Ville D, Kaminska A, Bahi-Buisson N, Biraben A, Plouin P, Telvi L, Dulac O, Chiron C. Early pattern of epilepsy in the ring chromosome 20 syndrome. Epilepsia 2006;47:543-549.
32. Locharernkul C, Ebner A, Promchainant C. Ring chromosome 20 with nonconvulsive status epilepticus: electroclinical correlation of a rare epileptic syndrome. Clin Electroencephalogr Neurosci 2005;36:151-160.
33. Biraben A, Semah F, Ribeiro MJ, Douaud G, Remy P, Depaulis A. PET evidence for a role of the basal ganglia in patients with ring chromosome 20 epilepsy. Neurology 2004;63; 63:73-77.
34. Aicardi J, Chevrie JJ. Atypical benign epilepsy of childhood. Dev Med Child Neurol 1982;24:281-292.
35. Hahn A. Atypical benign partial epilepsy/ pseudo-Lennox syndrome. Epileptic Disord 2000;2(Suppl 1):S11-S17.
36. Aicardi J. Atypical semiology of rolandic epilepsy in some related syndromes. Epileptic Disord 2000;2(Suppl 1):S5-S9.
37. Ferrie CD, Caraballo R, Covanis A, Demirbilek V, Dervent A, Fejerman N, Fusco L, Grünewald RA, Kanazawa O, Koutroumanidis M, Lada C, Livingston JH, Nicotra A, Oguni H, Martinovic Z, Nordli DR Jr, Parisi P, Scott RC, Specchio N, Verrotti A, Vigevano F, Walker MC, Watanabe K, Yoshinaga H, Panayiotopoulos CP. Autonomic status epilepticus in Panayiotopoulos syndrome and other childhood and adult epilepsies: a consensus view. Epilepsia 2007;48:1165-1172.
38. Panayiotopoulos CP. Panayiotopoulos Syndrome: a Common and Benign Childhood Epileptic Syndrome. London, England: John Libbey; 2002.
39. Kaplan PW. Prognosis in nonconvulsive status epilepticus. Epileptic Disord 2000;2:185-193.

40. Collins RC, Lothman EW, Olney JW. Status epilepticus in the limbic system: biochemical and pathological changes. In: Delgado-Escueta AV, Wasterlain CG, Treiman DM, Porter RJ, eds. Status Epilepticus: Mechanisms of Brain Damage and Treatment. Advances in Neurology. Vol 34. New York, NY: Raven Press; 1983:277-287.
41. Kramer RE, Lüders H, Lesser RP, Weinstein MR, Dinner DS, Morris HH, Wyllie E. Transient focal abnormalities of neuroimaging studies during focal status epilepticus. Epilepsia 1987;28:528-532.
42. Aicardi J, Arzimanoglou A. Images tomodensitométriques d'allure tumorale observées lors de certaines épilepsies de l'enfant. Journées Parisiennes de Pédiatrie. Paris, France: Flammarion; 1986:133-138.
43. Sammaritano M, Andermann F, Melanson D, Papius HM, Camfield P, Aicardi J, Sherwin A. Prolonged focal cerebral edema associated with partial status epilepticus. Epilepsia 1985;26: 334-339.
44. Browne TR, Penry JK. Benzodiazepines in the treatment of epilepsy. Epilepsia 1973;14:277-310.
45. Tassinari CA, Daniele O, Michelucci R, Bureau M, Dravet C, Roger J. Benzodiazepines: efficacy in status epilepticus. In: Delgado-Escueta AV, Wasterlain CG, Treiman DM, Porter RJ, eds. Status Epilepticus: Mechanisms of Brain Damage and Treatment. Advances in Neurology. Vol 34. New York, NY: Raven Press; 1983:465-475.
46. Cockerell OC, Walker MC, Sander JW, Shorvon SD. Complex partial status epilepticus: a recurrent problem. J Neurol Neurosurg Psychiatry

CHAPTER 22

# PROGNOSIS AND OUTCOMES OF ADULTS WITH NONCONVULSIVE STATUS EPILEPTICUS

NATHAN B. FOUNTAIN

Nonconvulsive status epilepticus (NCSE) is complicated in many ways, not the least of which is determining prognosis and outcome. This chapter addresses prognosis and outcome in adults only; prognosis and outcome for NCSE in children are considered in Chapter 21. It also focuses on clinical data, referencing animal data for discussions of pathophysiology, which are generally not available from human data. Classification, presentation, and terminology, although relevant for prognosis, are outlined elsewhere in this text and are not reviewed here.

Outcome is important for two reasons. First, it is clinically useful to know who is likely to die or develop long-term sequelae so that intervention can be provided to prevent those outcomes. This is especially important in NCSE because the usual treatment can cause serious iatrogenic morbidity and mortality, and adverse effects of treatment could outweigh its benefits for some types of patients. It is intuitive that aggressive therapies should be reserved for patients with significant risk of morbidity. Second, it is biologically important to know whether NCSE causes neuronal injury because this knowledge might be applicable to other electroclinical situations, such as nonconvulsive seizures or epileptic encephalopathies with continuous spike-and-wave in slow-wave sleep.

## METHODOLOGIC PROBLEMS

There are many methodologic problems with current studies of NCSE (1). Almost all studies are retrospective case series because NCSE is diagnosed at the time of the first EEG, although symptoms have usually been present prior to the EEG, sometimes for days or weeks. Most case series are small, so only very large differences between groups can be detected. Early studies did not characterize their populations well as to type or characteristics of NCSE and, thus, include heterogeneous populations. Conversely, some studies examined patients with only one particular etiology, making it difficult to generalize the findings to other cases of NCSE.

It is important to discern clearly the objective of each of these studies to determine whether there are sufficient data to support the conclusions and, then, whether the findings are applicable to NCSE in general or only to a limited set of patients. The most useful studies for determining mortality are large empiric observations, but studies of specific subgroups can inform treatment decisions. Of course, prospective intervention trials are necessary to determine whether outcome can be altered by our intervention.

Traditionally, NCSE was divided into absence status epilepticus (ASE) and complex partial status epilepticus (CPSE). ASE is conceptualized as a prolonged absence seizure, and CPSE is conceptualized as a prolonged complex partial seizure. There are certainly patients with CPSE who have complex partial seizures at other times and then have prolongation of their habitual seizures. There are also patients with absence epilepsy in an analogous situation, but this is much less common. Electrographically, most patients with NCSE do not have focal recurrent seizures or typical regular generalized spike-wave discharges. Instead, they usually have generalized rhythmic delta activity mixed with spikes, and thus, this activity cannot be classified electrographically as CPSE or ASE (2). Early reports of small case series could not distinguish CPSE from ASE (3,4). This is why the more generic term *NCSE* has become popular.

The inherent limitations of the traditional classification of NCSE are emphasized by studies of patients who ultimately proved to have frontal lobe status epilepticus. Five women with clinical ASE and generalized EEG discharges were later determined on prolonged EEG to have seizures with focal onset in the frontal region in four, and left hemisphere in one (5). A 5-year prospective study of patients with frontal NCSE identified 10 patients, three of whom had impaired consciousness associated with generalized EEG discharges (6). These results suggest that NCSE of focal onset can appear as generalized NCSE of the "absence" type. It is now generally agreed that most patients with NCSE do not fit neatly into the traditional category of CPSE or ASE, so outcome studies using this classification must be carefully reexamined.

The evolution of the definition of NCSE also has implications for understanding its outcome. The term *NCSE* was traditionally used to describe patients in "ictal confusion" or "spike-wave stupor" or "the wandering confused" (7). Some early NCSE studies gave little consideration to mortality because outcome was almost always perceived to be good. One of the first case series to identify the characteristics of NCSE included 10 patients with 1 to 10 years of follow-up; none died (3). Among critically ill patients in the intensive care unit, however, NCSE was not readily recognized until the recent advent of digital EEG that allows routine prolonged monitoring. Accordingly, presentation and outcome in the literature appear to be dichotomous: very good in the older literature concentrating on NCSE without other medical problems, but very poor in the more recent literature concentrating on the critically ill. New and old studies cannot be compared directly.

The studies of outcome and prognostication have special significance for NCSE because its "natural history" is still a matter of debate. Even determining acute mortality has been controversial. Prognostication has been elusive. It requires developing hypotheses about the influence of a factor on outcome and then prospectively measuring outcome based on the presence or severity of that factor. Factors determining prognosis are very important because they are likely to be points of intervention for treatment to prevent poor outcomes. There have been no studies of the prognostic value of any factors for outcome of NCSE, so we are left with correlations of outcome with various factors associated with NCSE and the inference that they provide prognostic information.

Poor outcome in NCSE has generally been defined as death—a simple measurable outcome that has clinical significance. In many case series, NCSE has high mortality, and it is important to know who is likely to die so as to prevent it. Other outcome measures have been neglected. NCSE could cause long-term sequelae from neuronal injury, e.g., impaired cognition or memory might result from cortical or hippocampal injury. Epilepsy could arise from a similar mechanism. These areas, however, have not been examined in detail.

## LESSONS FROM GENERALIZED CONVULSIVE STATUS EPILEPTICUS

Generalized convulsive status epilepticus (GCSE) has been studied extensively in humans and experimental animals. It seems reasonable to apply the lessons learned from GCSE to NCSE. The most important physiologic lesson has been that GCSE causes excitotoxic cell damage from activation of glutamate-mediated NMDA receptors (8). (See Chapter 7 on pathophysiology and animal models of NCSE.)

Mortality in GCSE results mainly from systemic physiologic alterations (8,9). Many patients die from physiologic changes that can be attributed to the extreme muscle exertion and catecholamine surge of convulsive motor activity. Because NCSE is not associated with extreme muscle activity, it is unlikely that these events contribute to death. Death later in GCSE or after its resolution, however, has other causes. GCSE is commonly associated with potentially serious electrocardiographic abnormalities (10), also reported in at least one case of NCSE (11). Death later in GCSE can also be due to respiratory complications of aspiration pneumonia or neurogenic pulmonary edema—which could also be caused by NCSE.

There are difficulties in applying findings from GCSE to NCSE. NCSE results from diverse etiologies, has diverse presentations, and is likely to result from diverse pathophysiologies. Therefore, it is unlikely that the pathophysiology of GCSE is universally applicable to NCSE (8). Indeed, ASE is more similar to a prolonged absence seizure than it is to a convulsion; the pathophysiology of NCSE in ASE is likely to be similar to the pathophysiology of an absence seizure. Absence seizures result from changes in recurrent thalamocortical inhibitory circuits that are not known to involve NMDA-mediated neurotransmission. Therefore, they are unlikely to cause excitotoxic cell damage. This is part of the reason for a generally good outcome after absence seizures in childhood absence epilepsy. In patients with absence epilepsy, ASE is unlikely to cause neuronal injury.

Examining NCSE that follows GCSE is similar to studying GCSE, since GCSE often eventually evolves to a nonconvulsive state. Refractory status epilepticus (RSE) usually starts as GCSE and thus often follows the natural history of GCSE. When these cases are grouped with cases of NCSE not preceded by GCSE, few appropriate conclusions can be drawn regarding the natural history, outcome, or prognosis of NCSE. There is a moderately large literature about RSE that includes NCSE of all types, but usually those following GCSE. There are good studies on the treatment of RSE that may help guide treatment, but they provide little information on the outcome of NCSE itself.

## OVERALL MORTALITY OF NONCONVULSIVE STATUS EPILEPTICUS

The mortality of NCSE is surprisingly similar to that of GCSE. We found an 18% mortality rate among 100 NCSE patients from an unselected retrospective consecutive case series (12). This is nearly identical to the mortality rate from a prospective population-based series of GCSE (13). It is also similar to the 25% mortality rate in another series of 33 patients with NCSE (14). Other studies have reported NCSE mortality rates that are much higher or lower, in selected populations. At one extreme, mortality was almost 100% in patients with subarachnoid hemorrhage (15,16). At the other extreme, almost no mortality was reported in NCSE case series without acute medical problems (3,17). These represent different selected subpopulations with different mortalities based on the underlying etiologies, so it is logical that mortality would be different.

## MORTALITY AND ETIOLOGY

Determining mortality based on classification of NCSE is inherently complicated (1). Classifying NCSE based on location, severity of illness, or presentation is problematic because patients with NCSE present across a spectrum of types and causes. Confining analysis to those with "critical illness" or "intensive care unit status" will exclude patients with milder medical problems, giving the appearance that NCSE has a higher mortality rate than it actually has. On the other hand, there is value in characterizing the outcome of patients with NCSE in these specific situations.

To avoid biases of classification, we examined an unselected 100-patient consecutive case series of all comers with NCSE and then retrospectively examined determinants of mortality (12). We found a strong statistical correlation of mortality with the presence of an acute medical etiology, severe mental status impairment, and the occurrence of complications during treatment. Prognosis of NCSE based on etiology is logical because NCSE is often caused by severe medical problems that have a high mortality of their own. Approaching mortality by etiology also clarifies much of the disparity in the literature.

Mortality is relatively high when NCSE is due to an acute medical problem. Mortality was 27% in the 52 patients with an acute medical cause in our series. Acute medical problems included primary neurologic problems, such as central nervous system infection, as well as systemic illnesses, such as sepsis. Mortality also rises with an increasing number of medical problems in the critically ill elderly (18).

NCSE occurring in critically ill patients in the intensive care unit has a poor prognosis. A case series of 23 such patients found a 33% mortality rate, and most correlated with duration of seizure activity and delay in diagnosis (19).

Mortality of NCSE occurring during the course of some specific etiologies has been reported. All 8 patients diagnosed with NCSE after subarachnoid hemorrhage died in one study, 11 of 12 in another, and 9 of 11 in a third (15,16,20). Among 94 patients monitored with continuous EEG after head trauma, only 6 cases of NCSE were found, but all 6 died (21). It is difficult to know whether these findings are pertinent for patients with NCSE of other etiologies.

Refractory status epilepticus, which often follows GCSE, has a consistently high mortality. NCSE follows GCSE in up to 48% of cases, so it is relatively common (22). In one series, RSE constituted 31% of 83 cases of status epilepticus (23). Rossetti and colleagues found that the outcome in 47 cases of RSE correlated with etiology, and not treatment choice, across several anesthetic agents (24). Claassen and colleagues found a 60% mortality rate in NCSE treated with midazolam, and mortality was 75% in the subgroup that presented as NCSE rather than as GCSE (25). Some of the morbidity and mortality in RSE is due to the preceding GCSE.

Mortality is very low when epilepsy is the etiology of NCSE. Status epilepticus occurs at some point during life in about 20% of patients with epilepsy (26). Thus, epilepsy is a relatively common cause, accounting for 31% of patients in our series. Despite the large number of patients with epilepsy, only one died. Many prior reports of small case series of patients with epilepsy did not report mortality, presumably because it did not occur or was thought to be low. None of the 10 patients reported by Guberman died (3). In another report of 10 patients with CPSE, 7 lived, but they had persistent cognitive problems (27).

When the etiology is unknown, prediction of mortality in NCSE remains an interesting problem. The cause can usually be determined and will probably be found more often as medical technology advances. The etiology was "cryptogenic" in 17% of our cases. Mortality was 18% in this group, intermediate between the higher mortality with an acute medical cause (27%) and the lower mortality with epilepsy (3%). On the other hand, a good outcome and no mortality was reported for de novo ASE in 10 cases (28). It is likely that some cases of NCSE labeled as cryptogenic have an unidentified acute medical cause with attendant increased mortality, whereas others do not, but the mortality in this group is primarily correlated with the severity of impairment of mental status.

## MORTALITY AND MENTAL STATUS

The prognosis of NCSE consistently correlates with the extent of altered mental status. Our study identified severely altered mental status in 72% of the 18 patients with NCSE who died, compared to the presence of severe altered mental status in just 24% of the 82 patients who lived. Drislane and Schomer examined the outcome of 48 patients with NCSE, astutely classifying them as in "electrographic status epilepticus" rather than using a clinical categorization (29). Mortality was 88% and correlated with the presence of coma, anoxia as the etiology, low-voltage EEG, and the presence of refractory seizures. In the studies of NCSE in the critically ill, essentially all patients have severely impaired mental status, and this likely contributes to their high mortality rates.

Altered mental status is often associated with acute and severe medical illness, so death is likely to result from a combination of the NCSE and the medical illness. An interaction analysis shows that both factors contribute independently to mortality (12). Depressed consciousness is likely to predispose to aspiration pneumonia because of impaired ability to clear secretions or refluxed stomach contents, regardless of etiology. This could be the cause of rare fatalities among NCSE patients with only epilepsy as the cause. Death from epilepsy-related NCSE is uncommon, likely because severely altered mental status is uncommon; the confusion due to NCSE alone is likely to be milder.

## MORTALITY AND OTHER FACTORS

Some have suggested that older age increases mortality in NCSE. Bottaro and colleagues found 50% had poor outcome among 19 elderly patients (mean age 80 years) with NCSE, compared with only 8% in a matched set of patients with similar altered mental status but without NCSE (30). Another study reported a 52% mortality rate in 24 critically ill elderly patients with NCSE (18). Age was not independently associated with outcome in our 100 patients with NCSE (12). Others have not reported a consistent correlation of mortality with age, but many have not examined the elderly as a specific group.

Some investigators have examined whether the EEG discharge pattern correlates with outcome. Litt and colleagues found mortality associated with a generalized EEG pattern in the critically ill elderly (18). We did not find a correlation of mortality with EEG pattern in a multiple variable analysis of 100 patients (12).

It might be logical to consider that the EEG appearance of NCSE should correlate with outcome (8). The reasoning is that, when NCSE results from excess excitatory neurotransmission, then it should have a higher morbidity or mortality, similar to the case with GCSE. When NCSE results from excess inhibitory neurotransmission, then it should have the morbidity of absence seizures. Therefore, NCSE associated with typical generalized spike-waves on EEG should have a better outcome because absence seizures do not cause neuronal injury. We have proposed a classification of status epilepticus based on the EEG presence of "spike-wave" or "non–spike-wave" (12). The improved prognosis of a generalized spike-wave pattern in this regard is for neuronal injury, but not necessarily for death. A decreased risk of neuronal injury does not protect patients from death due to aspiration associated with severely altered mental status or from other systemic problems. Severely impaired mental status is unlikely to occur in ASE with typical generalized spike-wave discharges, but, when present, it probably increases mortality. Thus, any beneficial effect on neuronal injury from the presence of generalized spike-wave discharges might be offset by the detrimental effect of impaired mental status.

## LONG-TERM PROGNOSIS

Determining long-term prognosis in NCSE is vitally important. Studies to date have demonstrated convincingly that mortality is low in some subgroups, such as those with prior epilepsy and mild mental status changes. These groups may still be at risk of neuronal injury.

There is circumstantial evidence of neuronal injury in NCSE. Neuron-specific enolase, a marker of cellular injury, is elevated during NCSE (31-33). Magnetic resonance imaging has demonstrated increased signal in the hippocampus after NCSE, but the findings are transient (34-36). A few autopsies on patients with NCSE have demonstrated focal neuronal loss. Three patients who died in focal motor status without other significant contributing factors had neuronal loss and gliosis in the hippocampus, amygdala, dorsomedial thalamus, Purkinje cells of the cerebellum, and piriform and entorhinal cortices (37). There is no large case series of mixed NCSE types to resolve the issue, however, and there is no compelling evidence that NCSE causes the severe injury that accompanies prolonged GCSE.

If NCSE causes neuronal injury, then it could manifest as cognitive impairment, but this is yet to be determined. There are few studies of this problem. A classic report by Krumholz and colleagues of 10 patients with CPSE demonstrated persistent memory and cognitive deficits in all 7 of the patients who lived (27). As noted by the authors, the report describes an association and does not establish cause. Seven of the patients had preceding disorders to NCSE, such as coma, convulsive status epilepticus, or viral encephalitis, which may each have contributed partially or completely to the cognitive and memory problems. Even in the more severe case of GCSE, there has been little evidence of cognitive impairment. Two studies have taken advantage of patients with epilepsy who had formal neuropsychologic testing as part of their routine evaluations and then happened to have an episode of status epilepticus. The authors performed follow-up neuropsychologic testing to determine whether there was evidence of injury. Dodrill and Wilensky reported a trend toward cognitive decline in 3 of 4 tests of mental ability administered after status epilepticus in 9 patients with epilepsy (38). Adachi and colleagues did not find a significant difference between IQ scores of 15 patients with epilepsy after status epilepticus. Such studies have not been performed in patients with NCSE alone (39).

Epilepsy might also follow NCSE as evidence of neuronal injury. The incidence of epilepsy following NCSE is not known. Recurrent NCSE is very common, reported in 2 of 10 patients with NCSE in one series and in approximately 60% in another (3,40). We found that epilepsy developed in 21% of 20 patients after NCSE in a preliminary evaluation of those without prior epilepsy and who did not die during NCSE (41). Whether an episode of NCSE was actually the first seizure in a patient who had already developed epilepsy or if NCSE caused the epilepsy is unknown, but both scenarios are plausible.

NCSE could cause mortality that is additive or synergistic with the underlying etiology. Stroke is synergistic with GCSE, such that the mortality of GCSE in the presence of stroke is higher than the mortality of each added together (42). The same could be true of NCSE, but this has not been examined. The etiologies of NCSE that are associated with high mortality also have high mortality when they occur without NCSE. This makes finding a greater increase in mortality with NCSE more difficult.

## IMPLICATIONS FOR TREATMENT

The goal of examining outcome and prognosis in NCSE is to identify points of possible intervention. The utility of any intervention in reducing mortality or preventing long-term sequelae is unknown. Future research should clearly identify points of intervention and test them. The most pressing need is to determine whether aggressive intervention with anesthetic-induced coma is more effective than less-aggressive treatment with standard antiepileptic drugs in reducing mortality or preventing sequelae.

The ultimate goal of prognostication is to define a treatment paradigm. There is currently insufficient evidence in studies of NCSE to provide any strong recommendations, but some inferences from the data are available. If the etiology of NCSE is epilepsy and mental status is not severely impaired, then the prognosis is very good; the patient is unlikely to die and already has epilepsy, so the risk of developing it is not a concern. In this case, it seems reasonable to start treatment with standard parenteral or oral antiepileptic drugs and avoid the iatrogenic risks of anesthetic coma if possible. If the etiology of NCSE is an acute medical condition, especially when accompanied by severely altered mental status, then more aggressive therapy with anesthetic coma (with strong vigilance for complications) seems reasonable. In this case, patients are likely to already be in the intensive care unit and are probably endotracheally intubated, so they are already exposed to these risks. Starting treatment with standard antiepileptic drugs is preferable, moving quickly to anesthetic coma if necessary. The group of greatest concern is the cryptogenic group, with heterogenous combinations of altered mental status and medical illnesses. This group probably warrants more aggressive therapy to avoid both mortality and the possibility of developing epilepsy or cognitive impairment. Whether this approach is ultimately appropriate will await randomized controlled clinical trials of therapy. See Chapter 20 on the treatment of NCSE.

## REFERENCES

1. Kaplan PW. Prognosis in nonconvulsive status epilepticus. Epileptic Disord 2000;2:185-193.
2. Granner MI, Lee SI. Nonconvulsive status epilepticus: EEG analysis in a large series. Epilepsia 1994;35:42-47.

3. Guberman A, Cantu-Reyna G, Stuss D, Broughton R. Nonconvulsive generalized status epilepticus: clinical features, neuropsychological testing, and long-term follow-up. Neurology 1986;36:1284-1291.
4. Tomson T, Svanborg E, Wedlund JE. Nonconvulsive status epilepticus: high incidence of complex partial status. Epilepsia 1986;27:276-285.
5. Kudo T, Sato K, Yagi K, Seino M. Can absence status epilepticus be of frontal lobe origin? Acta Neurol Scand 1995;92:472-477.
6. Thomas P, Zifkin B, Migneco O, Lebrun C, Darcourt J, Andermann F. Nonconvulsive status epilepticus of frontal origin. Neurology 1999;52:1174-1183.
7. Lee SI. Nonconvulsive status epilepticus. Ictal confusion in later life. Arch Neurol 1985;42: 778-781.
8. Fountain NB, Lothman EW. Pathophysiology of status epilepticus. J Clin Neurophysiol 1995;12:326-342.
9. Fountain NB. Status epilepticus: risk factors and complications. Epilepsia 2000;41(Suppl 2):S23-S30.
10. Boggs JG, Marmarou A, Agnew JP, Morton LD, Towne AR, Waterhouse EJ, Pellock JM, DeLorenzo RJ. Hemodynamic monitoring prior to and at the time of death in status epilepticus. Epilepsy Res 1998;31:199-209.
11. Spencer RG, Cox TS, Kaplan PW. Global T-wave inversion associated with nonconvulsive status epilepticus. Ann Intern Med 1998;129:163-164.
12. Shneker BF, Fountain NB. Assessment of acute morbidity and mortality in nonconvulsive status epilepticus. Neurology 2003;61:1066-1073.
13. DeLorenzo RJ, Hauser WA, Towne AR, Boggs JG, Pellock JM, Penberthy L, Garnett L, Fortner CA, Ko D. A prospective, population-based epidemiologic study of status epilepticus in Richmond, Virginia. Neurology 1996;46:1029-1035.
14. Camacho A, Perez-Martinez D, Villarejo A, Parrilla G, Floriach-Robert M, De La Pena P, Tejerina J. Nonconvulsive status epilepticus: experience in 33 patients. Neurologia 2001;16:394-398.
15. Dennis LJ, Claassen J, Hirsch LJ, Emerson RG, Connolly ES, Mayer SA. Nonconvulsive status epilepticus after subarachnoid hemorrhage. Neurosurgery 2002;51:1136-1143.
16. Little AS, Kerrigan JF, McDougall CG, Zabramski JM, Albuquerque FC, Nakaji P, Spetzler RF. Nonconvulsive status epilepticus in patients suffering spontaneous subarachnoid hemorrhage. J Neurosurg 2007;106:805-811.
17. Scholtes FB, Reiner WO, Meinardi H. Nonconvulsive status epilepticus: causes, treatment and outcome in 65 patients. J Neurol Neurosurg Psychiatry 1996;61:93-95.
18. Litt B, Wityk RJ, Hertz SH, Mullen PD, Weiss H, Ryan DD, Henry TR Nonconvulsive status epilepticus in the critically ill elderly. Epilepsia 1998;39:1194-1202.
19. Young GB, Jordan KG, Doig GS. An assessment of nonconvulsive seizures in the intensive care unit using continuous EEG monitoring: an investigation of variables associated with mortality. Neurology 1996;47:83-89.
20. Claassen J, Hirsch LJ, Frontera JA, Fernandez A, Schmidt M, Kapinos G, Wittman J, Connolly ES, Emerson RG, Mayer SA. Prognostic significance of continuous EEG monitoring in patients with poor-grade subarachnoid hemorrhage. Neurocrit Care 2006;4:103-112.
21. Vespa PM, Nuwer MR, Nenov V, Ronne-Engstrom E, Hovda DA, Bergsneider M, Kelly DF, Martin NA, Becker DP. Increased incidence and impact of nonconvulsive and convulsive seizures after traumatic brain injury as detected by continuous electroencephalographic monitoring. J Neurosurg 1999;91:750-760.
22. DeLorenzo RJ, Waterhouse EJ, Towne AR, Boggs JG, Ko D, DeLorenzo GA, Brown A, Garnett L. Persistent nonconvulsive status epilepticus after the control of convulsive status epilepticus. Epilepsia 1998;39:833-840.
23. Mayer SA, Claassen J, Lokin J, Mendelsohn F, Dennis LJ, Fitzsimmons BF. Refractory status epilepticus: frequency, risk factors, and impact on outcome. Arch Neurol 2002;59:205-210.
24. Rossetti AO, Logroscino G, Bromfield EB. Refractory status epilepticus: effect of treatment aggressiveness on prognosis. Arch Neurol 2005;62:1698-1702.
25. Claassen J, Hirsch LJ, Emerson RG, Bates JE, Thompson TB, Mayer SA. Continuous EEG monitoring and midazolam infusion for refractory nonconvulsive status epilepticus. Neurology 2001;57:1036-1042.
26. Hesdorffer DC, Logroscino G, Cascino G, Annegers JF, Hauser WA. Incidence of status epilepticus in Rochester, Minnesota, 1965-1984. Neurology 1998;50:735-741.
27. Krumholz A, Sung GY, Fisher RS, Barry E, Bergey GK, Grattan LM. Complex partial status epilepticus accompanied by serious morbidity and mortality. Neurology 1995;45:1499-1504.
28. Thomas P, Beaumanoir A, Genton P, Dolisi C, Chatel M. "De novo" absence status of late

onset: report of 11 cases. Neurology 1992;42:104-110.
29. Drislane FW, Schomer DL. Clinical implications of generalized electrographic status epilepticus. Epilepsy Res 1994;19:111-121.
30. Bottaro FJ, Martinez OA, Pardal MM, Bruetman JE, Reisin RC. Nonconvulsive status epilepticus in the elderly: a case-control study. Epilepsia 2007;48:966-972.
31. DeGiorgio CM, Gott PS, Rabinowicz AL, Heck CN, Smith T, Correale J. Neuron-specific enolase, a marker of acute neuronal injury, is increased in complex partial status epilepticus. Epilepsia 1996;37:606-609.
32. DeGiorgio CM, Heck CN, Rabinowicz AL, Gott PS, Smith T, Correale J. Serum neuron-specific enolase in the major subtypes of status epilepticus. Neurology 1999;52;746-749.
33. Rabinowicz AL, Correale J, Bracht KA, Smith, TD, DeGiorgio CM. Neuron-specific enolase is increased after nonconvulsive status epilepticus. Epilepsia 1995;36:475-479.
34. Henry TR, Drury I, Brunberg JA, Pennell PB, McKeever PE, Beydoun A. Focal cerebral magnetic resonance changes associated with partial status epilepticus. Epilepsia 1994;35:35-41.
35. Kramer RE, Lüders H, Lesser RP, Weinstein MR, Dinner DS, Morris HH, Wyllie E. Transient focal abnormalities of neuroimaging studies during focal status epilepticus. Epilepsia 1987;28:528-532.
36. Riela AR, Sires BP, Penry JK. Transient magnetic resonance imaging abnormalities during partial status epilepticus. J Child Neurol 1991;6:143-145.
37. Fujikawa DG, Itabashi HH, Wu A, Shinmei SS. Status epilepticus-induced neuronal loss in humans without systemic complications or epilepsy. Epilepsia 2000;41:981-991.
38. Dodrill CB, Wilensky AJ. Intellectual impairment as an outcome of status epilepticus. Neurology 1990;40(Suppl 2):23-27.
39. Adachi N, Kanemoto K, Muramatsu R, Kato M, Akanuma N, Ito M, Kawasaki J, Onuma T. Intellectual prognosis of status epilepticus in adult epilepsy patients: analysis with Wechsler Adult Intelligence Scale-revised. Epilepsia 2005;46:1502-1509.
40. Tomson T, Lindbom U, Nilson BY. Nonconvulsive status epilepticus in adults: thirty-two consecutive patients from a general hospital population. Epilepsia 1992;33:829-835.
41. Shneker B, Fountain NB. Epilepsy as chronic sequelae following nonconvulsive status epilepticus. [abstract] Epilepsia 2001;42(Suppl 7):147.
42. Waterhouse EJ, Vaughan JK, Barnes TY, Boggs JG, Towne AR, Kopec-Garnett L, DeLorenzo RJ. Synergistic effect of status epilepticus and ischemic brain injury on mortality. Epilepsy Res 1998;29:175-183.

# INDEX

www.ingramcontent.com/pod-product-compliance
Ingram Content Group UK Ltd.
Pitfield, Milton Keynes, MK11 3LW, UK
UKHW051912100926
8556IPUK00005B/853